Grains: Properties, Processing and Nutritional Content

Grains: Properties, Processing and Nutritional Content

Editor: Hayes Lawrence

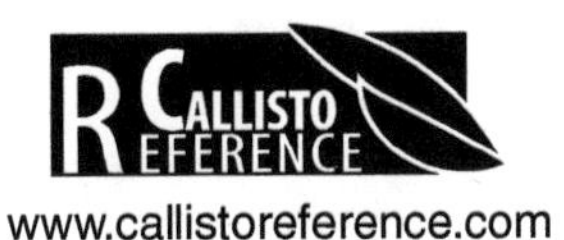

www.callistoreference.com

Callisto Reference,
118-35 Queens Blvd., Suite 400,
Forest Hills, NY 11375, USA

Visit us on the World Wide Web at:
www.callistoreference.com

ISBN: 978-1-64116-840-3 (Hardback)

Cataloging-in-Publication Data

Grains : properties, processing and nutritional content / edited by Hayes Lawrence.
p. cm.
Includes bibliographical references and index.
ISBN 978-1-64116-840-3
1. Grain. 2. Grain--Processing. 3. Cereals as food. 4. Nutrition. I. Lawrence, Hayes.
SB189 .G73 2023
633.1--dc23

Table of Contents

Preface

This book has been a concerted effort by a group of academicians, researchers and scientists, who have contributed their research works for the realization of the book. This book has materialized in the wake of emerging advancements and innovations in this field. Therefore, the need of the hour was to compile all the required researches and disseminate the knowledge to a broad spectrum of people comprising of students, researchers and specialists of the field.

Grains refer to the harvested seeds of grasses, including oats, corn, wheat and rice. Some other significant grains include millet, barley, sorghum and rye. All grains are rich in complex carbohydrates as well as certain essential minerals and vitamins. They are classified into three types, which include enriched grains, whole grains and refined grains. Whole grains contain high fibers and have been associated with health advantages such as a reduced risk of type 2 diabetes, heart disease, and colorectal cancer. Grains are processed industrially to prepare and manufacture food items such as pasta, oatmeal, pastries, crackers, breads, chips, breakfast cereals, tortillas and cookies. Furthermore, grains are also utilized to make sweeteners like rice syrup and high fructose corn syrup, which are commonly found in packaged foods. This book elucidates the properties, processing, and nutritional content of grains. It strives to provide a fair idea about this area of study and to help develop a better understanding of the latest advances within it. Researchers and students engaged in the study of grains will be assisted by this book.

At the end of the preface, I would like to thank the authors for their brilliant chapters and the publisher for guiding us all-through the making of the book till its final stage. Also, I would like to thank my family for providing the support and encouragement throughout my academic career and research projects.

Editor

1

Gluten-Free Bread with Cricket Powder—Mechanical Properties and Molecular Water Dynamics in Dough and Ready Product

Przemysław Łukasz Kowalczewski [1,*], Katarzyna Walkowiak [2], Łukasz Masewicz [2], Olga Bartczak [3], Jacek Lewandowicz [4], Piotr Kubiak [5] and Hanna Maria Baranowska [2]

1 Institute of Food Technology of Plant Origin, Poznań University of Life Sciences, 60-624 Poznań, Poland
2 Department of Physics and Biophysics, Poznań University of Life Sciences, 60-637 Poznań, Poland
3 Students' Scientific Club of Food Technologists, Poznań University of Life Sciences, 60-624 Poznań, Poland
4 Chair of Production Engineering and Logistics, Poznan University of Technology, 60-965 Poznań, Poland
5 Department of Biotechnology and Food Microbiology, Poznań University of Life Sciences, 60-627 Poznań, Poland
* Correspondence: przemyslaw.kowalczewski@up.poznan.pl

Abstract: Published data indicate that cricket powder (CP) is a good source of not only protein, fat and fiber, but also minerals. Due to the fact that this product naturally does not contain gluten, it is an interesting addition to the enrichment of gluten-free foods. This paper is a report on the results of starch substitution with CP (at 2%, 6% and 10%) on the properties of dough and bread. The rheology of dough and the texture of the final product were studied. While the changes caused in the dough by the introduction of CP were not pronounced, the bread obtained from it was characterized by significantly increased hardness and improved consistency. Analyses of water behavior at the molecular level with the use of ^{1}H Nuclear Magnetic Resonance (NMR) indicated that CP altered both the bound and bulk water fractions. Moreover, examination of water activity revealed a decreased rate of water transport in samples of bread that contained CP. These results indicate improved availability of water to the biopolymers of bread, which likely plays a role in shaping the textural properties of the product.

Keywords: gluten-free bread; edible insects; protein enrichment; rheology; texture; ^{1}H NMR; water behavior; water activity

1. Introduction

An increasing number of patients with celiac disease has led to increased interest in gluten-free (GF) products. Celiac disease is characterized by permanent gluten intolerance which, in turn, results in histopathological changes within the mucosa of the small intestine [1]. The only effective way to combat it is strict adherence to the GF diet [2,3]. It is estimated that about 1% of the population suffers from this disease [4–7]. Although the effectiveness of a gluten-free diet has not yet been proven for other diseases except celiac disease, it is also often recommended by doctors in other disease entities, such as non-celiac gluten sensitivity, Hashimoto's disease and irritable bowel syndrome [8]. Thus, the GF product market continues to grow.

Gluten is responsible for the retention of gases in dough, as well as for giving dough the right consistency. GF bread is characterized by structure and texture that is generally perceived as unattractive. In order to improve the properties of bread, including its aroma, additives, for example hydrocolloids, are used [9–12]. Moreover, GF bakery products are characterized by improper nutrient composition that results from the substitution of gluten containing flour with alternative starchy raw materials. Compared to traditional cereal products, GF breads have significantly lower nutritional value, especially in terms of decreased content of fiber, minerals and protein [9,13,14]. The additives used for the production of GF bread can supply the missing nutrients. Among such additives, edible insects can be distinguished.

In Africa, Latin America and Asia, edible insects have been known as a foodstuff for years [15,16]. As reported by the United Nations Food and Agriculture Organization, more than 1900 species of insects are eaten worldwide, including crickets, meal larvae, ants, grasshoppers and flies [17]. Research results published so far indicate that crickets, as well as cricket powder obtained from them, are a valuable source of protein, fat and minerals [18–20]. They also contain bioactive compounds [21,22]. Efforts have thus been undertaken to introduce them to the production of many food products [23–25]. To date, however, the impact of cricket powder (CP) on the characteristics of GF dough and the texture of GF bread has not been described. Therefore, the aim of the work was to assess the influence of cricket powder on the rheological properties of dough and the resulting texture of GF bread. Furthermore, water behavior in the tested bread samples was investigated with the use of low-field Nuclear Magnetic Resonance (NMR).

2. Materials and Methods

2.1. Materials

Corn starch was purchased from Glutenex (Sady, Poland), potato starch from PPZ Trzemeszno sp. z o.o. (Trzemeszno, Poland), guar gum from Limpio Chem LLP (Gujarat, India), pectin from Silvateam S.p.a. (via Torre, Italy), yeast from Lesaffre Polska (Wolczyn, Poland), sugar from Pfeifer & Langen Polska S.A. (Środa Wielkopolska, Poland), salt from Ciech Soda Polska S.A. (Janikowo, Poland) and rapeseed oil from ZT 'Kruszwica' S.A. (Kruszwica, Poland). The edible cricket powder was obtained from Crunchy Critters (Derby, United Kingdom). All chemicals and reagents used were of analytical grade.

2.2. Production of Bread

The recipe for reference gluten-free bread was as follows: 200 g corn starch, 50 g potato starch, 4.25 g guar gum, 4.25 g pectin, 15 g yeast, 5 g sugar, 4.25 g salt, 7.5 g rapeseed oil and 275 g distillated water [26]. Dough was prepared using the straight dough method. All the compounds, except oil, were mixed together with the use of KitchenAid mixer (model 5KPM5EWH, KitchenAid, Benton Harbor, MI, USA) for 2 min at a speed of 70 rpm, then oil was added, and mixing was continued for 6 min. Next, the dough was fermented in a fermentation chamber for 20 min (temperature 35 °C, relative humidity 85%) and punched. Each sample of dough was divided into two parts (280 g each) and placed in baking forms. The final fermentation was carried out for 15 min at 35 °C. Prepared dough was baked at 230 °C for 30 min (MIWE Michael Wenz GmbH, Amstein, Germany). Afterwards, the obtained breads were left at room temperature for 2 h to cool down, weighed and packed in polypropylene pouches. In the test samples, total starch was replaced with CP in three different quantities of 2%, 6% and 10%; the amounts of other components were unchanged. Reference dough and bread were denoted in the text as DB and RB, respectively. The dough samples containing cricket powder were named DCP2, DCP6, and DCP10 and the bread samples obtained from them were named BCP2, BCP6, and BCP10, respectively.

2.3. Rheological Properties of Dough

Viscoelastic properties were determined with the RheoStress1 rheometer (Haake Technik GmbH, Vreden, Germany) in controlled deformation mode (CD) with deformation set to 0.5%. Mechanical spectra were obtained within an angular velocity range of 0.1–100 rad·s^{-1}. The diameter parallel plate measurement geometrics (PP35 Ti) were 35 mm with a 1.0 mm gap. Complex viscosity (η^*), storage modulus (G′), and loss modulus (G″) were determined. The Ostwald de Waele equation (η*) and the power law equations (G′ and G″) were used to model the obtained spectra.

$$\eta^* = K^* \times \omega^{n^*-1}, \tag{1}$$

where η* is complex viscosity (Pa·s), K* is consistency index (Pa·s^n), ω is angular velocity (rad·s^{-1}) and n^* is flow behavior index (-).

$$G' = K' \times \omega^{n'}, \tag{2}$$

where G′ is storage modulus (Pa), K′ is the equation constant (Pa·s^n), ω is angular velocity (rad·s^{-1}), n' is the equation constant (-).

$$G'' = K'' \times \omega^{n''}, \tag{3}$$

where G″ is loss modulus (Pa), K″ is equation constant (Pa·s^n), ω is angular velocity (rad·s^{-1}), n'' is equation constant (-).

2.4. Texture Analysis

Texture profile analysis of bread was performed with a TA.XTplus texture analyzer (Stable Micro System Co. Ltd., Surrey, England) equipped with a 5 kg load cell [27]. Each sample was compressed twice with a cylindrical plunger probe with a 35 mm diameter. The test parameters were as follows: 10.0 mm s^{-1} pre-test speed, 5.0 mm s^{-1} test speed, 5.0 mm s^{-1} post-test speed, and 40% strain. Bread loaves were cut into slices (25 mm thick each and ends were discarded) and used to evaluate hardness, springiness, cohesiveness, chewiness and resilience. Texture analysis was repeated 15 times for each sample.

2.5. NMR Relaxometry

NMR measurements were performed according to Baranowska et al. [28]. Crumb or dough samples of 1.5 cm^3 were placed in measuring test tubes and sealed using Parafilm® (Bemis Company, Inc., Joplin, MO, USA). Measurements of the spin–lattice (T_1) and spin–spin (T_2) relaxation times were performed using a pulse NMR spectrometer MSL30 operating at 30 MHz (WL Electronics, Poznań, Poland). The samples were measured at 21.0 ± 0.5 °C. The inversion-recovery (180–t–90) [29] pulse sequence was used for measurements of the T_1 relaxation times. Distances between RF pulses (t) were changed within the range from 80 to 130 ms and the repetition time was 10 s. Each time, 32 free induction decay (FID) signals and 119 points for each FID signal were collected. Calculations of the spin–lattice relaxation time values were performed in CracSpin program using the 'spin grouping' approach. Marquardt's method of minimization was used for fitting multiexponential decays. Standard deviation was used to determine the accuracy of the analysis of relaxation parameters. Time changes of the current value of the FID signal amplitude in the employed frequency of impulses were described by the following formula:

$$M_z(t) = M_0\left\{1 - 2\exp\left(\frac{-t}{T_1}\right)\right\}, \tag{4}$$

where $M_z(t)$ is the actual magnetization value and M_0 is the equilibrium magnetization value.

Magnetization recovery was determined monoexponentially, which means that the system relaxes with one T_1 spin–lattice relaxation time. Measurements of the spin–spin (T_2) relaxation times were taken using the pulse train of the Carr–Purcell–Meiboom–Gill spin echoes ($\pi/2$–TE/2–$(\pi)_n$) [29]. The distance (τ) between 180 RF pulses amounted to 1 ms. The repetition time was 10 s. The number of spin echoes (n) amounted to 50. Eight accumulation signals were employed. To calculate the spin–spin relaxation time values, the authors applied adjustment of values of the echo amplitudes to the formula [30]:

$$M_{x,y}(\tau) = M_0 \sum_{i=1}^{n} p_i \exp\left[\frac{-\tau}{T_{2i}}\right], \tag{5}$$

where $M_{x,y}(\tau)$ is the echo amplitude, M_0 is the equilibrium amplitude, and p_i is the fraction of protons relaxing with the T_{2i} spin–spin time.

The calculations were performed using the dedicated software by application of the non-linear least-square algorithm. The accuracy of the relaxation parameters was estimated with standard deviation. The presence of two proton fractions was determined for all analyzed systems.

2.6. Measurements of Water Activity

Analyses of water activity a_w in the bread crumbs were conducted using a water diffusion and activity analyzer, ADA-7 (COBRABID, Poznań, Poland), with automatic recording of water evacuation from individual samples [31]. The thickness of the sample placed in the measurement chamber was 5 mm. Before the analysis, the temperature was stabilized at 21.0 ± 0.1 °C. The sample was then dried to the activity of 0.1000 ± 0.0005. The duration of each measurement was 1200 s. Water activity measurement results were used to describe water transport in breads with the use of the following phenomenological model [32]:

$$a_w(t) = a_r + \left(a_0 - a_p\right)e^{-V_D t} + \left(a_p - a_r\right)e^{-V_p t}, \tag{6}$$

where $a_w(t)$ is the temporary water activity value, a_0 is the initial water activity, a_p is the limit water activity (intermediate), a_r is the water activity at equilibrium condition (final), V_D is the transport rate, and V_p is the rate of the surface conduction.

2.7. Statistical Analysis

For every test, three independent measurements were taken, unless stated otherwise. One-way analysis of variance was performed independently for each dependent variable. Post-hoc Tukey HSD multiple comparison tests were used to identify statistically homogeneous subsets at $\alpha = 0.05$. Statistical analysis of the data was performed with Statistica 13 (Dell Software Inc., Round Rock, TX, USA) software.

3. Results and Discussion

3.1. Dough Rheology

The vast majority of food materials, including dough, exhibit rheological characteristics, which makes it impossible to classify their state as either solid or liquid. Such materials show both elastic and viscous properties [33]. Elastic properties are represented by the storage modulus (G′), which describes the energy temporarily stored in the sample that can be recovered, whereas viscous properties are described by the loss modulus (G″) that corresponds to the energy used for initiation of the flow that is irrevocably converted into shear heat [34]. Mechanical spectra of gluten-free doughs are presented in Figure S1.

Parameters of power law equations describing the visco-elastic properties of gluten-free dough enriched with cricket powder are presented in Table 1. The fit of the employed models to the experimental data was good, as indicated by the values of coefficient of determination (R^2), which exceeded 0.97. All investigated samples were characterized by the dominance of solid-like behavior indicated by the fact that the values of K′ were greater than K″. This is typical even for more sol-like materials, for example, starch paste [35]. Replacement of starch by cricket powder in amounts up to 6% resulted only in minor changes in rheological properties of the analyzed dough samples. The only relevant change observed was the decrease in complex viscosity (K*), which was a result of a decrease in both types of mechanical properties (K′ and K″). Similar values of n*, n′ and n″, determined for samples RD, DCP2 and DCP6, suggest that a minor decrease in viscosity was observed over a wide range of angular velocity values. This was the only change in the mechanical properties of the dough caused by replacement of starch by cricket powder in those samples. Further increase in the cricket powder to starch ratio in dough resulted in a significant decrease in viscosity along with an increase in all n equation parameters. This involved a stronger decrease in viscosity at higher shear forces compared to other dough samples.

Table 1. The viscoelastic properties of dough.

Sample	K *	n *	R^2	K′	n′	R^2	K″	n″	R^2
RD	51,550	0.347	0.994	55,460	0.135	0.965	12,750	0.121	0.984
DCP2	45,830	0.353	0.994	38,780	0.146	0.974	8877	0.125	0.989
DCP6	46,780	0.356	0.994	39,240	0.146	0.975	9570	0.123	0.983
DCP10	41,730	0.401	0.990	34,780	0.175	0.982	9054	0.146	0.979

RD—reference dough; DCP2, DCP6, DCP10—dough with 2, 6 and 10% substitution of starch with cricket powder.

3.2. Water Behavior of Dough and Crumb

Low-field NMR is a method used in food analysis since the 1990s. It allow one to measure the spin–lattice T_1 and spin–spin T_2 relaxation times, which characterize the molecular dynamics of water in a sample [30,31,36,37]. The parameters of molecular dynamics of water in the dough and crumb of bread were determined on the basis of the ^{1}H NMR tests and are presented in Table 2. The presence of two water fractions (bound and bulk) was found, which is a typical result for this type of material [38,39]. With the increase in the amount of starch substituted by CP, a significant decrease in the value of spin–net T_1 and both components of the spin–spin T_2 relaxation times was observed. This indicates that CP addition resulted in the decrease in the ratio of bulk-to-bound water fractions. The method of producing CP (roasting and grinding of insects) makes it hydrophobic instead of hydrophilic [40]. The results obtained therefore suggest that the introduction of CP leads to a greater availability of water for the biopolymers in the dough. This has influence on the viscoelastic properties of the dough—a network formed by starch and hydrocolloids (Table 1). The measurements of the relaxation time in the bread crumb show that after thermal processing the amount of bulk water fraction in relation to bound water fraction decreases with increasing amounts of CP additive. In the case of RB and BCP2, the value of the T_1 parameter was lower by approximately 15% after baking in comparison to RD and DCP2, respectively. The other two breads were characterized by a 20% decrease in the value of this relaxation time. There were no statistically significant changes in the value of the spin–spin relaxation time T_{22} for the crumb samples RB, BCP2 and BCP6 that would result from the presence of CP. At the same time, the comparison of the value of this parameter between dough and the respective crumbs shows a 3-fold decrease for the RB sample and a 2-fold decrease for the BCP10 sample. The fact that the T_{22} time was decreased in all the bread samples compared to the respective dough samples indicates that the baking process resulted in the removal of free water. The water available for biopolymers and hydrocolloids was largely retained in the structure. This can be evidenced by both a relatively small decrease in the T_1 value for crumbs and dough in individual samples and the absence of statistically significant changes in the value of both components of the spin–spin relaxation time.

There was no effect of the substitution of starch by CP on water activity at equilibrium condition (a_w) and limit water activity (a_p) of the crumb (Table 3). The transport rate (V_D) was lower in samples containing CP than in the reference bread. The transport rate limitation is the result of interactions between water and starch as well as between water and hydrocolloids. This confirms the previous suggestion based on the analysis of relaxation times that CP present in the bread crumb leads to increased availability of water to biopolymers. Also significantly lower was the rate of surface conduction (V_p) in samples that contained CP. Combined with the data obtained using low-field NMR, this result confirms the previously described changes in the molecular properties of water that are a consequence of the introduction of CP.

Table 2. Results of ^{1}H NMR study for dough and bread.

Sample	T_1 (ms)	T_{21} (ms)	T_{22} (ms)
RD	279.9 ± 3.1 ^{A}	5.24 ± 0.88 ^{A}	45.46 ± 0.76 ^{A}
DCP2	251.9 ± 2.3 ^{B}	3.16 ± 0.31 ^{B}	43.65 ± 0.56 ^{B}
DCP6	246.6 ± 0.9 ^{C}	2.25 ± 0.22 ^{C}	38.66 ± 0.30 ^{C}
DCP10	223.1 ± 0.9 ^{D}	2.17 ± 0.35 ^{C}	32.10 ± 0.19 ^{D}
RB	235.7 ± 1.5 ^{a}	1.39 ± 0.22 ^{c}	16.07 ± 0.41 ^{b}
BCP2	213.4 ± 0.6 ^{b}	2.43 ± 0.15 ^{a}	16.39 ± 0.31 ^{b}
BCP6	198.1 ± 0.8 ^{c}	2.52 ± 0.27 ^{a}	15.84 ± 0.32 ^{b}
BCP10	179.3 ± 0.6 ^{d}	2.83 ± 0.25 ^{a}	17.05 ± 0.84 ^{a}

Mean values denoted by different letters (uppercase for dough, lowercase for bread) differ statistically significantly ($p < 0.05$). NMR—Nuclear Magnetic Resonance; RD—reference dough; DCP2, DCP6, DCP10—dough with 2, 6 and 10% substitution of starch with cricket powder; RB—reference bread; BCP2, BCP6, BCP10—bread with 2, 6 and 10% substitution of starch with cricket powder.

Table 3. The results of water activity.

Sample	a_w (-)	a_p (-)	V_D (s^{-1})	V_p (s^{-1})
RB	0.925 ± 0.002 ^{a}	0.487 ± 0.013 ^{a}	0.024 ± 0.002 ^{a}	0.0030 ± 0.0001 ^{a}
BCP2	0.926 ± 0.003 ^{a}	0.503 ± 0.015 ^{a}	0.022 ± 0.002 ^{ab}	0.0026 ± 0.0001 ^{b}
BCP6	0.929 ± 0.006 ^{a}	0.641 ± 0.037 ^{a}	0.019 ± 0.004 ^{b}	0.0025 ± 0.0006 ^{b}
BCP10	0.910 ± 0.007 ^{a}	0.591 ± 0.016 ^{a}	0.019 ± 0.002 ^{b}	0.0018 ± 0.0002 ^{c}

Mean values denoted by different letters differ statistically significantly ($p < 0.05$). RB—reference bread; BCP2, BCP6, BCP10—bread with 2, 6 and 10% substitution of starch with cricket powder; a_p—limit water activity (intermediate); a_w—water activity at equilibrium condition (final); V_D—transport rate; V_p—rate of the surface conduction.

3.3. Crumb Texture

As commonly known, water content and activity have effects on the texture of bread. Texture profile analysis was conducted in order to evaluate these changes. The force required to squeeze the food between the teeth is a measure of the hardness, which is responsible for the perception of the freshness of food [41]. As stated in Table 4, the reference bread had the highest hardness and chewiness values. Moreover, the values of these parameters decreased with increasing amount of CP in the formula of the bread. Emulsifiers are used in baking technology to reduce crumb hardness [42]. The softening effect of CP could be connected with the emulsifying properties of cricket proteins. Similar effects on the structure of gluten-free crumbs were previously described by other authors who observed a decrease in crumb hardness after adding natural emulsifiers to dough [43–45]. Crumb cohesiveness, a parameter that describes the degree of deformation of the food structure before its breakage, significantly increased with the addition of CP. The increased consistency of the crumb in the case of CP-containing bread samples in comparison to the control sample is undoubtedly a desirable feature. GF breads usually have high susceptibility to fracture or crumbling [46]. Despite the fact that the springiness values did not differ significantly between the tested samples, CP incorporation significantly increased the ability of the crumb to return to its original state after compression, as evidenced by higher resilience values observed in all the enriched bread samples. This could be directly related to the high protein content in CP [18], which significantly affected the formation of the bread texture.

Table 4. Textural properties of breadcrumbs.

Sample	Hardness (N)	Springiness (%)	Cohesiveness (-)	Chewiness (-)	Resilience (-)
RB	37.21 ± 4.28 ^{a}	99.3 ± 1.5 ^{a}	0.556 ± 0.022 ^{b}	2238 ± 286 ^{a}	0.341 ± 0.028 ^{b}
BCP2	35.73 ± 1.53 ^{a}	99.3 ± 0.5 ^{a}	0.612 ± 0.068 ^{ab}	2096 ± 277 ^{ab}	0.400 ± 0.079 ^{a}
BCP6	25.08 ± 2.19 ^{b}	99.5 ± 2.2 ^{a}	0.645 ± 0.052 ^{a}	1726 ± 293 ^{b}	0.431 ± 0.035 ^{a}
BCP10	24.53 ± 1.79 ^{b}	99.9 ± 1.8 ^{a}	0.691 ± 0.062 ^{a}	1710 ± 77 ^{b}	0.443 ± 0.049 ^{a}

Mean values denoted by different letters differ statistically significantly ($p < 0.05$). RB—reference bread; BCP2, BCP6, BCP10—bread with 2, 6 and 10% substitution of starch with cricket powder.

4. Conclusions

While substitution of starch with CP may improve the nutritional value of gluten-free bread, it can also cause a number of changes in the properties of both the dough and the final product. Despite the fact that only small changes of macroscopic properties of dough were observed in these rheological analyses, the molecular-level analyses of water contained in the dough revealed that CP increases the availability of water for biopolymers, such as starch or hydrocolloids. This was probably an effect of binding the fat fraction. As a result, significant changes in water dynamics were also observed in the ready bread crumb samples. Moreover, it was shown that the introduction of CP leads to the reduction of hardness of the bread and improves its consistency. While the health-beneficial properties of edible insects are known, more research is needed in order to fully describe the health-promoting properties of bakery products supplemented with cricket powder.

Author Contributions: Conceptualization, P.K.; Investigation, P.K., K.W., Ł.M., O.B., J.L., P.K. and H.B.; Methodology, P.K. and H.B.; Supervision, P.K.; Writing original draft, P.K., J.L., P.K. and H.B..

Acknowledgments: The authors thank Paulina Sarbak and Krzysztof Smarzyński (Students' Scientific Club of Food Technologists, Poznań University of Life Sciences, Poznań, Poland) for their help with the preparation of bread and the analyses.

References

1. Green, P.H.R.; Cellier, C. Celiac Disease. *N. Engl. J. Med.* **2007**, *357*, 1731–1743. [CrossRef]
2. Van Heel, D.A. Recent advances in coeliac disease. *Gut* **2006**, *55*, 1037–1046. [CrossRef] [PubMed]
3. Armstrong, M.J.; Robins, G.G.; Howdle, P.D. Recent advances in coeliac disease. *Curr. Opin. Gastroenterol.* **2009**, *25*, 100–109. [CrossRef] [PubMed]
4. Niewinski, M.M. Advances in Celiac Disease and Gluten-Free Diet. *J. Am. Diet. Assoc.* **2008**, *108*, 661–672. [CrossRef] [PubMed]
5. Green, P.H.R. The many faces of celiac disease: Clinical presentation of celiac disease in the adult population. *Gastroenterology* **2005**, *128*, S74–S78. [CrossRef] [PubMed]
6. Lebwohl, B.; Sanders, D.S.; Green, P.H.R. Coeliac disease. *Lancet* **2018**, *391*, 70–81. [CrossRef]
7. Lindfors, K.; Ciacci, C.; Kurppa, K.; Lundin, K.E.A.; Makharia, G.K.; Mearin, M.L.; Murray, J.A.; Verdu, E.F.; Kaukinen, K. Coeliac disease. *Nat. Rev. Dis. Prim.* **2019**, *5*, 3. [CrossRef] [PubMed]
8. Zannini, E.; Arendt, E.K. Low FODMAPs and gluten-free foods for irritable bowel syndrome treatment: Lights and shadows. *Food Res. Int.* **2018**, *110*, 33–41. [CrossRef] [PubMed]
9. Torbica, A.; Hadnadev, M.; Dapčević, T. Rheological, textural and sensory properties of gluten-free bread formulations based on rice and buckwheat flour. *Food Hydrocoll.* **2010**, *24*, 626–632. [CrossRef]
10. Gujral, H.S.; Rosell, C.M. Improvement of the breadmaking quality of rice flour by glucose oxidase. *Food Res. Int.* **2004**, *37*, 75–81. [CrossRef]
11. Lazaridou, A.; Duta, D.; Papageorgiou, M.; Belc, N.; Biliaderis, C.G. Effects of hydrocolloids on dough rheology and bread quality parameters in gluten-free formulations. *J. Food Eng.* **2007**, *79*, 1033–1047. [CrossRef]
12. Pacyński, M.; Wojtasiak, R.Z.; Mildner-Szkudlarz, S. Improving the aroma of gluten-free bread. *LWT-Food Sci. Technol.* **2015**, *63*, 706–713. [CrossRef]
13. Rybicka, I.; Doba, K.; Bińczak, O. Improving the sensory and nutritional value of gluten-free bread. *Int. J. Food Sci. Technol.* **2019**. [CrossRef]
14. Rybicka, I.; Gliszczyńska-Świgło, A. Minerals in grain gluten-free products. The content of calcium, potassium, magnesium, sodium, copper, iron, manganese, and zinc. *J. Food Compos. Anal.* **2017**, *59*, 61–67. [CrossRef]
15. Raheem, D.; Carrascosa, C.; Oluwole, O.B.; Nieuwland, M.; Saraiva, A.; Millán, R.; Raposo, A. Traditional consumption of and rearing edible insects in Africa, Asia and Europe. *Crit. Rev. Food Sci. Nutr.* **2018**, 1–20. [CrossRef] [PubMed]
16. Ghosh, S.; Jung, C.; Meyer-Rochow, V.B. What Governs Selection and Acceptance of Edible Insect Species. In *Edible Insects in Sustainable Food Systems*; Springer International Publishing: Cham, Switzerland, 2018; pp. 331–351.

17. Van Huis, A. Potential of Insects as Food and Feed in Assuring Food Security. *Annu. Rev. Entomol.* **2013**, *58*, 563–583. [CrossRef] [PubMed]
18. Montowska, M.; Kowalczewski, P.Ł.; Rybicka, I.; Fornal, E. Nutritional value, protein and peptide composition of edible cricket powders. *Food Chem.* **2019**, *289*, 130–138. [CrossRef] [PubMed]
19. Zielińska, E.; Baraniak, B.; Karaś, M.; Rybczyńska, K.; Jakubczyk, A. Selected species of edible insects as a source of nutrient composition. *Food Res. Int.* **2015**, *77*, 460–466. [CrossRef]
20. Kulma, M.; Kouřimská, L.; Plachý, V.; Božik, M.; Adámková, A.; Vrabec, V. Effect of sex on the nutritional value of house cricket, Acheta domestica L. *Food Chem.* **2019**, *272*, 267–272. [CrossRef]
21. Zielińska, E.; Baraniak, B.; Karaś, M. Identification of antioxidant and anti-inflammatory peptides obtained by simulated gastrointestinal digestion of three edible insects species (Gryllodes sigillatus, Tenebrio molitor, Schistocerca gragaria). *Int. J. Food Sci. Technol.* **2018**, *53*, 2542–2551. [CrossRef]
22. Zielińska, E.; Baraniak, B.; Karaś, M. Antioxidant and Anti-Inflammatory Activities of Hydrolysates and Peptide Fractions Obtained by Enzymatic Hydrolysis of Selected Heat-Treated Edible Insects. *Nutrients* **2017**, *9*, 970. [CrossRef] [PubMed]
23. Pauter, P.; Różańska, M.; Wiza, P.; Dworczak, S.; Grobelna, N.; Sarbak, P.; Kowalczewski, P.Ł. Effects of the replacement of wheat flour with cricket powder on the characteristics of muffins. *Acta Sci. Pol. Technol. Aliment.* **2018**, *17*, 227–233. [PubMed]
24. Smarzyński, K.; Sarbak, P.; Musiał, S.; Jeżowski, P.; Piatek, M.; Kowalczewski, P.Ł. Nutritional analysis and evaluation of the consumer acceptance of pork pâté enriched with cricket powder-preliminary study. *Open Agric.* **2019**, *4*, 159–163. [CrossRef]
25. Duda, A.; Adamczak, J.; Chełmińska, P.; Juszkiewicz, J.; Kowalczewski, P. Quality and Nutritional/Textural Properties of Durum Wheat Pasta Enriched with Cricket Powder. *Foods* **2019**, *8*, 46. [CrossRef] [PubMed]
26. Korus, J.; Juszczak, L.; Ziobro, R.; Witczak, M.; Grzelak, K.; Sójka, M. Defatted strawberry and blackcurrant seeds as functional ingredients of gluten-free bread. *J. Texture Stud.* **2012**, *43*, 29–39. [CrossRef]
27. Kowalczewski, P.; Różańska, M.; Makowska, A.; Jeżowski, P.; Kubiak, P. Production of wheat bread with spray-dried potato juice: Influence on dough and bread characteristics. *Food Sci. Technol. Int.* **2019**, *25*, 223–232. [CrossRef] [PubMed]
28. Baranowska, H.M.; Masewicz, Ł.; Kowalczewski, P.Ł.; Lewandowicz, G.; Piątek, M.; Kubiak, P. Water properties in pâtés enriched with potato juice. *Eur. Food Res. Technol.* **2018**, *244*, 387–393. [CrossRef]
29. Brosio, E.; Gianferri, R.R. An analytical tool in foods characterization and traceability. In *Basic NMR in Foods Characterization*; Research Signpost: Kerala, India, 2009; pp. 9–37.
30. Baranowska, H.M. Water Molecular Properties in Forcemeats and Finely Ground Sausages Containing Plant Fat. *Food Biophys.* **2011**, *6*, 133–137. [CrossRef]
31. Płowaś-Korus, I.; Masewicz, Ł.; Szwengiel, A.; Rachocki, A.; Baranowska, H.M.; Medycki, W. A novel method of recognizing liquefied honey. *Food Chem.* **2018**, *245*, 885–889. [CrossRef]
32. Masewicz, L.; Lewandowicz, J.; Le Thanh-Blicharz, J.; Kempka, M.; Baranowska, H.M. Diffusion of water in potato starch pastes. In Proceedings of the 12th International Conference on Polysaccharides-Glycoscience, Prague, Czech Republic, 19–21 October 2016; pp. 193–195.
33. Abang Zaid, D.N.; Chin, N.L.; Yusof, Y.A. A Review on Rheological Properties and Measurements of Dough and Gluten. *J. Appl. Sci.* **2010**, *10*, 2478–2490. [CrossRef]
34. Yan, H.; Yayuan, Z.; Ling, Z.; Zhengbiao, G. Study on physicochemical characteristics of waxy potato starch in comparison with other waxy starches. *Starch-Stärke* **2011**, *63*, 754–759. [CrossRef]
35. Lewandowicz, J.; Baranowska, H.M.; Szwengiel, A.; Le Thanh-Blicharz, J. Molecular structure vs. Functional properties of waxy and normal corn starch. In Proceedings of the 12th International Conference on Polysaccharides-Glycoscience, Prague, Czech Republic, 19–21 October 2016; pp. 53–57.
36. Makowska, A.; Baranowska, H.M.; Michniewicz, J.; Chudy, S.; Kowalczewski, P.Ł. Triticale extrudates—Changes of macrostructure, mechanical properties and molecular water dynamics during hydration. *J. Cereal Sci.* **2017**, *74*, 250–255. [CrossRef]
37. Piątek, M.; Baranowska, H.M.; Krzywdzińska-Bartkowiak, M. Microstructure and water molecular dynamics in meat after thawing. *Fleischwirtschaft* **2013**, *93*, 100–104.
38. van Nieuwenhuijzen, N.H.; Tromp, R.H.; Mitchell, J.R.; Primo-Martín, C.; Hamer, R.J.; van Vliet, T. Relations between sensorial crispness and molecular mobility of model bread crust and its main components as measured by PTA, DSC and NMR. *Food Res. Int.* **2010**, *43*, 342–349. [CrossRef]

39. Curti, E.; Bubici, S.; Carini, E.; Baroni, S.; Vittadini, E. Water molecular dynamics during bread staling by Nuclear Magnetic Resonance. *LWT-Food Sci. Technol.* **2011**, *44*, 854–859. [CrossRef]
40. Bassett, F. Comparison of Functional, Nutritional, and Sensory Properties of Spray-Dried and Oven-Dried Cricket (Acheta Domesticus) Powder. Master's Thesis, Brigham Young University, Provo, UT, USA, 2018.
41. Giannou, V.; Tzia, C. Frozen dough bread: Quality and textural behavior during prolonged storage—Prediction of final product characteristics. *J. Food Eng.* **2007**, *79*, 929–934. [CrossRef]
42. Gray, J.A.; Bemiller, J.N. Bread Staling: Molecular Basis and Control. *Compr. Rev. Food Sci. Food Saf.* **2003**, *2*, 1–21. [CrossRef]
43. Conte, P.; Del Caro, A.; Balestra, F.; Piga, A.; Fadda, C. Bee pollen as a functional ingredient in gluten-free bread: A physical-chemical, technological and sensory approach. *LWT* **2018**, *90*, 1–7. [CrossRef]
44. Alvarez-Jubete, L.; Auty, M.; Arendt, E.K.; Gallagher, E. Baking properties and microstructure of pseudocereal flours in gluten-free bread formulations. *Eur. Food Res. Technol.* **2010**, *230*, 437–445. [CrossRef]
45. Demirkesen, I.; Mert, B.; Sumnu, G.; Sahin, S. Rheological properties of gluten-free bread formulations. *J. Food Eng.* **2010**, *96*, 295–303. [CrossRef]
46. Onyango, C.; Mutungi, C.; Unbehend, G.; Lindhauer, M.G. Modification of gluten-free sorghum batter and bread using maize, potato, cassava or rice starch. *LWT-Food Sci. Technol.* **2011**, *44*, 681–686. [CrossRef]

2

Composition, Protein Profile and Rheological Properties of Pseudocereal-Based Protein-Rich Ingredients

Loreto Alonso-Miravalles and James A. O'Mahony *

School of Food and Nutritional Sciences, University College Cork, Cork T12 Y337, Ireland; 116221127@umail.ucc.ie

* Correspondence: sa.omahony@ucc.ie

Abstract: The objectives of this study were to investigate the nutrient composition, protein profile, morphology, and pasting properties of protein-rich pseudocereal ingredients (quinoa, amaranth, and buckwheat) and compare them to the more common rice and maize flours. Literature concerning protein-rich pseudocereal ingredients is very limited, mainly to protein profiling. The concentrations of macronutrients (i.e., ash, fat, and protein, as well as soluble, insoluble and total dietary fibre) were significantly higher for the protein-rich variants of pseudocereal-based flours than their regular protein content variants and the rice and maize flours. On profiling the protein component using sodium dodecyl sulfate–polyacrylamide gel electrophoresis (SDS-PAGE), all samples showed common bands at ~50 kDa and low molecular weight bands corresponding to the globulin fraction (~50 kDa) and albumin fraction (~10 kDa), respectively; except rice, in which the main protein was glutelin. The morphology of the starch granules was studied using scanning electron microscopy with quinoa and amaranth showing the smallest sized granules, while buckwheat, rice, and maize had the largest starch granules. The pasting properties of the ingredients were generally similar, except for buckwheat and amaranth, which showed the highest and lowest final viscosity, respectively. The results obtained in this study can be used to better understand the functionality and food applications of protein-rich pseudocereal ingredients.

Keywords: pseudocereal; cereal; protein-rich ingredients; macronutrient; protein profile; morphology; rheological properties

---

1. Introduction

The global protein demand for the 7.3 billion inhabitants of the world is approximately 202 million tonnes annually [1]. The expected continuous growth of the global population to 9.6 billion people by 2050 is creating an ever-greater need to identify and develop sustainable solutions for provision of high-quality food protein [2,3]. Plant-based protein ingredients are becoming more popular due to their contribution to environmental sustainability and to food security challenges, in addition to their cost-effectiveness, compared with animal-based proteins [4]. However, replacing animal-based protein ingredients with plant-origin material is not easy due mainly to important differences in composition and taste/flavour [5]. Moreover, applications of plant proteins are poorly studied and commercially limited due mainly to their techno-functional properties (e.g., poor solubility), anti-nutritional components, off-flavour, and colour [6,7].

Quinoa, amaranth, and buckwheat are non-conventional sources of protein that have been the subject of limited studies in recent years, although their cultivation goes back thousands of years [8,9]. They are gluten-free dicotyledonous grains, referred to as pseudocereals, with somewhat similar composition and nutritional value to cereals, such as rice and maize [10,11]. Quinoa and amaranth are cultivated in South America, and buckwheat, originally from Central Asia, is now also cultivated in Central and Eastern Europe [12]. Their main compositional component is starch [13] which forms semi-crystalline structures referred to as "starch granules", and depending on the botanical source, these granules vary in size, shape, and amylose:amylopectin ratio [14], which consequently influences the techno-functional properties of the flour ingredients [15,16]. Protein, fibre, fat, minerals, and vitamins are the remaining macro- and micro-nutrients that constitute pseudocereals [9,17]. The protein content of amaranth, buckwheat, and quinoa, has been reported to be 12.0%–18.9% and the concentrations of essential amino acids, particularly, cysteine and methionine, are known to be higher than in some common cereals such as rice and maize [12].

Regarding classification of pseudocereal proteins, the literature in this area is often inconsistent and contradictory [17]. Several authors [18,19] have reported globulins and albumins to be the main proteins in quinoa, amaranth, and buckwheat, in contrast to other cereals, such as rice, where the main proteins are glutelin and prolamins [20]. Amaranth, quinoa, and buckwheat are also good sources of dietary fibre, which has proven effects in promoting desirable physiological outcomes, such as lowering blood cholesterol and increased satiety, due to its resistance to digestion and absorption in the small intestine, followed by complete or partial fermentation in the large intestine [21–23]. In addition, pseudocereals are rich in micro-nutrients such as calcium, magnesium, and iron and good sources of vitamin E and riboflavin [24].

These macro- and micro-nutrients are located in different parts of the grain (Figure 1). In amaranth and quinoa seeds, the embryo or germ, which is circular in shape, surrounds the starch-rich perisperm, and together with the seed coat, represent the bran fraction, which is relatively rich in fat and protein [25]. In contrast, in buckwheat seeds, starch reserves are stored in the endosperm, as in common cereals, and the embryo, rich in fat and protein, extends through the starchy endosperm [26]. Protein-enriched fractions can be prepared from such pseudocereal grains using two principal approaches—dry or wet fractionation techniques [27]. Dry fractionation employs mechanical forces (milling and air/size classification) and is a more sustainable means of obtaining protein-rich fractions, while wet fractionation techniques use large quantities of water, chemicals (e.g., for pH adjustment), and a final drying step that consumes energy [4,28]. Therefore, protein-rich fractions from pseudocereals can offer unique nutritional and technological properties that have not yet been fully investigated or tested in food applications [29–31].

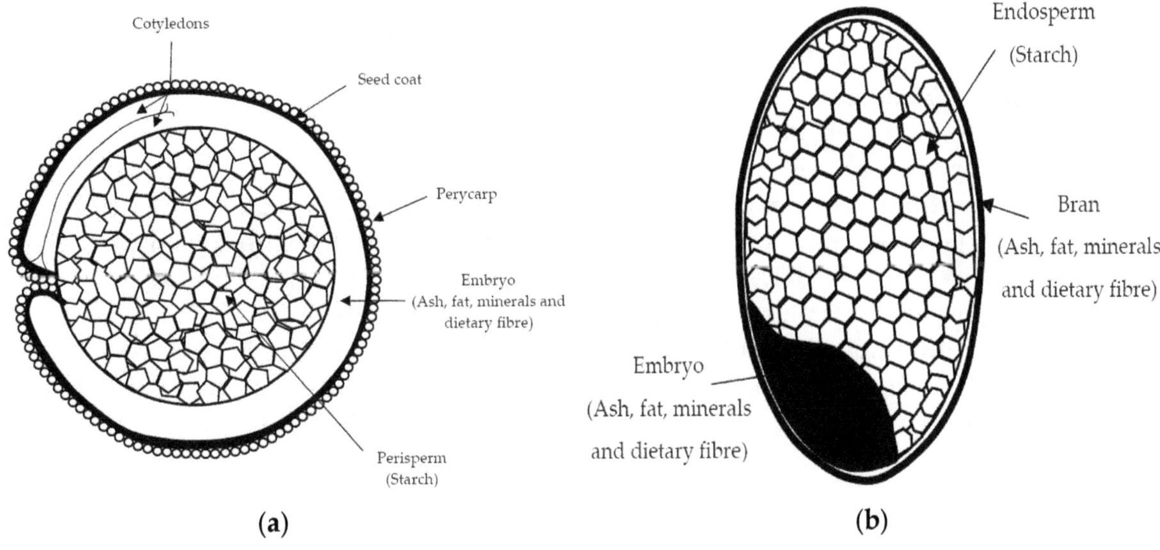

Figure 1. *Cont.*

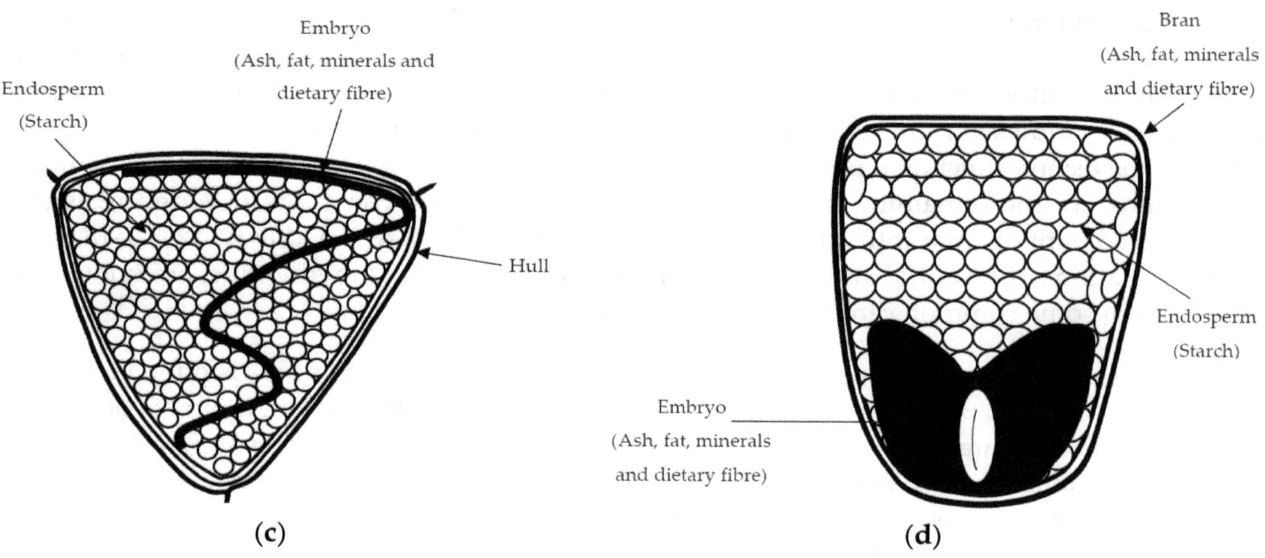

Figure 1. Schematic representation of grain structure of quinoa and amaranth (**a**); rice (**b**); buckwheat (**c**); and maize (**d**).

The aim of this work was to determine systematically the nutritional composition, protein profile, and physical properties of several novel protein-enriched ingredients from quinoa, amaranth, and buckwheat and compare them to regular protein content pseudocereal and cereal flours. These protein-rich fractions have great potential as ingredients, not only for their nutritional value (e.g., rich in protein and fibre) but also for their technological functionality (e.g., starch pasting properties). Scientific information on pseudocereal protein-rich fractions is scarce in the literature, thus, the results of this original and novel study can help with our understanding of the potential applications of these plant-based protein-rich ingredients in food formulations.

2. Materials and Methods

2.1. Cereal and Pseudocereal Flour Ingredients

Ten different regular and protein-rich cereal and pseudocereal flours/ingredients were analysed in this study. Seven of the flours were of pseudocereal origin: quinoa wholegrain flour (QWGF), quinoa dehulled flour (QDF), quinoa protein-rich flour (QPRF), amaranth wholegrain flour (AWGF), amaranth protein-rich flour (APRF), buckwheat dehulled flour (BDF), and buckwheat protein-rich flour (BPRF). Protein enrichment in the protein-rich flours was achieved using a dry milling approach. In brief, the grains were milled using either an impact or a jet mill, with different screen inserts used to produce flour and seed fragments; only buckwheat was milled using a jet mill. All grains, except amaranth, were sourced from commercial suppliers and had been de-hulled prior to milling. After milling, the protein-rich fractions were separated from the milled flours using size-based dry sieve classification. Rice flour (RF), rice protein concentrate (RPC), and maize flour (MF) were included in the study as comparator flour ingredients and were of cereal origin. All of the pseudocereal flours were provided by the Fraunhofer Institut (Munich, Germany) except the QWGF, which was purchased from Ziegler & Co. (Wunsiedel, Germany). The RF and RPC ingredients were purchased from Beneo (Tienen, Belgium) and the MF was purchased from the Quay Co-op (Cork, Ireland).

2.2. Chemical Composition

Moisture, ash, fat, and protein contents of samples were determined according to the standard methods of the Association of Analytical Chemists [32]. Moisture was determined by oven drying at 103 °C for 5 h (AOAC 925.10). The ash content was analysed by dry ashing in a muffle furnace at

500 °C for 5 h (AOAC 923.03). Fat determination was carried out following AOAC 922.06, using a Soxtec 2055 (Foss, Ballymount, Co., Dublin, Ireland). Total nitrogen content was determined by the Kjeldahl method (AOAC 930.29) using the following nitrogen-to-protein conversion factors: 6.25 for quinoa, buckwheat, and maize [12,33], 5.85 for amaranth [24], and 5.95 for rice ingredients [12]. Total carbohydrate was calculated by difference (i.e., 100—sum of protein, fat, ash, and moisture). Total starch (AOAC Methods 996.11 and AACC Method 76-13.01), damaged starch as a % of total starch (AACC method 76-31.01 and ICC method No. 164), and soluble (SDF), insoluble (IDF), and total dietary fibre (TDF) (AOAC Method 991.43 and AACC Method 32-07.01) contents were determined using enzyme kits (Megazyme, Bray, Co., Wicklow, Ireland). β-glucan, casein, and high-amylose maize starch were used as controls in dietary fibre analysis (K-TDFC; Megazyme, Wicklow, Ireland).

2.3. *Electrophoretic Protein Profile Analysis*

The protein profile was assessed by sodium dodecyl sulphate-polyacrylamide gel electrophoresis (SDS-PAGE) using precast gels (Mini-PROTEAN TGX, Bio-Rad Laboratories, Hercules, CA, USA) under non-reducing (method **I** and **II**) and reducing conditions (method **III**). The sample loading buffer contained 65.8 mM Tris-HCl (pH 6.8), 26.3% glycerol, 2.1% sodium dodecyl sulfate (SDS) and 0.01% bromophenol blue. The running buffer (10× Tris/Glycine/SDS, Bio-Rad Laboratories, Hercules, CA, USA) had a composition of 25 mM Tris, 192 mM glycine, and 0.1% SDS (*w*/*v*), pH 8.3. The staining solution used was Coomassie Brilliant Blue R-250 (Bio-Rad Laboratories, Hercules, CA, USA). The target final protein concentration was, in all cases, 1 mg/mL, and 10 μL of sample solution loaded into each well of the gel. For the preparation of the samples, three different methods were used. For method **I**, the approach of Abugoch et al. [34] was followed, with slight modifications. Briefly, the powder samples were mixed directly with the sample loading buffer at a concentration of 1 mg/mL, vortexed for 1 min until the powder was fully suspended and mixed over 2 h at 20 °C and at 250 rpm. For methods **II** and **III**, the approach of Amagliani et al. [20] was followed, with the modification that the powders were mixed with the protein extracting buffer overnight, and 1,4-dithiothreitol (DTT; 1%) was used in method **III** as a reducing agent.

2.4. *Microstructural Analysis*

The powders were mounted on aluminium stubs using double-sided adhesive carbon tape, and sputter coated with a 5 nm layer of gold/palladium (Au:Pd = 80:20) using a Quorum Q150R ES Sputter Coating Unit (Quorum Technologies Ltd., Sussex, UK). Subsequently, the samples were loaded into a sample tube and examined using a JSM-5510 scanning electron microscope (JEOL Ltd., Tokyo, Japan), operated at an accelerating voltage of 5 kV.

2.5. *Pasting Behaviour*

Pasting properties were studied using an AR-G2 controlled-stress rheometer equipped with a starch pasting cell (AR-G2; TA Instruments Ltd., Waters LLC, Leatherhead, UK). The internal diameter of the cell was 36.0 mm, the diameter of the rotor was 32.4 mm, and the gap between the two elements at the geometry base was 0.55 mm. A heating and cooling cycle described by Li et al. [35] was applied to 16% (*w*/*w*) suspensions of flours ingredients at a fixed shear rate of 17 rad/s.

2.6. *Statistical Analysis*

All the analyses were conducted in triplicate. The data generated was subjected to one-way analysis of variance (ANOVA) using R i386 version 3.3.1 (R foundation for statistical computing, Vienna, Austria). A Tukey's paired comparison test was used to determine statistically significant differences ($p < 0.05$) between mean values for different samples, at a 95% confidence level.

3. Results and Discussion

3.1. Chemical Composition

The dry matter that remains after moisture removal is commonly referred to as total solids [36]. Protein-rich samples had higher total solids ($p < 0.05$) content than their regular flour counterparts. The higher total solids content of these protein-rich ingredients can be an advantage from a microbiological and chemical stability perspective [37]. Ash refers to substances resulting from the incineration of dry matter in a powder sample and is directly related to the mineral content of the sample [38]. The protein-rich ingredients, QPRF, APRF, BPRF, and RPC showed higher ash contents (3.6%, 6.9%, 3.0%, and 3.4%, respectively) than the regular flours QWGF, QDF, AWGF, BDF, RF, and MF (2.3%, 1.8%, 2.4%, 1.5%, 0.8%, and 0.7%, respectively). Protein-rich flours are usually produced using dry fractionation approaches [28], classifying the parts of the grain that are rich in protein (e.g., embryo fraction) which results in a concomitant increase in other components such as minerals [5,25,39]. These pseudocereal protein-rich fractions with higher ash content would be expected to be enriched in selected minerals such as phosphorus, magnesium, and potassium that are located in embryonic tissues [33,40].

The fat content of the protein-rich ingredients QPRF, APRF, and BPRF (12.8%, 16.6%, and 4.8%, respectively) was significantly higher ($p < 0.05$) than the regular flours (Table 1). The higher fat content of the protein-rich ingredients was expected taking into consideration that the dry fractionation process classifies fractions rich in fat along with protein. Arendt and Zannini [40], reported that in quinoa, 49% of the total fat content is located in the embryo. Gamel et al. [41], reported 45% higher fat content in amaranth protein-rich flours, in comparison with a regular flour, and related it with the association of fat with cell wall materials and protein bodies during the protein enrichment process. BPRF showed the lowest value for fat (4.7%) among the protein-rich ingredients. In this study, the low fat content of BDF is most likely due to its relatively low level of protein enrichment (20%) which suggests lower enrichment in the embryo fraction where most of the fat is located. Also, Alvarez-Jubete et al. [26] stated that the fat content in quinoa and amaranth is two to three times higher than in buckwheat and common cereals. The fact that these pseudocereals have high levels of fat reduce the need for adding fat when these protein-rich flours are used as ingredients (e.g., baked products) where fat plays an important role in texture and flavour [41].

The protein-rich flour ingredients, QPRF, APRF, and BPRF, had values for protein of 33.3%, 38.6%, and 20.5%, respectively. The protein contents for pseudocereal flours ranged from 13.1% to 15.7% which are higher than the protein values for RF (8.2%) and MF (6.4%). These values are in accordance with the study of Mota et al. [12], who reported a protein content for pseudocereals significantly higher than in common cereals such as rice and maize. Moreover, a recent review by Navruz et al. [42] reported the nutritional and health benefits of quinoa, such as protein digestibility values similar to casein and higher lysine levels than other grains.

The values for starch in protein-rich samples were lower (21.4–47.3%) than those for the regular flours (50.5–61.6%). The lower values for starch in the protein-rich ingredients were expected as protein-rich ingredients are more enriched in the embryo fraction (rich in proteins), while the perisperm (quinoa and amaranth) or endosperm (buckwheat) where the starch granules are located, are less abundant. The level of starch damage is related to the process and the conditions (e.g., pressure or shear) used to obtain the protein-rich flour ingredients [43]. Such damage changes the granular structure of starch and influences the rheological and functional properties of the starch granules by modulating their water sorption and swelling capacity [43]. QWGF, QDF, QPRF, AWGF, RF, and MF showed similar levels of damaged starch (~7–12% of total starch); while APRF, BDF, and BPRF had the lowest levels of starch damage (~2%) (Table 1). The differences in damaged starch between the samples are usually related to the severity of the extraction process employed [20]. RPC showed the highest damaged starch content (88.3%), which might have arisen from the use of chemicals and aggressive environmental conditions (temperature and pH) in obtaining high protein levels in the final product [4].

Table 1. Macronutrient composition of quinoa wholegrain flour (QWGF), quinoa dehulled flour (QDF), quinoa protein-rich flour (QPRF), amaranth wholegrain flour (AWGF), amaranth protein-rich flour (APRF), buckwheat dehulled flour (BDF), buckwheat protein-rich flour (BPRF), rice flour (RF), rice protein concentrate (RPC), and maize flour (MF;. Total dietary fibre (TDF). Values are means ± standard deviations of data from triplicate analysis.

	Moisture	Ash	Protein (% *w*/*w*)	Fat	Carbohydrate	Starch	Damaged Starch (% Total Starch)	TDF (% *w*/*w*)
Quinoa								
QWGF	9.01 ± 0.10^{d}	2.30 ± 0.00^{c}	13.1 ± 0.10^{b}	6.54 ± 0.07^{d}	69.0 ± 0.27^{d}	60.0 ± 2.58^{d}	10.6 ± 0.47^{d}	11.4 ± 1.10^{b}
QDF	8.86 ± 0.25^{d}	1.80 ± 0.10^{b}	15.7 ± 0.30^{b}	5.36 ± 0.61^{d}	68.3 ± 1.26^{d}	50.5 ± 1.40^{bc}	11.7 ± 0.32^{e}	9.75 ± 1.17^{b}
QPRF	5.25 ± 0.25^{a}	3.60 ± 0.19^{e}	33.3 ± 1.10^{d}	12.8 ± 0.73^{e}	45.0 ± 2.27^{b}	21.4 ± 0.81^{a}	10.4 ± 0.40^{d}	18.8 ± 0.23^{c}
Amaranth								
AWGF	8.94 ± 0.05^{d}	2.40 ± 0.02^{c}	14.6 ± 0.30^{b}	6.04 ± 0.10^{d}	68.1 ± 0.47^{d}	52.8 ± 1.45^{c}	12.2 ± 0.35^{e}	11.3 ± 0.86^{b}
APRF	7.76 ± 0.12^{b}	6.86 ± 0.18^{f}	38.6 ± 1.74^{e}	16.6 ± 0.08^{f}	30.2 ± 2.12^{a}	20.3 ± 0.31^{a}	2.61 ± 0.01^{b}	24.0 ± 2.56^{d}
Buckwheat								
BDF	8.75 ± 0.11^{d}	1.51 ± 0.31^{b}	14.2 ± 0.06^{b}	2.77 ± 0.05^{bc}	72.8 ± 0.53^{e}	61.6 ± 0.12^{d}	1.52 ± 0.06^{a}	10.3 ± 1.72^{b}
BPRF	6.86 ± 0.17^{c}	3.05 ± 0.10^{d}	20.5 ± 0.90^{c}	4.76 ± 0.15^{cd}	64.8 ± 1.32^{c}	47.3 ± 1.20^{b}	2.22 ± 0.07^{ab}	19.0 ± 0.48^{c}
Rice								
RF	8.89 ± 0.19^{d}	0.85 ± 0.05^{a}	8.22 ± 0.14^{a}	0.71 ± 0.08^{a}	81.3 ± 0.46^{f}	78.5 ± 0.82^{e}	10.7 ± 0.14^{f}	1.12 ± 0.20^{a}
RPC	6.24 ± 0.08^{a}	3.42 ± 0.24^{d}	75.0 ± 0.38^{f}	0.79 ± 0.00^{a}	14.6 ± 0.7^{g}	6.50 ± 0.71^{f}	88.3 ± 0.11^{g}	5.83 ± 0.41^{e}
Maize								
MF	12.2 ± 0.31^{e}	0.74 ± 0.04^{a}	6.42 ± 0.21^{a}	1.66 ± 0.02^{ab}	79.0 ± 0.58^{f}	76.0 ± 2.26^{e}	7.21 ± 0.25^{c}	2.00 ± 0.40^{a}

Values followed by different superscript letters (a–f) in the same column are significantly different ($p < 0.05$).

Dietary fibre denotes carbohydrate polymers which are not hydrolysed by the endogenous enzymes in the small intestine of humans [21,22]. Total dietary fibre (TDF) is divided into two categories, based on differences in solubility in water: soluble (SDF) and insoluble (IDF) dietary fibre. Protein-rich cereal ingredients showed significantly higher levels (19–24%) ($p < 0.05$) of TDF than the regular protein containing ingredients (1.1–11.5%) (Table 1 and Figure 2). Among the pseudocereal flours there were no significant differences ($p < 0.05$) in TDF, but they showed higher contents of TDF ($p < 0.05$) in comparison with RF and MF. These results were expected on comparison with literature data: Nascimento et al. [33], reported that pseudocereals can have seven times more fibre than common grains such as rice. The TDF values were similar to those found in other studies for quinoa [33,44,45] where values for TDF of 10.4%, 11.7%, and 12.7%, respectively, were reported, whereas Alvarez-Jubete et al. [26] reported slightly higher values for TDF (14.2%). The value for AWGF is in line with Nascimento et al. [33] who reported a TDF content of 11.3% for amaranth. Other authors, such as Repo-Carrasco et al. [46], reported slightly higher values (ranging from 14% to 16%) for amaranth (*Amaranthus caudatus*) flours. Regarding the soluble and insoluble dietary fibre fractions, the IDF fraction was higher than the SDF fraction in all the ingredients except for RF. This is in accordance with values reported in the literature for quinoa [47,48] and amaranth [19]. However, the IDF content of AWGF was slightly lower than that reported previously by Repo-Carrasco et al. [46] for the varieties Oscar Blanco (12.15%) and Centenario (13.92%). RPC had the lowest values for TDF, SDF, and IDF, which might be explained by the higher protein enrichment levels for this sample, which was in turn, associated with lower levels of other components such as starch, fat, and dietary fibre.

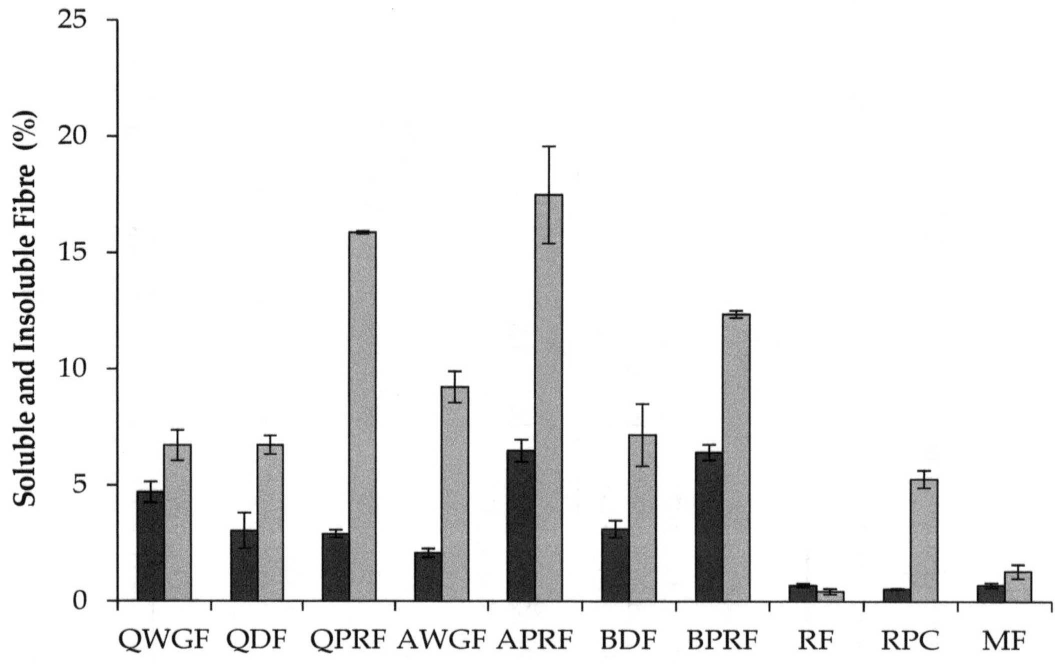

Figure 2. Soluble (■) and insoluble (□) dietary fibre content (% *w*/*w*) of quinoa wholegrain flour (QWGF), quinoa dehulled flour (QDF), quinoa protein-rich flour (QPRF), amaranth wholegrain flour (AWGF), amaranth protein-rich flour (APRF), buckwheat dehulled flour (BDF), buckwheat protein-rich flour (BPRF), rice flour (RF), rice protein concentrate (RPC), and maize flour (MF).

3.2. Protein Profile by SDS-PAGE Electrophoresis

SDS-PAGE analyses under non-reducing conditions (Figure 3a,b) and reducing conditions (Figure 3c) were performed using methods **I**, **II**, and **III**, respectively, as outlined in Section 2.3. All samples, except maize, showed common protein bands at ~50 kDa under non-reducing conditions (Figure 3a,b). This band corresponds to the globulin and glutelin fraction in pseudocereals and rice, respectively. For quinoa samples (QWGF, QDF, and QPRF), bands at ~50 kDa (Figure 3a,b) correspond to the 11S globulin fraction, also commonly referred to as chenopodin. Chenopodin consists of ~49 and 57 kDa subunits that are associated into a hexamer by non-covalent interactions [18,49]. When quinoa proteins are treated directly with the sample loading buffer (Figure 3a), two bands with molecular weight (MW) lower and higher than ~50 kDa can be observed. The higher intensity of the lower MW band (Figure 3a,b), suggests that this subunit is predominant in chenopodin protein. When the sample was treated with the protein extracting buffer containing SDS, urea, and thiourea (i.e., under non-reducing conditions; method **II** and Figure 3b), the chenopodin (~50 kDa) did not dissociate into bands of lower MW suggesting that disulphide bonds are the principal linkage between the subunits. In a similar manner to quinoa, the amaranth samples (AWGF and APRF), showed a band at ~50 kDa (Figure 3a,b), which corresponds to the hexameric 11S globulin or amarantin [17]. This major band might also be attributed to another glutelin-type protein which has similar molecular characteristics to those of amaranth 11S globulin [50]. Buckwheat samples, showed a main band at ~50 kDa, which may correspond to the major storage protein of buckwheat, the 13S legume-like globulin, and the minor storage protein, the trimer 8S vicilin-like globulin [51]. Rice samples also showed a major band at ~50 kDa (Figure 3a,b) which corresponds to the glutelin precursor [20].

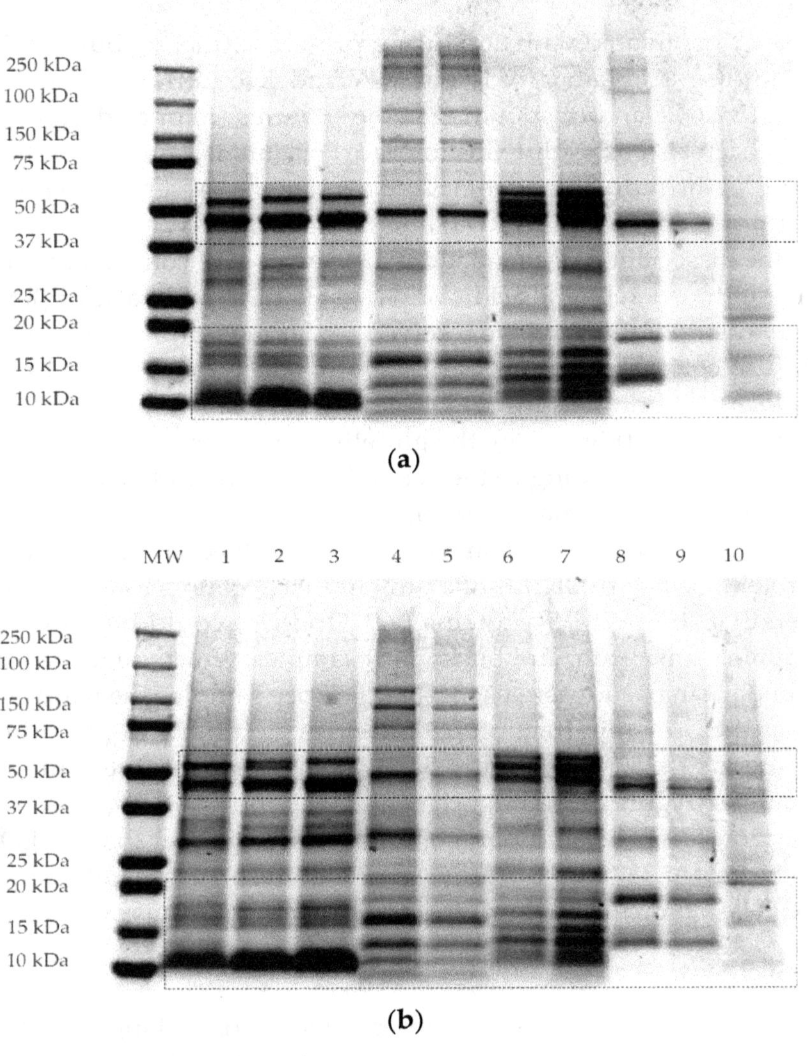

Figure 3. *Cont.*

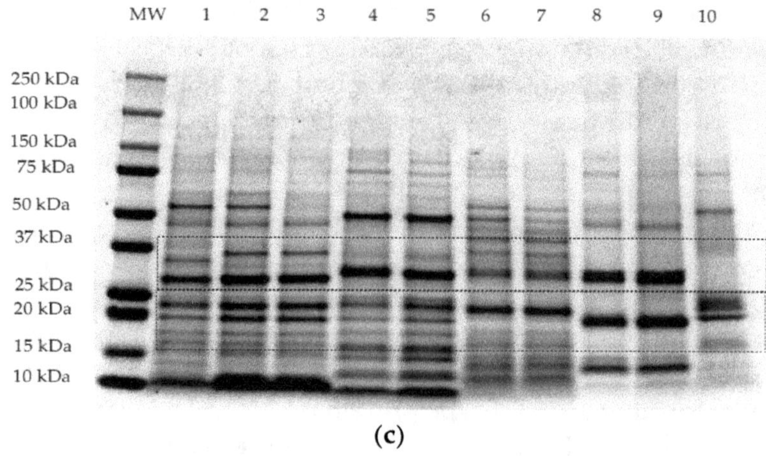

(c)

Figure 3. Representative sodium dodecyl sulphate–polyacrylamide gel electrophoresis (SDS-PAGE) patterns of quinoa wholegrain flour (1), quinoa dehulled flour (2), quinoa protein-rich flour (3), buckwheat dehulled flour (4), buckwheat protein-rich flour (5), amaranth wholegrain flour (6), amaranth protein-rich flour (7), rice flour (8), rice protein concentrate (9), and maize flour (10). The first lane of each gel contains the molecular weight marker. Samples were prepared according to methods I, II, and III for gel (**a**–**c**), respectively, as explained in Section 2.3.

When the samples were treated with a reducing protein extracting buffer (Figure 3c), the 50 kDa band was disrupted into several bands of lower MW and two of those bands were predominantly around 25–30 kDa and 15–20 kDa, corresponding to the subunits (α- or acidic and β- or basic) that form the globulins for pseudocereals or the glutelins for rice. For quinoa samples treated with the extracting buffer containing DTT as the reducing agent (Figure 3c), it was observed that the disulphide bonds that link the acidic or α- (MW ~28 and 34 kDa) and basic or β- (MW ~17 and 19 kDa) subunits were disrupted, leading to the dissociation of chenopodin into lower MW constituent proteins [28]. The same was observed for amaranth, whereby the acidic or α- (34–36 kDa) and basic or β- (22–24 kDa) subunits of amarantin linked by disulphide bonds are resolved under reducing conditions [17]. Buckwheat 13S legume-like globulin also consists of a small basic subunit (16–29 kDa) linked by a disulphide bond to a large acidic (30–38 kDa) subunit (Figure 3c) [52]. In the case of rice proteins, when the samples are treated with the reducing agent (Figure 3c), the glutelin precursor is disrupted into two main bands with MW ~30 and 20 kDa corresponding to the acidic (α-glutelin) and basic (β-glutelin) subunits that are linked by disulphide bonds. For maize proteins, when the sample was treated with the reducing extracting buffer (Figure 3c), two main protein bands were resolved around 20 kDa that may be related to the main maize protein, zein, a prolamin-like protein that accounts for 60% of the total protein [53].

Bands corresponding to low MW proteins (~10–15 kDa) could be observed in the three gels (Figure 3a–c) for all quinoa, amaranth, and buckwheat samples, which might be related to the albumin fraction, which is abundant in pseudocereals [54–56]. For rice samples the band evident at 13 kDa was reported previously as the prolamin fraction [20]. Besides globulin and albumin proteins, amaranth showed high MW proteins (~250 kDa; Figure 3a,b) which were resolved into bands of lower MW under reducing conditions (Figure 3c). Abugoch et al. [34], reported that amaranth glutelin contained an appreciable proportion of aggregated polypeptides of MW greater than 60 kDa. It is possible that the band evident on the gels at ~37 kDa for AWGF sample, and which is not disrupted under reducing conditions, might be the albumin-1 fraction, reported previously to have a MW of 34 kDa [17,55].

3.3. Starch Granules: Shape and Size

Different sizes, shapes, and structures were observed for flour and ingredient powder morphology and ultra-structure using scanning electron microscopy (SEM) analysis (Figure 4). Quinoa samples presented the smallest sized granules (1–1.20 μm) among all samples and had a polygonal shape.

The protein-rich flour (QPRF) showed granules covered and linked to other types of substances. This embryo-rich fraction is rich in protein, fibre, and fat which suggests that the starch granules are embedded in a matrix formed by these compounds. Li and Zhu [57] observed that some starch aggregates appeared to be coated with a film-like substance surrounded by a protein matrix. Amaranth samples, AWGF and APRF, showed circular granules with a size of ~2.5–3 μm. Amaranth seed is one of the few sources of small-granule starch, typically 1 to 3 μm in diameter, with a regular granule size [19]. The starch granules in APRF also appeared to be embedded within a matrix as observed for QPRF. Buckwheat starch granules showed the largest size (5 to 7.5 μm) among the pseudocereal samples with a mixture of spherical and polygonal structures. Christa et al. [58], also observed spherical, oval, and polygonal granules with a size distribution from 2 to 6 μm for buckwheat starch. Analysis of the granule structure and matrix positioning showed other components attached which may be protein and fat [59]. The BPRF samples, similar to that observed for QPRF and APRF, also had starch granules embedded in a matrix of other components. Analysis of RF ultrastructure showed starch granules with diameter between 4 and 5 μm, with an angular shape, while maize flour exhibited the largest starch granules (15 μm) with both circular and rod-shapes. These results are in agreement with Nienke et al. [60], who categorized starch granules into different sizes and defined the starch granules for amaranth and quinoa as very small, rice and buckwheat as small, and maize as generally having relatively large granules. The small size of the starch granules of some pseudocereals, such as quinoa, can offer advantages (e.g., altered emulsion stabilisation properties) in respect of incorporation into product formulations [57,61].

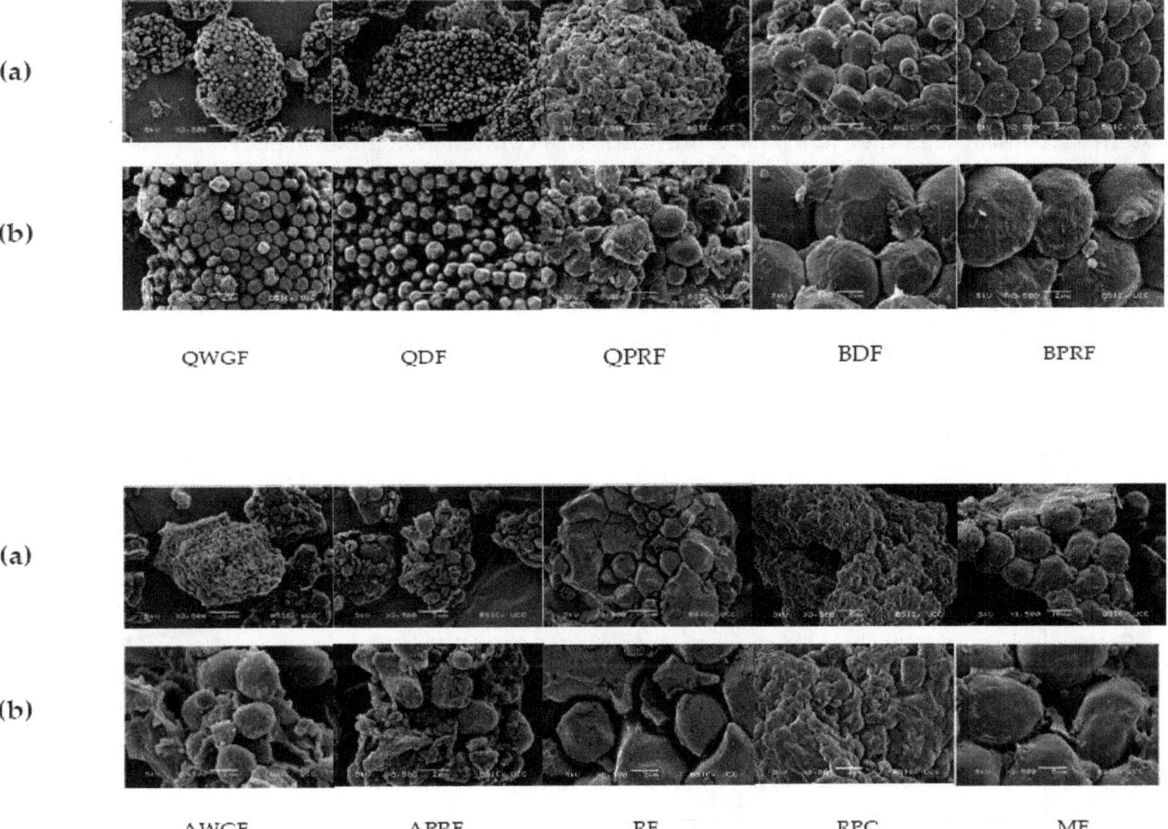

Figure 4. Scanning electron micrographs of quinoa wholegrain flour (QWGF), quinoa dehulled flour (QDF), quinoa protein-rich flour (QPRF), buckwheat dehulled flour (BDF), buckwheat protein-rich flour (BPRF), amaranth wholegrain flour (AWGF), amaranth protein-rich flour (APRF), rice flour (RF), rice protein concentrate (RPC), and maize flour (MF). *Magnification* row (**a**) ×3500; (**b**) ×8500. *Scale bars* row (**a**) 5 μm; (**b**) 2 μm.

3.4. Pasting Properties

The mean values for the initial, peak and final viscosity at the end of the holding stage at 95 °C, on completion of cooling to 50 °C, and at the end of the final holding period at 50 °C were recorded during pasting and are presented in Table 2. The shape of the pasting curves differed depending on the type of flour/ingredient (Figure 5a,b). Among the regular protein content flour samples, BDF and RF had the highest viscosity and AWGF the lowest. QWGF and QDF showed slight differences, with QDF having the lowest viscosity; this may be explained by the lower content of starch (50.5%) in QDF than in QWGF (60%). The peak time was very similar for all the flours (~12 min) tested, except MF and BDF which required a shorter time (~10.5 min) to reach peak viscosity, most likely due to the lower extent of absorption and swelling of their starch granules [62]. During the holding period at 95 °C, the material slurries were subjected to high temperature and mechanical shear stress, which further disrupted the starch granules, resulting in the leaching out from starch granules, and alignment, of amylose. It was observed that all the samples displayed a decrease in viscosity, especially so for BDF, RF, and MF, which had the more pronounced decreases in viscosity during the holding period at 95 °C (Figure 5a). The decrease in viscosity during the holding period is often correlated with high peak viscosity: it can be seen how BDF, RF and MF had the highest peak viscosities (Figure 5a). During cooling, re-association between starch molecules, especially amylose chains, will result in the formation of a gel structure and, therefore, viscosity will increase due to retrogradation and reordering of starch molecules. BDF (13.0 Pa·s) and AWGF (1.72 Pa·s) showed the highest and lowest final viscosity, respectively, while QWGF, QDF, RF, and MF showed broadly similar final viscosity values (5.83, 4.40, 4.31, and 5.07 Pa·s, respectively). Regarding the rheological profile of the protein-rich ingredients (Figure 5b), a similar pattern was observed as for the regular protein-content flours in respect of the initial, peak and final viscosities, but with considerably lower viscosity values observed overall. This can be explained by the lower content of starch and the higher content of dietary fibre in the protein-rich samples (Table 2). The water binding capacity of dietary fibre is greatly increased by the presence of high amounts of hydroxyl groups and can be related to a reduction in water availability, which could impact viscosity and pasting properties [63]. Also, the protein-rich flour ingredients are rich in ash, protein, and fat, which have been shown previously to influence the functionality of starch and impact on rheological behaviour of starch dispersions during pasting [59].

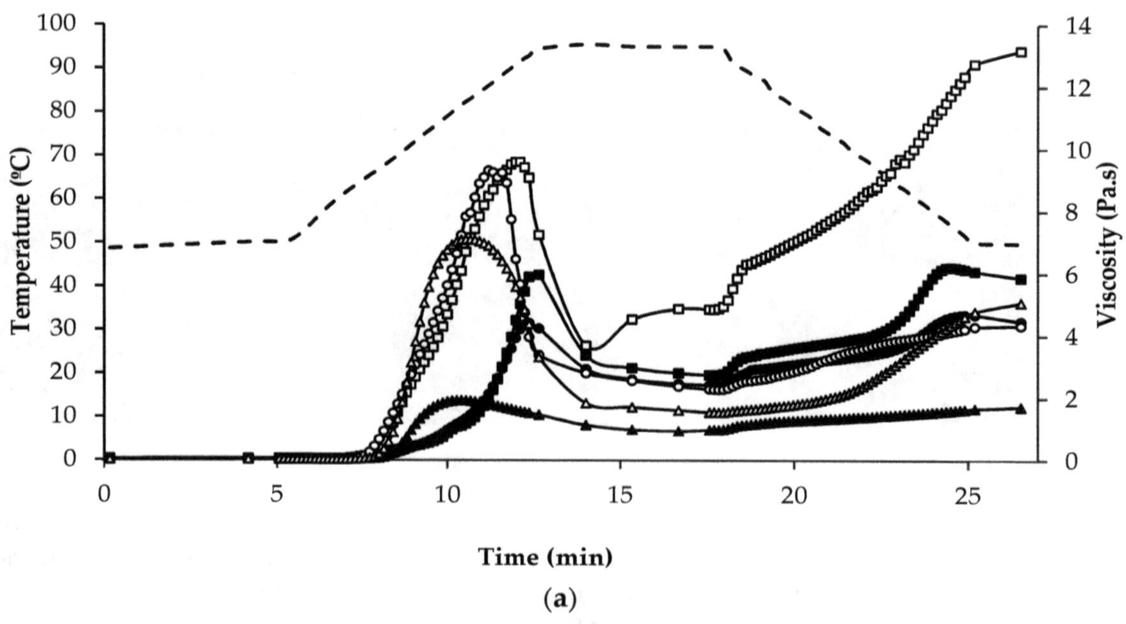

(a)

Figure 5. *Cont.*

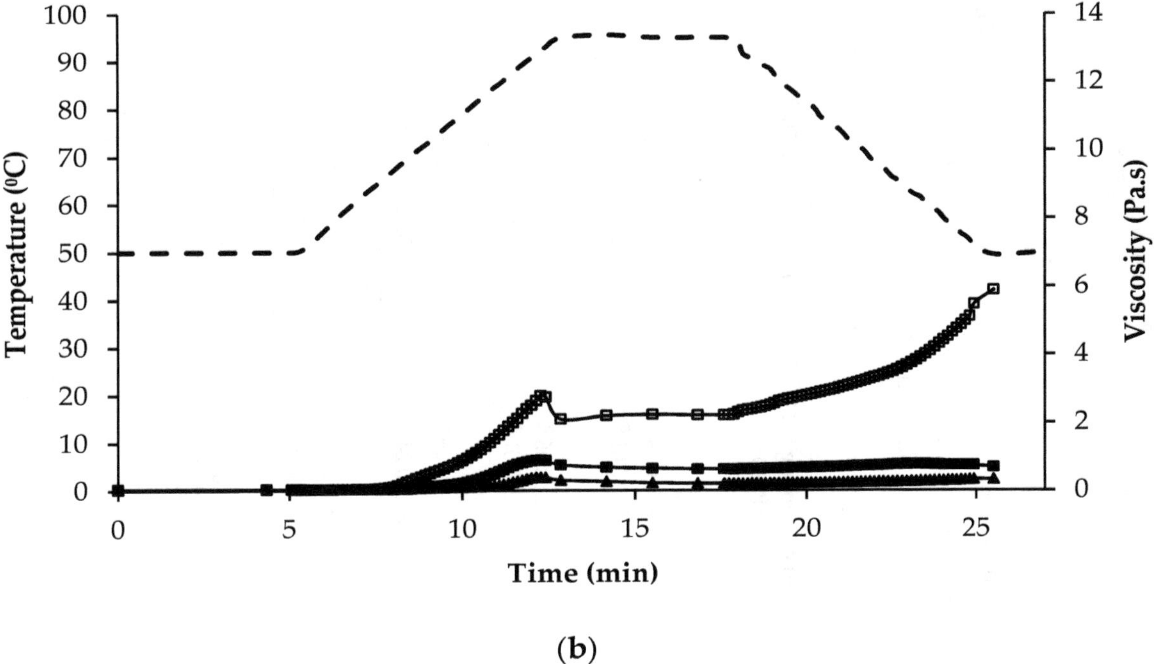

(b)

Figure 5. Temperature (dashed line) and viscosity (symbols) at various stages of the pasting regime of (**a**) regular protein containing flours: quinoa wholegrain flour (—▪—), quinoa dehulled flour (—•—), amaranth wholegrain flour (—▲—), buckwheat dehulled flour (BDF) (—◻—), rice flour (RF) (—○—), and maize flour (—△—); (**b**) of protein enriched flour ingredients: quinoa protein-rich flour (—▪—), amaranth protein-rich flour (—▲—), buckwheat protein-rich flour (—◻—).

Of particular interest, were the high and low viscosity values recorded during pasting for buckwheat and amaranth, respectively. These differences can be related to several factors associated with the starch component of the ingredients, namely the proportion and type of crystalline organization (amylose:amylopectin ratio), size and ultra-structure of the starch granule and extent of starch damage. The amylose content of amaranth and quinoa starch, a component which is related to a stronger and more cohesive gel with higher final paste viscosity [62,64], has been reported to be much lower than that found in buckwheat, rice, or maize [9]. In the case of quinoa starch, the amylose content ranges from 3.5% to 19.6% of total starch, while in amaranth seeds amylose levels have been reported to be lower than 8% [26]. In contrast, the amylose content of buckwheat has been reported to be as high as 57% [58]. Therefore, for buckwheat a higher final viscosity would be expected than for quinoa or amaranth. The starch granule size also influences the pasting temperature, whereby smaller granules have been associated with lower pasting temperatures [60]. BDF had the largest starch granules among the pseudocereal samples analysed in this study (Figure 4) while quinoa and amaranth had the smallest. Yoshimoto et al. [65], reported a higher granule swelling and gelling capacity for buckwheat starches compared with cereal starches. Another factor that can impact the pasting properties is the resistance of starch to digestion by α-amylase during the heating process; Izydorczyk et al. [66] associated the ability of buckwheat to form strong gels with the high resistance of the starch component to digestion by α-amylase. In addition, Lu et al. [67] associated reduced enzyme digestibility of cooked buckwheat groats with retrogradation and formation of resistant starch.

The understanding of the heat-induced rheological behaviour of these protein-rich ingredients is of great importance for the development of tailored nutritional products (e.g., low viscosity in plant-based milk substitutes or high viscosity in yogurt-type products).

Table 2. Viscosity of quinoa wholegrain flour (QWGF), quinoa dehulled flour (QDF), quinoa protein-rich flour (QPRF), amaranth wholegrain flour (AWGF), amaranth protein-rich flour (APRF), buckwheat dehulled flour (BDF), buckwheat protein-rich flour (BPRF), rice flour (RF), rice protein concentrate (RPC), and maize flour (MF) dispersions at various stages of the pasting regime. Values are means ± standard deviations of data from triplicate analysis.

	Stage of Pasting					
	Initial Viscosity (mPa·s)	**Peak Viscosity (Pa·s)**	**Peak Time (min)**	**End of Holding at 95 °C (Pa·s)**	**End of Cooling to 50 °C (Pa·s)**	**Final Paste at 50 °C (Pa·s)**
Quinoa						
QWGF	$18.4 \pm 0.76^{a,b}$	6.25 ± 0.18^{e}	12.5	2.74 ± 0.34^{e}	6.07 ± 0.30^{e}	5.83 ± 0.43^{e}
QDF	$24.8 \pm 1.05^{b,c}$	4.39 ± 0.16^{d}	12.5	2.41 ± 0.24^{c}	4.68 ± 0.19^{c}	4.40 ± 0.22^{c}
QPRF	$24.1 \pm 0.12^{b,c}$	0.91 ± 0.03^{ab}	12.5	0.63 ± 0.01^{a}	0.75 ± 0.01^{a}	0.67 ± 0.01^{a}
Amaranth						
AWGF	29.1 ± 1.32^{c}	$1.92 \pm 0.07^{b,c}$	10.3	0.98 ± 0.03^{b}	1.64 ± 0.06^{b}	1.72 ± 0.07^{b}
APRF	26.4 ± 0.84^{c}	0.29 ± 0.03^{a}	12.5	0.13 ± 0.01^{a}	0.19 ± 0.01^{a}	0.19 ± 0.01^{a}
Buckwheat						
BDF	48.4 ± 2.64^{e}	9.60 ± 0.46^{f}	12.1	4.84 ± 0.90^{f}	12.5 ± 0.47^{f}	13.0 ± 0.35^{f}
BPRF	37.5 ± 2.21^{d}	2.81 ± 0.10^{c}	12.5	2.23 ± 0.07^{d}	5.35 ± 0.24^{d}	5.92 ± 0.24^{e}
Rice						
RF	15.5 ± 0.06^{a}	9.37 ± 1.43^{f}	11.2	2.28 ± 0.23^{c}	4.24 ± 0.15^{c}	4.31 ± 0.13^{c}
RPC	17.9 ± 0.13^{a}	n.d.	n.d.	0.02 ± 0.00^{g}	0.02 ± 0.00^{g}	0.02 ± 0.00^{g}
Maize						
MF	16.4 ± 0.02^{a}	7.11 ± 0.20^{e}	10.6	1.54 ± 0.15^{cd}	4.67 ± 0.30^{cd}	5.07 ± 0.33^{d}

Values followed by different superscript letters (a–g) in the same column are significantly different ($p < 0.05$). n.d. = not detected.

4. Conclusions

In this study, the nutrient composition, protein profile, and rheological properties of a range of novel protein-rich pseudocereal flour ingredients were studied and compared to regular protein content pseudocereal, maize, and rice flours. The protein-rich flour ingredients had higher levels of ash, fat, and dietary fibre, and lower levels of starch. An integrated proteomic approach was implemented to gain enhanced clarity on the ingredient's protein profiles, with two strong protein extracting buffers being used for the first time, to allow the complete solubilization and characterization of the proteins in the pseudocereal ingredients. The results showed common bands under non-reducing and reducing conditions that corresponded to the globulin and albumin fractions. The predominance of globulins and albumins in pseudocereals is technologically significant since they are highly soluble in water and dilute salt solutions, which can be an advantage for food formulation purposes, in particular for the production of plant-based beverages. Buckwheat and amaranth had the highest and lowest final viscosity, respectively; while the protein-rich flours had considerably lower viscosity than their regular protein content counterparts. This study provides essential and much-needed new fundamental and applied knowledge on the compositional, structural, and functional properties of protein-rich pseudocereal ingredients to assist in further developing their utilisation in nutritious, functional, and stable food formulations.

Author Contributions: James A. O'Mahony and Loreto Alonso-Miravalles conceived and designed the experiments; Loreto Alonso-Miravalles performed the experiments, collated and analysed the data; James A. O'Mahony and Loreto Alonso-Miravalles prepared the manuscript.

Acknowledgments: This study was part of the PROTEIN2FOOD project. This project has received funding from the European Union's Horizon 2020 research and innovation programme under grant agreement No. 635727. The authors would like to acknowledge Juergen Bez (Fraunhofer Institut, Munich, Germany) for providing the protein-rich ingredients.

References

1. Henchion, M.; Hayes, M.; Mullen, A.M.; Fenelon, M.; Tiwari, B. Future protein supply and demand: strategies and factors influencing a sustainable equilibrium. *Foods* **2017**, *6*, 53. [CrossRef] [PubMed]
2. Day, L. Proteins from land plants—Potential resources for human nutrition and food security. *Trends Food Sci. Technol.* **2013**, *32*, 25–42. [CrossRef]
3. Nations, U. *Revision of World Population Prospects*; United Nations: New York, NY, USA, 2015.
4. Aiking, H. Future protein supply. *Trends Food Sci. Technol.* **2011**, *22*, 112–120. [CrossRef]
5. Schutyser, M.A.I.; Pelgrom, P.J.M.; van der Goot, A.J.; Boom, R.M. Dry fractionation for sustainable production of functional legume protein concentrates. *Trends Food Sci. Technol.* **2015**, *45*, 327–335. [CrossRef]
6. Wouters, A.G.B.; Rombouts, I.; Fierens, E.; Brijs, K.; Delcour, J.A. Relevance of the functional properties of enzymatic plant protein hydrolysates in food systems. *Compr. Rev. Food Sci. Food Saf.* **2016**, *15*, 786–800. [CrossRef]
7. Alting, A.C.; Van De Velde, F. Proteins as clean label ingredients in foods and beverages. In *Natural Food Additives, Ingredients and Flavourings*; Baines, D., Seal, R., Eds.; Woodhead Publishing Limited: Cambridge, UK, 2012; pp. 197–211. ISBN 978-1-84-569811-9.
8. Jacobsen, S.E.; Sørensen, M.; Pedersen, S.M.; Weiner, J. Feeding the world: Genetically modified crops versus agricultural biodiversity. *Agron. Sustain. Dev.* **2013**, *33*, 651–662. [CrossRef]
9. Haros, C.M.; Schoenlechner, R. *Pseudocereals: Chemistry and Technology*, 1st ed.; Wiley Blackwell: Chichester, UK, 2017; ISBN 978-1-11-893825-6.
10. Schoenlechner, R.; Siebenhandl, S.; Berghofer, E. Pseudocereals. In *Gluten-Free Cereal Product and Beverages*; Arendt, E.K., Dal Bello, F., Eds.; Elsevier: New York, NY, USA, 2008; pp. 149–190. ISBN 978-0-12-373739-7.
11. Taylor, J.; Awika, J. *Gluten-Free Ancient Grains. Cereals, Pseudocereals, and Legumes: Sustainable, Nutritious, and Health-Promoting Foods for the 21st Century*, 1st ed.; Taylor, J., Awika, J., Eds.; Woodhead Publishing Limited: Duxford, UK, 2017; ISBN 978-0-08-100866-9.

12. Mota, C.; Santos, M.; Mauro, R.; Samman, N.; Matos, A.S.; Torres, D.; Castanheira, I. Protein content and amino acids profile of pseudocereals. *Food Chem.* **2016**, *193*, 55–61. [CrossRef] [PubMed]
13. Tester, R.F.; Karkalas, J.; Qi, X. Starch—Composition, fine structure and architecture. *J. Cereal Sci.* **2004**, *39*, 151–165. [CrossRef]
14. Steadman, K.J.J.; Burgoon, M.S.S.; Lewis, B.A.A.; Edwardson, S.E.E.; Obendorf, R.L.L. Buckwheat seed milling fractions: Description, macronutrient composition and dietary fibre. *J. Cereal Sci.* **2001**, *33*, 271–278. [CrossRef]
15. Schirmer, M.; Höchstötter, A.; Jekle, M.; Arendt, E.; Becker, T. Physicochemical and morphological characterization of different starches with variable amylose/amylopectin ratio. *Food Hydrocoll.* **2013**, *32*, 52–63. [CrossRef]
16. Horstmann, S.; Belz, M.M.; Heitmann, M.; Zannini, E.; Arendt, E. Fundamental study on the impact of gluten-free starches on the quality of gluten-free model breads. *Foods* **2016**, *5*, 30. [CrossRef] [PubMed]
17. Janssen, F.; Pauly, A.; Rombouts, I.; Jansens, K.J.A.; Deleu, L.J.; Delcour, J.A. Proteins of amaranth (*Amaranthus* spp.), buckwheat (*Fagopyrum* spp.), and quinoa (*Chenopodium* spp.): A food science and technology perspective. *Compr. Rev. Food Sci. Food Saf.* **2017**, *16*, 39–58. [CrossRef]
18. Mäkinen, O.E.; Zannini, E.; Koehler, P.; Arendt, E.K. Heat-denaturation and aggregation of quinoa (*Chenopodium quinoa*) globulins as affected by the pH value. *Food Chem.* **2016**, *196*, 17–24. [CrossRef] [PubMed]
19. Venskutonis, P.R.; Kraujalis, P. Nutritional components of amaranth seeds and vegetables: A review on composition, properties, and uses. *Compr. Rev. Food Sci. Food Saf.* **2013**, *12*, 381–412. [CrossRef]
20. Amagliani, L.; O'Regan, J.; Kelly, A.L.; O'Mahony, J.A. Composition and protein profile analysis of rice protein ingredients. *J. Food Compos. Anal.* **2016**, *59*, 18–26. [CrossRef]
21. DeVries, J.W. *Dietary Fibre: New Frontiers for Food and Health*; van der Kamp, J.W., Jones, J.M., McCleary, B.V., Topping, D.L., Eds.; Wageningen Academic Publishers: Wageningen, The Netherlands, 2010; ISBN 978-9-08-686128-6.
22. Codex Alimentarius Commission. *Report of the 27th Session of the Codex Committee on Nutrition and Foods for Special Dietary Uses*; Codex Alimentarius Commission: Rome, Italy, 2005.
23. Foschia, M.; Peressini, D.; Sensidoni, A.; Brennan, C.S. The effects of dietary fibre addition on the quality of common cereal products. *J. Cereal Sci.* **2013**, *58*, 216–227. [CrossRef]
24. Alvarez-Jubete, L.; Arendt, E.K.; Gallagher, E. Nutritive value and chemical composition of pseudocereals as gluten-free ingredients. *Int. J. Food Sci. Nutr.* **2009**, *60*, 240–257. [CrossRef] [PubMed]
25. Burrieza, H.P.; Lopez-Fernandez, M.P.; Maldonado, S. Analogous reserve distribution and tissue characteristics in quinoa and grass seeds suggest convergent evolution. *Front. Plant Sci.* **2014**, *5*, 546. [CrossRef] [PubMed]
26. Alvarez-Jubete, L.; Arendt, E.K.; Gallagher, E. Nutritive value of pseudocereals and their increasing use as functional gluten-free ingredients. *Trends Food Sci. Technol.* **2010**, *21*, 106–113. [CrossRef]
27. Nosworthy, M.G.; Tulbek, M.C.; House, J.D. Does the concentration, isolation, or deflavoring of pea, lentil, and faba bean protein alter protein quality? *Cereal Foods World* **2017**, *62*, 139–142. [CrossRef]
28. Avila Ruiz, G.; Arts, A.; Minor, M.; Schutyser, M. A hybrid dry and aqueous fractionation method to obtain protein-rich fractions from quinoa (*Chenopodium quinoa* Willd). *Food Bioprocess Technol.* **2016**, *9*, 1502–1510. [CrossRef]
29. Berghout, J.A.M.; Pelgrom, P.J.M.; Schutyser, M.A.I.; Boom, R.M.; van der Goot, A.J. Sustainability assessment of oilseed fractionation processes: A case study on lupin seeds. *J. Food Eng.* **2015**, *150*, 117–124. [CrossRef]
30. Boukid, F.; Folloni, S.; Sforza, S.; Vittadini, E.; Prandi, B. Current trends in ancient grains-based foodstuffs: insights into nutritional aspects and technological applications. *Compr. Rev. Food Sci. Food Saf.* **2018**, *17*, 123–136. [CrossRef]
31. Pelgrom, P.J.M.; Boom, R.M.; Schutyser, M.A.I. Functional analysis of mildly refined fractions from yellow pea. *Food Hydrocoll.* **2015**, *44*, 12–22. [CrossRef]
32. AOAC. *Official Methods of Analysis of the Association of Official Analytical Chemists*, 18th ed.; AOAC: Washington, DC, USA, 2010.
33. Nascimento, A.C.; Mota, C.; Coelho, I.; Gueifão, S.; Santos, M.; Matos, A.S.; Gimenez, A.; Lobo, M.; Samman, N.; Castanheira, I. Characterisation of nutrient profile of quinoa (*Chenopodium quinoa*), amaranth (*Amaranthus caudatus*), and purple corn (*Zea mays* L.) consumed in the North of Argentina: Proximates, minerals and trace elements. *Food Chem.* **2014**, *148*, 420–426. [CrossRef] [PubMed]

34. Abugoch James, L.E. Quinoa (*Chenopodium quinoa* Willd.): Composition, chemistry, nutritional, and functional properties. *Adv. Food Nutr. Res.* **2009**, *58*, 1–31. [CrossRef] [PubMed]
35. Li, G.; Wang, S.; Zhu, F. Physicochemical properties of quinoa starch. *Carbohydr. Polym.* **2016**, *137*, 328–338. [CrossRef] [PubMed]
36. Bradley, R.L. Moisture and Total Solids Analysis. In *Food Analysis*; Nielsen, S., Ed.; Springer: West Lafayette, IN, USA, 2010; pp. 85–104. ISBN 1441914781.
37. Roudaut, G.; Debeaufort, F. Moisture loss, gain and migration in foods. In *Food and Beverage Stability and Shelf Life*; Elsevier: New York, NY, USA, 2011; pp. 63–105. ISBN 978-1-84-569701-3.
38. Schuck, P.; Dolivet, A.; Jeantet, R. Determination of Dry Matter and Total Dry Matter. In *Analytical Methods for Food and Dairy Powders*; Schuck, P., Dolivet, A., Jeantet, R., Eds.; John Wiley & Sons, Ltd.: Hoboken, NJ, USA, 2012; pp. 45–57. ISBN 978-1-11-830739-7.
39. Tyler, R.T.; Youngs, C.G.; Sosulski, F.W. Air Classification of legumes. I. Separation efficiency, yield, and composition of the starch and protein fractions. *Cereal Chem.* **1981**, *58*, 144–148.
40. Arendt, E.K.; Zannini, E. *Cereal Grains for the Food and Beverage Industries*, 1st ed.; Woodhead Publishing Limited: Cambridge, UK, 2013; ISBN 978-0-85-709413-1.
41. Gamel, T.H.; Mesallam, A.S.; Damir, A.A.; Shekib, L.A.; Linssen, J.P. Characterization of amaranth seeds oil. *J. Food Lipids* **2007**, *14*, 323–334. [CrossRef]
42. Navruz-Varli, S.; Sanlier, N. Nutritional and health benefits of quinoa (*Chenopodium quinoa* Willd.). *J. Cereal Sci.* **2016**, *69*, 371–376. [CrossRef]
43. Barrera, G.N.; Bustos, M.C.; Iturriaga, L.; Flores, S.K.; Leon, A.E.; Ribotta, P.D. Effect of damaged starch on the rheological properties of wheat starch suspensions. *J. Food Eng.* **2013**, *116*, 233–239. [CrossRef]
44. Nowak, V.; Du, J.; Charrondière, U.R. Assessment of the nutritional composition of quinoa (*Chenopodium quinoa* Willd.). *Food Chem.* **2016**, *193*, 47–54. [CrossRef] [PubMed]
45. Ando, H.; Chen, Y.-C.; Tang, H.; Mayumi, S.; Watanabe, K.; Mitsunaga, T. Food components in fractions of quinoa seed. *Food Sci. Technol. Res.* **2002**, *8*, 80–84. [CrossRef]
46. Repo-Carrasco, R.; Peña, J.; Kallio, H.; Salminen, S. Dietary fiber and other functional components in two varieties of crude and extruded kiwicha (*Amaranthus caudatus*). *J. Cereal Sci.* **2009**, *49*, 219–224. [CrossRef]
47. Ruales, J.; Grijalva, Y.; Lopez-Jaramillo, P.; Nair, B. The nutritional quality of an infant food from quinoa and its effect on the plasma level of insulin-like growth factor-1 (IGF-1) in undernourished children. *Int. J. Food Sci. Nutr.* **2002**, *53*, 143–154. [CrossRef] [PubMed]
48. Repo-Carrasco, R.; Astuhuaman Serna, L. Quinoa (*Chenopodium quinoa*, Willd.) as a source of dietary fiber and other functional components. *Food Sci. Technol.* **2009**, *31*, 225–230. [CrossRef]
49. Mir, N.A.; Riar, C.S.; Singh, S. Nutritional constituents of pseudo cereals and their potential use in food systems: A review. *Trends Food Sci. Technol.* **2018**, *75*, 170–180. [CrossRef]
50. Vasco-Méndez, N.L.; Paredes-López, O. Antigenic homology between amaranth glutelins and other storage proteins. *Food Biochem.* **1994**, *18*, 227–238. [CrossRef]
51. Milisavljević, M.D.; Timotijević, G.S.; Radović, S.R.; Brkljačić, J.M.; Konstantinović, M.M.; Maksimović, V.R. Vicilin-like storage globulin from buckwheat (*Fagopyrum esculentum* Moench) seeds. *J. Agric. Food Chem.* **2004**, *52*, 5258–5262. [CrossRef] [PubMed]
52. Choi, S.M.; Ma, C.Y. Conformational study of globulin from common buckwheat (*Fagopyrum esculentum* Moench) by fourier transform infrared spectroscopy and differential scanning calorimetry. *J. Agric. Food Chem.* **2005**, *53*, 8046–8053. [CrossRef] [PubMed]
53. Anderson, T.J.; Lamsa, B.P. Zein extraction from corn, corn products, and coproducts and modifications for various applications: A review. *Cereal Chem.* **2011**, *88*, 159–173. [CrossRef]
54. Valencia-Chamorro, S.A. Quinoa. In *Encyclopedia of Food Sciences and Nutrition*; Elsevier: Amsterdam, The Netherlands, 2003; pp. 4895–4902.
55. Gorinstein, S.; Pawelzik, E.; Delgado-Licon, E.; Haruenkit, R.; Weisz, M.; Trakhtenberg, S. Characterisation of pseudocereal and cereal proteins by protein and amino acid analyses. *J. Sci. Food Agric.* **2002**, *82*, 886–891. [CrossRef]
56. Radovic, R.S.; Maksimovic, R.V.; Brkljacic, M.J.; Varkonji Gasic, I.E.; Savic, P.A. 2S albumin from buckwheat (*Fagopyrum esculentum* Moench) seeds. *J. Agric. Food Chem.* **1999**, *47*, 1467–1470. [CrossRef] [PubMed]
57. Li, G.; Zhu, F. Molecular structure of quinoa starch. *Carbohydr. Polym.* **2017**, *158*, 124–132. [CrossRef] [PubMed]

58. Christa, K.; Soral-Smietana, M.; Lewandowicz, G. Buckwheat starch: Structure, functionality and enzyme in vitro susceptibility upon the roasting process. *Int. J. Food Sci. Nutr.* **2009**, *60*, 140–154. [CrossRef] [PubMed]
59. Debet, M.R.; Gidley, M.J. Three classes of starch granule swelling: Influence of surface proteins and lipids. *Carbohydr. Polym.* **2006**, *64*, 452–465. [CrossRef]
60. Nienke, L.; Chang, P.R.; Tyler, R.T. Analytical, biochemical and physicochemical aspects of starch granule size, with emphasis on small granule starches: A review. *Starch Stärke* **2004**, *56*, 89–99. [CrossRef]
61. Rayner, M.; Timgren, A.; Sjoo, M.; Dejmek, P. Quinoa starch granules: A candidate for stabilising food-grade pickering emulsions. *J. Sci. Food Agric.* **2012**, *92*, 1841–1847. [CrossRef] [PubMed]
62. Ragaee, S.; Abdel-Aal, E.S.M. Pasting properties of starch and protein in selected cereals and quality of their food products. *Food Chem.* **2006**, *95*, 9–18. [CrossRef]
63. Bulut-Solak, B.; Alonso-Miravalles, L.; O'Mahony, J.A. Composition, morphology and pasting properties of Orchis anatolica tuber gum. *Food Hydrocoll.* **2016**, *69*, 483–490. [CrossRef]
64. Wang, S.; Li, C.; Copeland, L.; Niu, Q.; Shuo, W. Starch retrogradation: A comprehensive review. *Compr. Rev. Food Sci. Food Saf.* **2015**, *14*, 568–585. [CrossRef]
65. Yoshimoto, Y.; Egashira, T.; Hanashiro, I.; Ohinata, H.; Takase, Y.; Takeda, Y. Molecular structure and some physicochemical properties of buckwheat starches. *Cereal Chem.* **2004**, *81*, 515–520. [CrossRef]
66. Izydorczyk, M.S.; McMillan, T.; Bazin, S.; Kletke, J.; Dushnicky, L.; Dexter, J. Canadian buckwheat: A unique, useful and under-utilized crop. *Can. J. Plant Sci.* **2013**, *94*, 509–524. [CrossRef]
67. Lu, L.; Murphy, K.; Baik, B.K. Genotypic variation in nutritional composition of buckwheat groats and husks. *Cereal Chem.* **2013**, *90*, 132–137. [CrossRef]

3

The Potential of Modulating the Reducing Sugar Released (and the Potential Glycemic Response) of Muffins using a Combination of a Stevia Sweetener and Cocoa Powder

Jingrong Gao [1,2,3,*], Xinbo Guo [1,4], Margaret A. Brennan [2,3], Susan L. Mason [2], Xin-An Zeng [1,4] and Charles S. Brennan [1,2,3,4,*]

1 School of Food Science and Engineering, South China University of Technology, Guangzhou 510640, China; guoxinbo@scut.edu.cn (X.G.); xazeng@scut.edu.cn (X.-A.Z.)
2 Department of Wine, Food and Molecular Biosciences, Lincoln University, Christchurch 7647, New Zealand; margaret.brennan@lincoln.ac.nz (M.A.B.); Sue.mason@lincoln.ac.nz (S.L.M.)
3 Riddet Research Institute, Palmerston North 4442, New Zealand
4 Overseas Expertise Introduction Center for Discipline Innovation of Food Nutrition and Human Health (111 Center), Guangzhou 510640, China
* Correspondence: gaojingrong@scut.edu.cn (J.G.); charles.brennan@lincoln.ac.nz (C.S.B.)
† The article is part of Ph.D. Thesis of Jingrong Gao.

Abstract: Muffins are popular bakery products. However, they generally contain high amounts of sugar. The over-consumption of muffins may therefore result in a high calorie intake and could lead to increased health risks. For this reason, muffins were prepared substituting sucrose with two levels of a base of stevia (Stevianna®). In addition, cocoa powder and vanilla were added to the muffin formulation with and without Stevianna® to mask any potential off flavors. Results illustrate that muffins with 50% Stevianna® replacement of sucrose were similar to the control samples in terms of volume, density and texture. However, replacement of sugar with 100% Stevianna® resulted in reductions in height (from 41 to 28 mm), volume (from 63 to 51 mL), and increased firmness (by four-fold) compared to the control sample. Sugar replacement significantly reduced the in vitro predictive glycemic response of muffins (by up to 55% of the control sample). This work illustrates the importance of sugar in maintaining muffin structure as well as controlling the rate of glucose release during simulated digestions.

Keywords: muffin; in vitro starch digestibility; glycemic index; stevia; sugar replacement

---

1. Introduction

In recent years, consumers have gained an increasing awareness regarding the effect of dietary carbohydrates on the nutritional quality of foods. In particular, attention has been focused on the relationship between the various types of carbohydrate containing foods and the different postprandial glucose responses by these foods post ingestion [1–7]. The glycemic index (GI) is a physiological classification widely accepted for carbohydrate foods based on their ability to raise the concentration of glucose in the blood [7–9]. Bakery foods, muffins for example, are regarded as a high glycemic impact food due to the high concentration of sugar contained in the muffins. Previous research [10,11] has shown that the over-consumption of sucrose can lead to a number of metabolic complications including hyperinsulinemia, hyperglycemia, hypertension and insulin resistance, as well as being related to dyslipidemia and ectopic lipid deposition in healthy subjects with diabetes [12]. Indeed, high GI food products are quickly digested and their carbohydrate is rapidly absorbed, resulting in higher blood glucose levels [13]. On the contrary, the health benefits of the low GI products are thought to be derived from the slower the rate of carbohydrate absorption, consequently leading to a gradual rise in blood glucose level and better glycemic control [14].

The food industry has focused on reducing the calorific content of food to promote a healthier diet. Therefore, different natural sweeteners have been used in sugar-reduced or sugar-free products based on their multiple potential health benefits and functional properties, including maintaining sweetness and acceptable texture [15–18].

Steviol glycosides have been extracted and purified from the leaves of *Stevia rebaudiana* Bertoni, commonly known as stevia; they are naturally sweet-tasting, have good solubility in water, good temperature and pH stability [19–21] as well as having no calorific value [22], allowing them to be used as a sugar substitute or natural sweetener. Stevioside and rebaudioside A are the major glycoside constituents responsible for sweetness and are the most abundant glycosides in the *Stevia rebaudiana* Bertoni plant [23–25]. They are very useful as a food additive due to their relative sweetness being 250–300 times sweeter than table sugar [26].

Extracts from stevia have broad health-promoting properties for blood glucose and insulin levels in human studies [27]. Steviol glycosides are not hydrolyzed by human digestive enzymes of the mouth, stomach, and small intestine [28]. However, rebaudioside A and stevioside are hydrolyzed (in vitro and in vivo) to aglycone steviol by colon microflora through the successive removal of glucose units [29]. Chang et al. [27] reported that insulin sensitivity is increased due to stevia consumption in rodent models, and thus does not increase blood glucose and insulin levels [22]. Furthermore, previous work has found that a reduction in the predicted glycemic response was observed due to 50% or 100% replacement of sucrose with Stevianna® in muffins during in vitro digestion experiments [30]. Therefore, stevia has the potential to be a low-cost natural sweetener due to important pro-health properties, such as being non-calorific, non-fermentable and non-toxic as well as having a high-intensity sweetness [31], and it is also recommended as a treatment for diabetics and obese persons [23].

However, several studies have shown that the utilization of stevia as a sugar replacer in baking leads to a negative effect on appearance, compactness, moisture and texture of the bakery products structure [17,32,33]. These results have indicated that stevia is not acceptable to replace sucrose completely in bakery products as stevia exhibits high-intensity sweetness but does not possess the necessary bulking characteristics [34]. That is why Stevianna® (product code ST001 SE supplied by Stevianna® NZ) is used for our study, as it incorporates rebaudioside A (98% steviol glycoside; 1%) with erythritol (99%).

Erythritol is a four-carbon sugar alcohol or polyol with approximately 60% to 80% of the sweetness of sucrose [35]. It is not only a sweetener but also a bulking agent, and thus can be used as a sugar replacer in bakery products. Partial replacement of sucrose with erythritol had no negative influence on physical quality characteristics in a baked product [34,36]. In addition, previous studies reported that erythritol is useful as a non-glycemic and low-calorie sweetener that is safe for diabetics [37,38]. Erythritol has been demonstrated to have a small molecular size, thus it is rapidly absorbed by the small intestine and does not undergo systemic metabolism by the human body [37,39]. Some research has shown that the combination of a high-intensity sweetener with bulking agents or fibers in sugar-reduced formulations of food resulted in bakery products with acceptable physical quality [26,29,40,41].

None of these previous studies assessed a complex food sweetener to replace traditional sugar in bakery products. The aim of the study was to evaluate the replacement of sugar with Stevianna® (1 × sweetness of sucrose) and the addition of cocoa powder and/or vanilla to muffins for their physical properties and glycemic response, compared with a control muffin formulation with no added Stevianna®, cocoa powder, or vanilla.

2. Materials and Methods

2.1. Raw Materials

Wheat flour (Medal Premium baker flour, Champion, Auckland, New Zealand), white sugar (Chelsea, Auckland, New Zealand), baking powder (Edmonds, Christchurch, New Zealand), iodized table salt (Cerebos, Auckland, New Zealand), skim milk powder (Pams, Auckland, New Zealand), 100% cocoa powder (Cadbury, Dunedin, New Zealand), vanilla (Hansells, Sydney, Australia), canola oil (Pams, Auckland, New Zealand), and fresh eggs were purchased from a local supermarket and tap water was used. Muffins were prepared containing 0%, 50% and 100% Stevianna® (produce code ST001_SE; Stevianna®, Auckland, New Zealand) as a replacement for sucrose. Stevianna® utilizes Reb-A 98% steviol glycoside as the main sugar substitute along with erythritol.

2.2. Muffin Preparation

The muffin recipe was adapted from a previous study [30] and is given in Table 1. The Stevianna® was dissolved in the water and mixed with liquid whole egg and oil. After that, the dry ingredients were added into the liquid components and mixed for 5 min. The batter was poured into a paper baking case in a muffin pan. The muffins were baked for 18 min in a preheated Simpson Gemini Atlas series oven at 180 °C set to fan bake. Baked muffins were cooled at room temperature for 1 h, then packed in plastic resealable bags and stored in a refrigerator at 4 °C until physical analysis.

2.3. Muffin Height

The muffin product was taken out from the paper baking case, and the muffin height was measured with an electronic caliper (INSIZE) from the highest point of the muffin to the bottom of the muffin.

2.4. Moisture Content

A domestic kitchen food chopper (Zyliss®) was used to crush and homogenize the muffin (crust and crumb) of each formulation. Approximately 4 g was dried in an air oven at 105 °C for 16 h, until no further weight change.

The moisture content (MC) was calculated using the following equation:

$$\mathrm{MC}\ (\%) = (\mathrm{W}_{\text{before drying}} - \mathrm{W}_{\text{after drying}}/\mathrm{W}_{\text{before drying}}) \times 100 \quad (1)$$

where W denotes weight (g).

2.5. Muffin Volume

The volume of the muffins was measured by the rapeseed displacement method. Each muffin was placed in a plastic beaker of known volume (total volume, Vt), and the remaining space in the plastic beaker was then filled with rapeseed; the volume of the rapeseed required (Vs) was then determined by graduated cylinder. Muffin volume was calculated as the difference between the total volume and volume of rapeseed—the muffin volume = Vt − Vs [36].

2.6. Muffin Texture

A texture analyzer (TA.XT. Plus, Stable Microsystems, Surrey, UK) was used to measure the texture profile of muffins in terms of the firmness and springiness of the samples. The samples were compressed to a strain of 25% of the original height using a 75 mm cylindrical probe and a 50 kg load cell, and a test speed of 1.0 mm/s was used. Data was obtained from the Texture expert software (Stable Microsystems, Surrey, UK). Firmness and springiness values were calculated as the overall force of compression required and the resistance post compression.

Table 1. Formulas for muffins at two Stevianna levels, with or without cocoa powder and/or vanilla.

Formulation [a]	C	V	CP	CP + V	50S	50S + V	50S + CP	50S + CP + V	100S	100S + V	100S + CP	100S + CP + V
Ingredients	**Mass (g)**											
Wheat flour	138.4	138.4	115.3	115.3	138.4	138.4	115.3	115.3	138.4	138.4	115.3	115.3
Sugar	92.2	92.2	92.2	92.2	46.1	46.1	46.1	46.1	0	0	0	0
Baking powder	6.5	6.5	6.5	6.5	6.5	6.5	6.5	6.5	6.5	6.5	6.5	6.5
Salt	1.4	1.4	1.4	1.4	1.4	1.4	1.4	1.4	1.4	1.4	1.4	1.4
Skim milk powder	8.7	8.7	8.7	8.7	8.7	8.7	8.7	8.7	8.7	8.7	8.7	8.7
Oil	77.6	77.6	77.6	77.6	77.6	77.6	77.6	77.6	77.6	77.6	77.6	77.6
Liquid whole egg	34.6	34.6	34.6	34.6	34.6	34.6	34.6	34.6	34.6	34.6	34.6	34.6
Top water	97.6	97.6	97.6	97.6	97.6	97.6	97.6	97.6	97.6	97.6	97.6	97.6
Cocoa powder	0	0	23.1	23.1	0	0	23.1	23.1	0	0	23.1	23.1
Vanilla	0	3	0	3	0	3	0	3	0	3	0	3
Stevia	0	0	0	0	46.1	46.1	46.1	46.1	92.2	92.2	92.2	92.2

[a] Sample name of formulation: Control (C); Vanilla (V); Cocoa Powder (CP); Cocoa + Vanilla (CP + V); 50% Stevianna (50S); 50% Stevianna + Vanilla (50S + V); 50% Stevianna + Cocoa (50S + CP); 50% Stevianna + Cocoa + Vanilla (50S + CP + V); 100% Stevianna (100S); 100% Stevianna + Vanilla (100S + V); 100% Stevianna + Cocoa (100S + CP); 100% Stevianna + Cococa + Vanilla (100S + CP + V).

2.7. *Muffin Total Starch*

Total starch analysis was carried out according to the official American Association of Cereal Chemists method 76.13 [42], using Megazyme (Bray, Dublin, Ireland) total starch kit.

2.8. *In Vitro Predictive Glycemic Response Digestion Analysis*

The procedure used for the determination of potential glycemic response is the same as that reported previously by [30]. This procedure measures the breakdown of carbohydrates to sugars by the action of amylase enzymes added to the baked muffin. Whole muffins were chopped with a domestic kitchen food chopper (Zyliss®) to stimulate particle size reduction which occurs during natural mastication for at least one minute of steady chopping until a fine crumb was achieved. A 3.5 g sample was used to determine the predictive glycemic response.

Triplicate samples of product (approximate 1 g of cooked muffin) were each placed into the 60 mL plastic pots and 30 mL of distilled water added, and duplicate blank samples. These pots were inserted to a pre-heated 15 place magnetic heated stirring block (IKAMAG® RT15, IKA®-WERKE Gmblt & Co., Staufen, Germany) preheated to 37 °C, on each pot one magnetic stirrer, followed by 0.8 mL of 1 M aqueous HCl. Then, 1 mL of a 10% pepsin (Acros Organics, New Jersey, NJ, USA CAS: 901-75-6) solution in 0.05 M HCl was added in order to replicate gastric digestion. The sample was incubated at 37 °C for 30 min with slow constant stirring (130 rpm) to simulate gastric digestion conditions. In vitro stomach digestion was halted by the addition of 2 mL $NaHCO_3$. Small intestine digestion was mimicked by the addition of 5 mL 0.1 M Na maleate buffer pH 6. An aliquot (1 mL) was withdrawn (Time 0) and added to 4 mL absolute ethanol to stop any further enzyme reaction. A 0.1 mL dose of amyloglucosidase (A.niger, Megazyme, E-AMGDF; 3260 U/mL) was added to prevent end-product inhibition of pancreatic amylase. A 5 mL 2.5% pancreatin (EC: 232-468-9, CAS: 8049-47-6, activity: 42362 FIP-U/g, Applichem GmbH, Darmstadt, Germany) in 0.1 M Na maleate buffer pH 6 followed by the volume being made to 53 mL with continued stirring and heat maintained at 37 °C for 120 min. Triplicate 1 mL aliquots were withdrawn at 0, 20, 60, 120 min and added to 4 mL absolute ethanol. Reducing sugar content was analyzed by dinitrosalicyclic (DNS) colorimetry, and the area under the curve (AUC) was calculated by dividing the graph into trapezoids as described elsewhere [30]. The reducing sugar content was regarded as an indicator for the predictive glycemic response.

2.9. *Statistical Analyses*

All analyses were conducted in triplicate. Analysis of variance (one-way ANOVA) was performed on the data, and Tukey's comparison test ($p < 0.05$) was used to determine the significance. These analyses were performed using Minitab (Minitab Pty Ltd., Sydney, Australia).

3. Results and Discussion

3.1. *Moisture Content*

Table 2 shows that the moisture content of muffin samples ranged from 19% to 27%. The moisture content of the muffin samples produced was higher when cocoa powder or/and vanilla was used. In addition, Figure 1 shows that moisture content values increased significantly ($p < 0.05$) when sucrose was replaced by Stevianna®—in particular the moisture content of 100% Stevianna® samples were higher than the full-sucrose muffin samples. Sucrose plays an important role in water retention that results in reduced moisture loss during the baking of the muffins [43]. However, the moisture content increased when sucrose was replaced because the Stevianna® acted as a humectant and prevented water from escaping during baking. Research using other types of sugar replacers has shown similar results. Martínez-Cervera et al. [44] used erythritol in muffins for its water retention properties. Ghosh and Sudha [45] showed that the use of the polyol sorbitol was reflected in a significantly higher moisture content ($p < 0.05$). Due to the high water-binding capacity of formulations with carbohydrate-based sugar replacers, a greater amount of water is required in cereal products.

Table 2. Effect of Stevianna on texture profile analysis and total starch in muffins with or without cocoa powder and/or vanilla.

Product	Firmness (g)	Springiness (%)	Total Starch (%)
C	746.06 ± 44.10 [b]	51.29 ± 0.44 [ab]	26.83 ± 1.92 [abc]
V	763.51 ± 51.48 [b]	51.66 ± 0.09 [a]	27.93 ± 0.42 [ab]
CP	680.99 ± 30.33 [b]	49.26 ± 0.54 [ab]	26.14 ± 0.60 [abcd]
CP + V	662.97 ± 68.46 [b]	49.99 ± 0.43 [ab]	24.43 ± 1.06 [bcde]
50S	906.07 ± 111.09 [b]	51.51 ± 0.62 [ab]	28.50 ±0.85 [a]
50S + V	1102.18 ± 102.10 [b]	51.49 ± 0.78 [a]	29.03 ± 0.36 [a]
50S + CP	987.03 ± 68.00 [b]	48.67 ± 0.52 [a]	22.72 ± 0.39 [de]
50S + CP + V	890.78 ± 76.18 [b]	49.59 ± 0.54 [b]	23.40 ± 0.09 [cde]
100S	4512.78 ± 399.65 [a]	45.07 ± 0.71 [c]	26.60 ± 0.94 [abc]
100S + V	4419.70 ± 409.69 [a]	45.44 ± 0.56 [c]	29.09 ± 2.56 [a]
100S + CP	3868.00 ± 300.87 [a]	44.74 ± 1.12 [c]	22.62 ± 1.42 [e]
100S + CP + V	3839.94 ± 522.34 [a]	43.11 ± 1.36 [c]	26.17 ± 1.14 [abcd]

Control (C); Vanilla (V); Cocoa Powder (CP); Cocoa+Vanilla (CP + V); 50% Stevianna (50S); 50% Stevianna + Vanilla (50S + V); 50% Stevianna + Cocoa (50S + CP); 50% Stevianna + Cocoa + Vanilla (50S + CP + V); 100% Stevianna (100S); 100% Stevianna + Vanilla (100S + V); 100% Stevianna + Cocoa (100S + CP); 100% Stevianna + Cococa + Vanilla (100S + CP + V). All measurements are the mean values ± SD of triplicate determinations. Means in the same column with different letters are significantly different ($p < 0.05$).

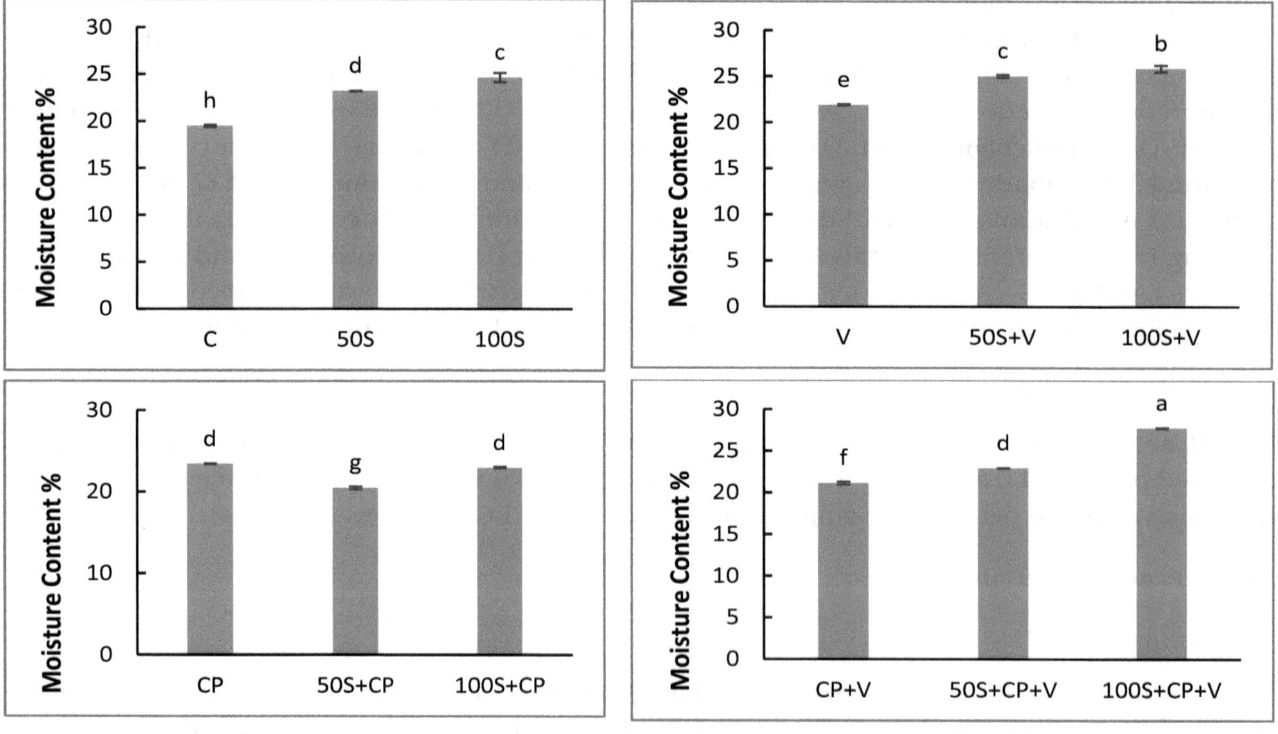

Figure 1. Moisture content for muffins of formulation made from two levels of Stevianna without/with cocoa powder and/or vanilla. Control (C); Vanilla (V); Cocoa Powder (CP); Cocoa + Vanilla (CP + V); 50% Stevianna (50S); 50% Stevianna + Vanilla (50S + V); 50% Stevianna + Cocoa (50S + CP); 50% Stevianna + Cocoa + Vanilla (50S + CP + V); 100% Stevianna (100S); 100% Stevianna + Vanilla (100S + V); 100% Stevianna + Cocoa (100S + CP); 100% Stevianna + Cococa + Vanilla (100S + CP + V). Values with different letters are significantly different to one another $p < 0.05$.

Moisture content in bakery products is an important factor as it has a direct impact on the texture attributes and a strong correlation has been found between moisture content and firmness [46]. As can be seen from the Table 2, muffin firmness increased as moisture content increased. As reported by Rößle et al. [47], this must be related to the replacement of the sugar by Stevianna®, affecting the formation of muffin structure.

3.2. *The Impact of Sugar Replacement on Product Physico-Chemical Characteristics*

The height of the muffins prepared with the different levels of Stevianna® with/without cocoa powder and/or vanilla is shown in Figure 2. The full-sucrose muffin was significantly higher ($p < 0.05$) than the muffins that were prepared using Stevianna®. The lowest height was found in the 100% Stevianna® muffin samples. The full-sucrose muffin with cocoa powder and/or vanilla group had a greater height than the control and other samples (Figure 2). These results indicate that the decrease in muffin height was associated with an absence of interconnectivity of a more compact structure and with a low number of air cells for levels of sucrose replacement higher than 50% (Figure 3).

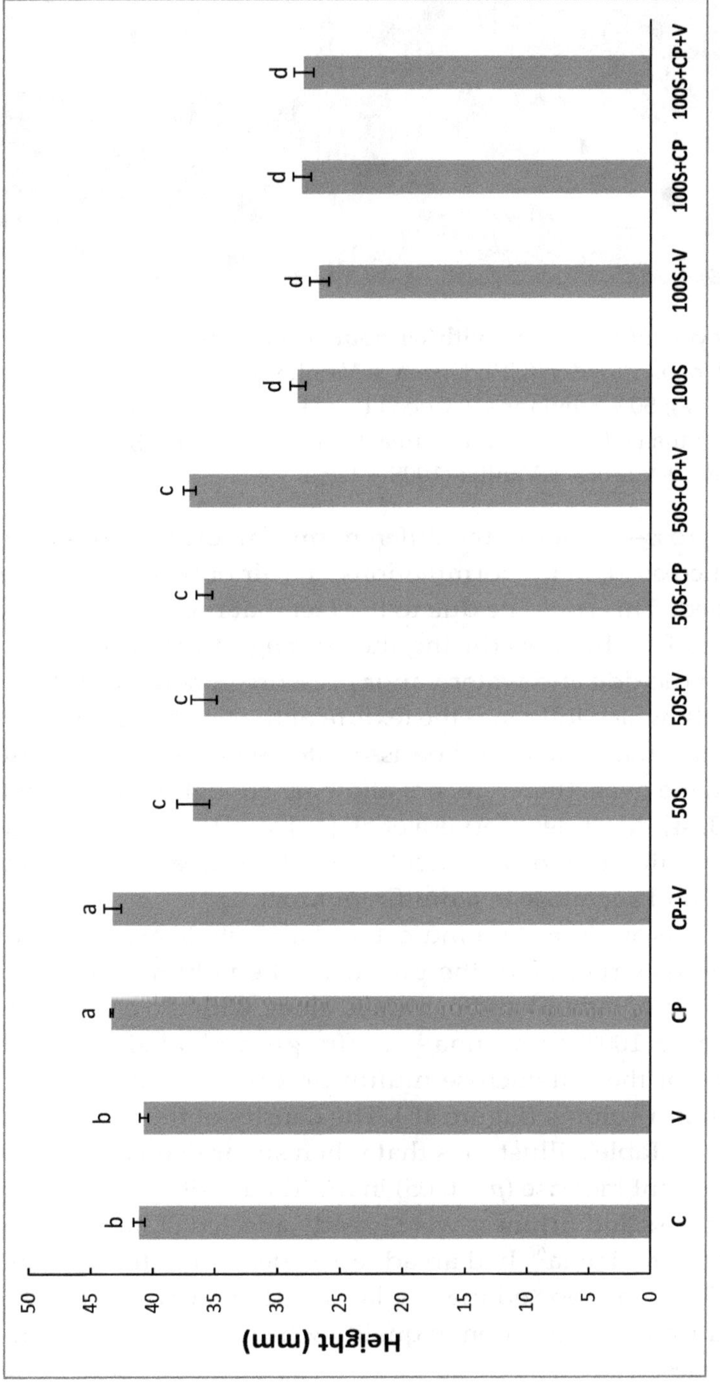

Figure 2. Effect of Stevianna without/with cocoa powder and/or vanilla on the height of muffin. Control (C); Vanilla (V); Cocoa Powder (CP); Cocoa + Vanilla (CP + V); 50% Stevianna (50S); 50% Stevianna + Vanilla (50S + V); 50% Stevianna + Cocoa (50S + CP); 50% Stevianna + Cocoa + Vanilla (50S + CP + V); 100% Stevianna (100S); 100% Stevianna + Vanilla (100S + V); 100% Stevianna + Cocoa (100S + CP); 100% Stevianna + Cococa + Vanilla (100S + CP + V). Values with different letters are significantly different to one another $p < 0.05$.

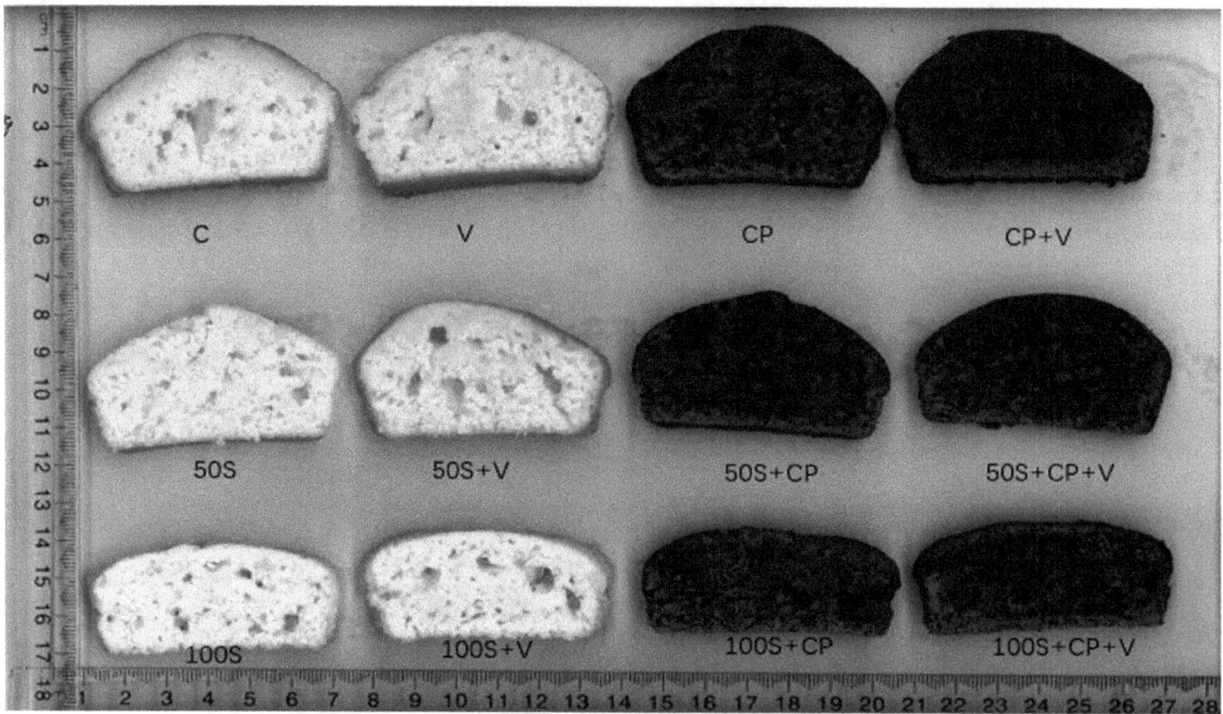

Figure 3. Effect of two levels of Stevianna with/without cocoa powder and/or vanilla in muffins: Control (C); Vanilla (V); Cocoa Powder (CP); Cocoa + Vanilla (CP + V); 50% Stevianna (50S); 50% Stevianna + Vanilla (50S + V); 50% Stevianna + Cocoa (50S + CP); 50% Stevianna + Cocoa + Vanilla (50S + CP + V); 100% Stevianna (100S); 100% Stevianna + Vanilla (100S + V); 100% Stevianna + Cocoa (100S + CP); 100% Stevianna + Cococa + Vanilla (100S + CP + V).

Photographs of vertical cross-sections of the different muffin formulations are shown in Figure 3. As the Stevianna® content increased, in the formulations, the air bubbles became smaller and the air channels gradually diminished. This could be due to the fact that muffins with a full sucrose content gained an increased number of air bubbles during the beating of the batter, and these air bubbles are then expanded by carbon dioxide and water vapor pressure generated during baking, resulting in the formation of air channels, which influence the texture of the finished muffin product. The lack of air channels as the sucrose was replaced may also be associated with earlier thermosetting of the batter during the heating process in the oven, therefore, not allowing enough time for bubble expansion and formation of air channels [43,44]. Martínez-Cervera et al. [44] also found that the number of small air bubbles increased, air channels diminished, and circular bubbles increased with an increase in sucrose replacement by polydextrose and sucralose in a muffin product.

The volume of the muffin is an important indicator of air bubble expansion during baking and consequently also of the porous structure of the product. The volumes of muffins prepared with different levels of Stevianna® with/without and/or vanilla along with the control muffin are presented in Figure 4A. The samples with 100% Stevianna® muffin group had significantly lower volumes ($p < 0.05$) compared to those of the full-sucrose muffin products. Muffin density appeared to be negatively correlated with muffin volume (Figure 4B). The density of the muffins was calculated from mass and volume after baking. Table 2 illustrates that when sugar was completely substituted with Stevianna®, there was a significant increase ($p < 0.05$) in muffin density. Additionally, product quality characteristics such as springiness and firmness were greatly affected (Table 2). These results indicate that an increase in the level of Stevianna® had an adverse effect on volume, density and texture of the muffin. Manisha et al. [26] also reported that replacement of sucrose with 100% stevioside and liquid sorbitol caused a significant deterioration in quality which decreased volume and resulted in a firmer texture in cake properties.

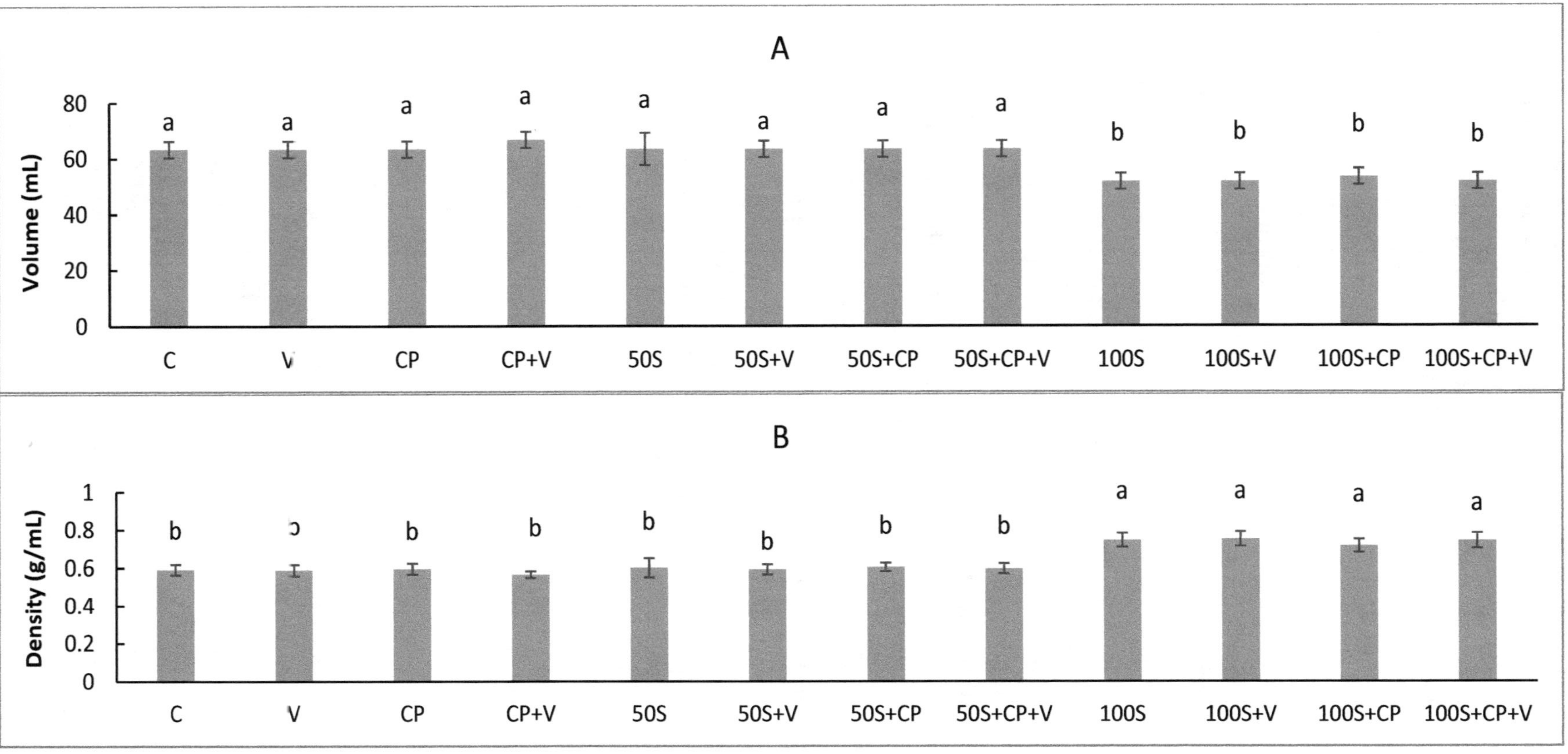

Figure 4. Volume (**A**) and density (**B**) values for muffins containing two levels of Stevianna as sugar replacer with or without cocoa powder and vanilla. Control (C); Vanilla (V); Cocoa Powder (CP); Cocoa + Vanilla (CP + V); 50% Stevianna (50S); 50% Stevianna + Vanilla (50S + V); 50% Stevianna + Cocoa (50S + CP); 50% Stevianna + Cocoa + Vanilla (50S + CP + V); 100% Stevianna (100S); 100% Stevianna + Vanilla (100S + V); 100% Stevianna + Cocoa (100S + CP); 100% Stevianna + Cococa + Vanilla (100S + CP + V). Values with different letters are significantly different to one another $p < 0.05$.

A function of sugar during cake baking is that it delays starch gelatinization, thus contributing to the aeration of the batter and the optimum quality of sugar will affect formation of the cake structure and improve crumb texture and tenderness [26]. The decrease in sugar-free muffin expansion is the result of less air bubble incorporation and reduced air holding capacity during baking [48]. In addition, starch gelatinization temperature seems to contribute to volume development due to different interactions between the Stevianna® and starch and proteins of the batter, and these interactions affect starch gelatinization and protein denaturation temperatures. These results are in agreement with Ronda et al. [49]'s findings which showed that a decrease in starch gelatinization and protein denaturation temperatures in sorbitol cakes is expected to cause a premature thermosetting of protein or starch matrix—this process will start at the crust due to direct contact with the heating medium. Therefore, this lowers the heat transfer rate, and produces a vapor pressure build-up, resulting in inadequate expansion of individual bubbles. Additionally, Ronda et al. [49] found that high-fructose corn syrup (HFCS) mainly contributed to the early gelatinization of starch during the baking process and restricted the volume of baked products compared to sucrose.

However, the 50% Stevianna® used had no significant effect on the volume and density of muffin compared to the full-sucrose muffin samples (Figure 4). These results suggest that muffin samples containing half the amount of Stevianna® have a similar ability, compared with muffins with full sucrose, to retain air. These results are consistent with those of Lin et al. [38], who found no significant differences among the volume estimates for 50% erythritol cakes. Furthermore, the addition of the 50% Stevianna® in muffin samples exhibited a texture close to that of the full-sucrose muffin samples (Table 2), which conferred an appearance of firmness and springiness. The results were consistent with previous research [30].

3.3. The Impact of Sugar Replacement on the In Vitro Predictive Glycemic Response

The total starch of modified muffins was measured and compared with the control sample (Table 2). Compared to the control muffin, 50% or 100% sucrose replacement with Stevianna® with added cocoa powder samples had significantly lower amounts of total starch. Similar levels of total starch were observed in control and full-sucrose muffin samples—50% and 100% Stevianna® with/without cocoa powder and/or vanilla muffin samples. Thus, the presence of cocoa powder with Stevianna® in muffin had a significant effect on total starch contents.

The effects of Stevianna® on in vitro starch digestion in muffin and chocolate muffin products were investigated by measuring the glucose released during starch digestion. Figure 5 shows the reducing sugars curves of two levels of Stevianna® with/without cocoa powder and/or vanilla muffin samples that were compared with full-sucrose with/without cocoa powder and/or vanilla samples, respectively. These two levels of Stevianna® used in this study were found to decrease reducing sugars released by digestive enzymes, compared with the full-sucrose muffin samples. The rate and extent of reducing sugars released were the highest in the control muffin, followed by 50% Stevianna® with/without cocoa powder and/or vanilla muffin products, and 100% Stevianna® with/without cocoa powder and/or vanilla muffins (Figure 5). In particular, muffins with Stevianna® showed a significant decrease in terms of reducing sugars released throughout the 120 min starch digestion process.

The total area under the hydrolysis curve (AUC) relates the total glucose release to the digestion time of 120 min. The concentration of the Stevianna® had a significant effect on the AUC values ($p < 0.05$), which demonstrated that the replacement of sucrose with 100% Stevianna® resulted in the lowest AUC value of muffin samples in a dose response (Figure 6). It is of interest that the additions of vanilla and/or cocoa powder with muffin production did not lead to a significant reduction of in vitro digestion values compared to the full-sucrose—50% Stevianna®, and 100% Stevianna® samples, respectively. These results are consistent with the previous report by Gao et al. [30].

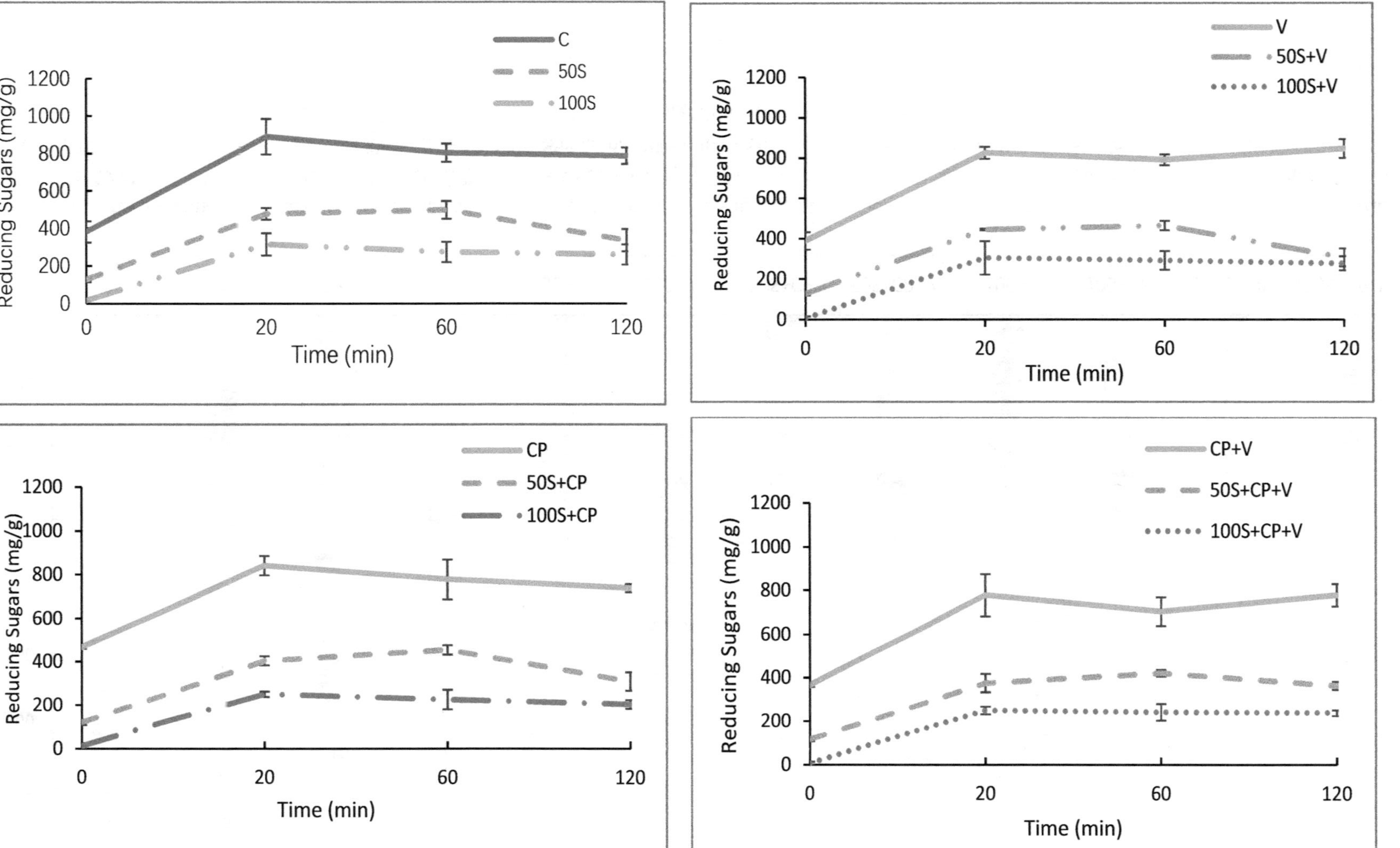

Figure 5. Amount of reducing sugars released per g of food material during in vitro digestion. Control (C); Vanilla (V); Cocoa Powder (CP); Cocoa + Vanilla (CP + V); 50% Stevianna (50S); 50% Stevianna + Vnilla (50S + V); 50% Stevianna + Cocoa (50S + CP); 50% Stevianna + Cocoa + Vanilla (50S + CP + V); 100% Stevianna (100S); 100% Stevianna + Vanilla (100S + V); 100% Stevianna + Cocoa (100S + CP); 100% Stevianna + Cococa + Vanilla (100S + CP + V).

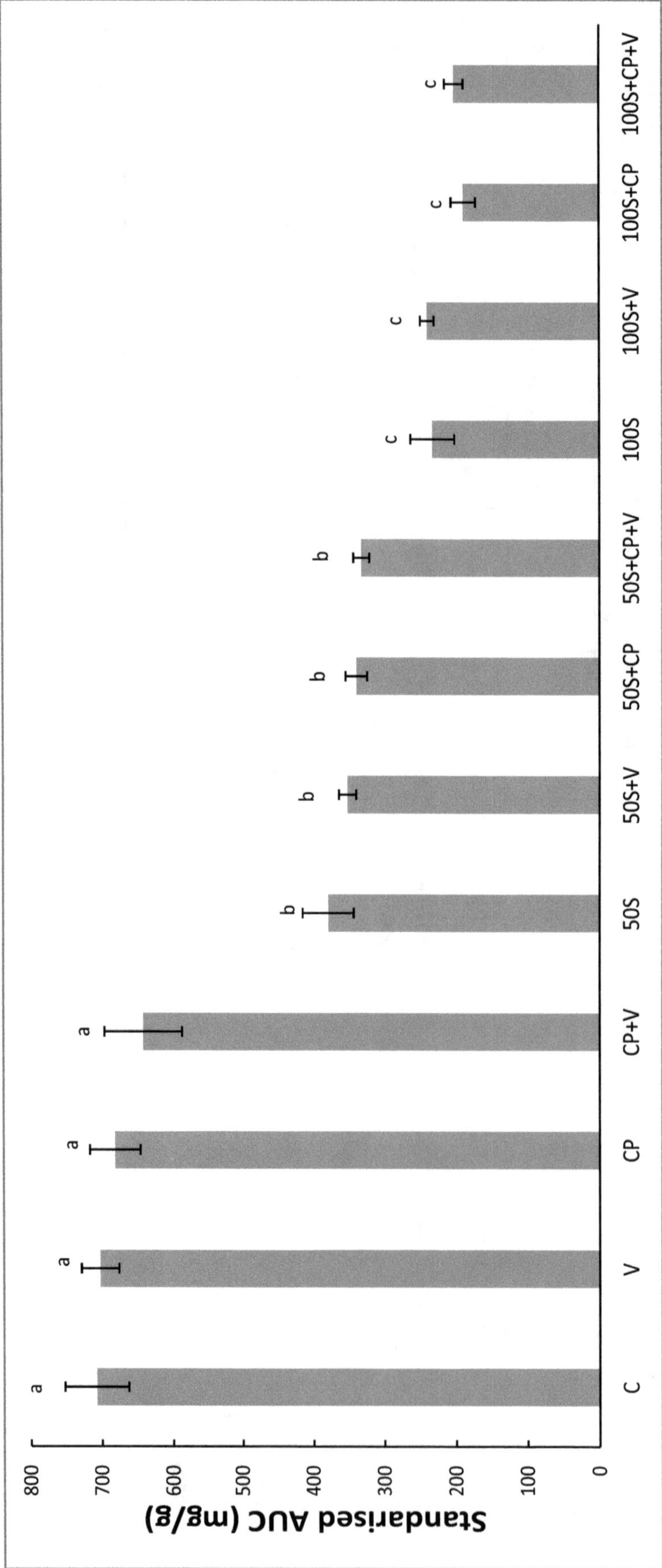

Figure 6. Values for area under the curve (AUC) comparing the control and other low-sugar muffins made with two levels of Stevianna with/without cocoa powder and/or vanilla. Control (C); Vanilla (V); Cocoa Powder (CP); Cocoa + Vanilla (CP + V); 50% Stevianna (50S); 50% Stevianna + Vanilla (50S + V); 50% Stevianna + Cocoa (50S + CP); 50% Stevianna + Cocoa + Vanilla (50S + CP + V); 100% Stevianna (100S); 100% Stevianna + Vanilla (100S + V); 100% Stevianna + Cocoa (100S + CP); 100% Stevianna + Cococa + Vanilla (100S + CP + V). Values with different letters are significantly different to one another $p < 0.05$.

This study did not focus on the impact of sweeteners on in vitro starch digestion analysis of bakery products. However, several research projects have been designed to test the effects of the stevia or erythritol on postprandial glucose and insulin levels in vivo and in vitro digestion methods as compared to sucrose [50,51].

The breakdown or disruption of starch granules that results from salivary amylase causes a greater susceptibility of the granule to further enzyme degradation. This process will lead to more readily digestible starch, and hence create a higher blood glucose response [52]. The level of postprandial blood glucose is a major factor in predicting the profile of insulin resistance. Alizadeh et al. [50] found that there were differing effects on postprandial blood insulin levels that were dependent on the type and amount of sweetener consumed. The effect of the consumption of beverages containing stevia has been tested by measuring the in vivo glycemic impact [53], and it was found that postprandial glucose and insulin levels were significantly reduced in the stevia beverages compared to the sucrose beverages. These effects on postprandial glucose levels are mainly due to the lack of calories and carbohydrate content of Stevianna®, and thus there are no reducing sugars released. A similar trend has been observed in that the postprandial insulin levels were reduced in stevia ice cream samples compared to full-sucrose ice cream samples [50], and this is most likely due to the functional properties of stevia that results in no contribution to the available carbohydrate and glycemic response in food products. In addition, Roberts and Renwick [54] illustrated that steviol glycosides are not readily absorbed by the upper small intestine when it is administered orally to normal rat or human subjects. There are no human digestive enzymes present in the small intestine to hydrolyze the β-glycosidic linkages, resulting in limited small intestine digestion.

Lin et al. [36] illustrated that 0%–100% sugar replacement with erythritol in cookies decreased the carbohydrate contents by in vivo digestion. Since the calorie value of erythritol is approximately 0.4 kcal/g [39], it provides no energy to the body and thus it is not systemically metabolized nor fermented in the colon [37]. It has been suggested that the consumption of erythritol does not raise postprandial glycemic and insulin levels by oral ingestion in healthy human subjects [28]. In a previous study [39], more than 90% of erythritol is rapidly absorbed by the small intestine when eaten and is excreted unchanged in the urine.

The Stevianna® used in our study was composed of rebaudioside A (stevia) and erythritol and, therefore, the observations made are consistent with those made by the above studies. Our experiment results showed that under in vitro conditions a lower reducing sugar liberation took place when sucrose was replaced by Stevianna® in muffins, and consequently this can be beneficial to as it will decrease the postprandial blood glucose. Additionally, it is probable that the intake of these muffins decreases the rate of intestine absorption of glucose and delays gastric emptying.

4. Conclusions

The stevia-containing product, Stevianna®, has been shown to be a suitable sucrose replacement for a low-sucrose formulation of muffins. The results showed that 50% sugar replacement with Stevianna® had similar physical quality characteristics in terms of volume, density and texture to a control muffin. However, when the sugar was replaced by 100% Stevianna®, the muffin quality showed a reduction in volume, an increase in textural firmness and a correspondingly high density of the product when compared to the control muffin samples. Furthermore, Stevianna® was able to simulate sucrose functionality in muffins, producing an increase in moisture content in comparison with the full-sucrose muffins. The negative effect of Stevianna® on muffin properties can be associated with the fact that as the Stevianna® level was raised, it led to a reduction of air bubble expansion during the heating process (possibly due to the weakening of the starch–protein–sugar interface of the muffin, allowing for greater structural collapse) and thus a corresponding reduction in height. This research illustrates that Stevianna® is a major factor impacting on the physical characteristics of muffins. The addition of cocoa powder and/or vanilla did not affect the quality of muffins significantly.

In relation to the nutritional quality of the muffin products, the effect of Stevianna® inclusion on the predicted glycemic impact as determined by in vitro digestion illustrated the role of sugar in elevating the glycemic response during digestion. The replacement of sugar with increasing levels of Stevianna® was found to significantly decrease the potential glycemic response values, and this is most likely to be attributed to the fact that Stevianna® was not degraded into glucose units and acted as an inert filler within the muffin samples. Therefore the inclusion of cocoa powder and/or vanilla powder did not have a significant change to the predicted glycemic response values of the muffins.

The breakdown or disruption of starch granules that results from salivary amylase causes a greater susceptibility of the granule to further enzyme degradation. This process will lead to more readily digestible starch, and hence create a higher blood glucose response [52]. The level of postprandial blood glucose is a major factor in predicting the profile of insulin resistance. Alizadeh et al. [50] found that there were differing effects on postprandial blood insulin levels that were dependent on the type and amount of sweetener consumed. The effect of the consumption of beverages containing stevia has been tested by measuring the in vivo glycemic impact [53], and it was found that postprandial glucose and insulin levels were significantly reduced in the stevia beverages compared to the sucrose beverages. These effects on postprandial glucose levels are mainly due to the lack of calories and carbohydrate content of Stevianna®, thus there are no reducing sugars released. A similar trend has been observed in that the postprandial insulin levels were reduced in stevia ice cream samples compared to full-sucrose ice cream samples [50], and this is most likely due to the functional properties of stevia that results in no contribution to the available carbohydrate and glycemic response in food products. In addition, Roberts and Renwick [54] illustrated that steviol glycosides are not readily absorbed by the upper small intestine when it is administered orally to normal rat or human subjects. There are no human digestive enzymes present in the small intestine to hydrolyze the β-glycosidic linkages, resulting in limited small intestine digestion.

Lin et al. [36] illustrated that 0%–100% sugar replacement with erythritol in cookies decreased the carbohydrate contents by in vivo digestion. Since the calorie value of erythritol is approximately 0.4 kcal/g [39], it provides no energy to the body and thus it is not systemically metabolized nor fermented in the colon [37]. It has been suggested that the consumption of erythritol does not raise postprandial glycemic and insulin levels by oral ingestion in healthy human subjects [28]. In a previous study [39], more than 90% of erythritol is rapidly absorbed by the small intestine when eaten and is excreted unchanged in the urine.

Finally, it can be seen that a partial replacement of Stevianna® for sucrose with/without cocoa powder and/or vanilla in muffins gave a product with quality characteristics close to that of the full-sucrose muffin sample. At the same time, the reduction in potential glycemic response values was greater than would have been expected with 50% sucrose reduction and consequently providing a quality muffin that produces a lowered postprandial response with the potential associated health benefits.

Author Contributions: J.G., M.A.B., C.S.B., X.G. and X.-A.Z. conceived and designed the experiments; J.G. and X.G. performed the experiments; J.G., M.A.B., S.L.M. and C.S.B. analyzed the data; J.G., C.S.B. and M.A.B. were responsible for writing the manuscript.

References

1. Giuberti, G.; Gallo, A. Reducing the glycaemic index and increasing the slowly digestible starch content in gluten-free cereal-based foods: A review. *Int. J. Food Sci. Technol.* **2018**, *53*, 50–60. [CrossRef]
2. Sopade, P.A. Cereal processing and glycaemic response. *Int. J. Food Sci. Technol.* **2017**, *52*, 22–37. [CrossRef]

3. Connolly, A.; O'Keeffe, M.B.; Nongonierma, A.B.; Piggott, C.O.; FitzGerald, R.J. Isolation of peptides from a novel brewers spent grain protein isolate with potential to modulate glycaemic response. *Int. J. Food Sci. Technol.* **2017**, *52*, 146–153. [CrossRef]
4. Brennan, C.S. Dietary fibre, glycaemic response, and diabetes. *Mol. Nutr. Food Res.* **2005**, *49*, 560–570. [CrossRef]
5. Jenkins, D.J.; Wolever, T.M.; Taylor, R.H.; Barker, H.M.; Fielden, H.; Jenkins, A.L. Effect of guar crispbread with cereal products and leguminous seeds on blood glucose concentrations of diabetics. *Br. Med. J.* **1980**, *281*, 1248–1250. [CrossRef]
6. Monro, J.A. Faecal bulking efficacy of Australasian breakfast cereals. *Asia Pac. J. Clin. Nutr.* **2002**, *11*, 176–185. [CrossRef]
7. Monro, J.A.; Shaw, M. Glycemic impact, glycemic glucose equivalents, glycemic index, and glycemic load: Definitions, distinctions, and implications. *Am. J. Clin. Nutr.* **2008**, *87*, 237S–243S. [CrossRef]
8. Gao, J.; Wang, Y.; Dong, Z.; Zhou, W. Structural and mechanical characteristics of bread and their impact on oral processing: A review. *Int. J. Food Sci. Technol.* **2018**, *53*, 858–872. [CrossRef]
9. Klunklin, W.; Savage, G. Physicochemical, antioxidant properties and in vitro digestibility of wheat–purple rice flour mixtures. *Int. J. Food Sci. Technol.* **2018**, *53*, 1962–1971. [CrossRef]
10. Barros, C.M.M.R.; Lessa, R.Q.; Grechi, M.P.; Mouço, T.L.M.; Souza, M.; das, G.C.; Wiernsperger, N.; Bouskela, E. Substitution of drinking water by fructose solution induces hyperinsulinemia and hyperglycemia in hamsters. *Clinics* **2007**, *62*, 327–334. [CrossRef]
11. Bartkiene, E.; Sakiene, V.; Bartkevics, V.; Wiacek, C.; Rusko, J.; Lele, V.; Ruzauskas, M.; Juodeikiene, G.; Klupsaite, D.; Bernatoniene, J.; et al. Nutraceuticals in gummy candies form prepared from lacto-fermented lupine protein concentrates, as high-quality protein source, incorporated with *Citrus paradise* L. essential oil and xylitol. *Int. J. Food Sci. Technol.* **2018**, *53*, 2015–2025. [CrossRef]
12. Lê, K.A.; Ith, M.; Kreis, R.; Faeh, D.; Bortolotti, M.; Tran, C.; Tappy, L. Fructose overconsumption causes dyslipidemia and ectopic lipid deposition in healthy subjects with and without a family history of type 2 diabetes. *Am. J. Clin. Nutr.* **2009**, *89*, 1760–1765. [CrossRef] [PubMed]
13. Burton, P.; Lightowler, H.J. Influence of bread volume on glycaemic response and satiety. *Brit. J. Nutr.* **2006**, *96*, 877–882. [CrossRef] [PubMed]
14. Bae, I.Y.; Jun, Y.; Lee, S.; Lee, H.G. Characterization of apple dietary fibers influencing the in vitro starch digestibility of wheat flour gel. *LWT Food Sci. Technol.* **2016**, *65*, 158–163. [CrossRef]
15. Baeva, M.R.; Panchev, I.N.; Terzieva, V.V. Comparative study of texture of normal and energy reduced sponge cakes. *Nahrung* **2000**, *44*, 242–246. [CrossRef]
16. Karp, S.; Wyrwisz, J.; Kurek, M.A.; Wierzbicka, A. Combined use of cocoa dietary fibre and steviol glycosides in low-calorie muffins production. *Int. J. Food Sci. Technol.* **2017**, *52*, 944–953. [CrossRef]
17. Kulthe, A.A.; Pawar, V.D.; Kotecha, P.M.; Chavan, U.D.; Bansode, V.V. Development of high protein and low calorie cookies. *Int. J. Food Sci. Technol.* **2014**, *51*, 153–157. [CrossRef]
18. Livesey, G. Health potential of polyols as sugar replacers, with emphasis on low glycaemic properties. *Nutr. Res. Rev.* **2003**, *16*, 163–191. [CrossRef]
19. Oehme, A.; Wüst, M.; Wölwer-Rieck, U. Steviol glycosides are not altered during commercial extraction and purification processes. *Int. J. Food Sci. Technol.* **2017**, *52*, 2156–2162. [CrossRef]
20. Azevedo, B.M.; Morais-Ferreira, J.M.; Luccas, V.; Bolini, H.M. Bittersweet chocolates containing prebiotic and sweetened with stevia (*Stevia rebaudiana* Bertoni) with different Rebaudioside A contents: Multiple time-intensity analysis and physicochemical characteristics. *Int. J. Food Sci. Technol.* **2017**, *52*, 1731–1738. [CrossRef]
21. Wardy, W.; Jack, A.R.; Chonpracha, P.; Alonso, J.R.; King, J.M.; Prinyawiwatkul, W. Gluten-free muffins: Effects of sugar reduction and health benefit information on consumer liking, emotion, and purchase intent. *Int. J. Food Sci. Technol.* **2018**, *53*, 262–269. [CrossRef]
22. Gregersen, S.; Jeppesen, P.B.; Holst, J.J.; Hermansen, K. Antihyperglycemic effects of stevioside in type 2 diabetic subjects. *Metabolism* **2004**, *53*, 73–76. [CrossRef] [PubMed]
23. Goyal, S.K.; Goyal, R.K. Stevia (*Stevia rebaudiana*) a bio-sweetener: A review. *Int. J. Food Sci. Nutr.* **2010**, *61*, 1–10. [CrossRef] [PubMed]

24. Phimolsiripol, Y.; Siripatrawan, U.; Teekachunhatean, S.; Wangtueai, S.; Seesuriyachan, P.; Surawang, S.; Laokuldilok, T.; Regenstein, J.M.; Henry, C.J. Technological properties, *in vitro* starch digestibility and *in vivo* glycaemic index of bread containing crude malva nut gum. *Int. J. Food Sci. Technol.* **2017**, *52*, 1035–1041.
25. Quiles, A.; Llorca, E.; Schmidt, C.; Reißner, A.-M.; Struck, S.; Rohm, H.; Hernando, I. Use of berry pomace to replace flour, fat or sugar in cakes. *Int. J. Food Sci. Technol.* **2018**, *53*, 1579–1587. [CrossRef]
26. Manisha, G.; Soumya, C.; Indrani, D. Studies on interaction between stevioside, liquid sorbitol, hydrocolloids and emulsifiers for replacement of sugar in cakes. *Food Hydrocoll.* **2012**, *29*, 363–373. [CrossRef]
27. Chang, J.C.; Wu, M.C.; Liu, I.M.; Cheng, J.T. Increase of insulin sensitivity by stevioside in fructose-rich chow-fed rats. *Horm. Metab. Res.* **2005**, *37*, 610–616. [CrossRef]
28. O'Donnell, K.; Kearsley, M. *Sweeteners and Sugar Alternatives in Food Technology*, 2nd ed.; Wiley-Blackwell: Oxford, UK, 2012; pp. 215–218.
29. Wheeler, A.; Boileau, A.C.; Winkler, P.C.; Compton, J.C.; Prakash, I.; Jiang, X.; Mandarino, D.A. Pharmacokinetics of rebaudioside A and stevioside after single oral doses in healthy men. *Food Chem. Toxicol.* **2008**, *46*, S54–S60. [CrossRef]
30. Gao, J.; Brennan, M.A.; Mason, S.L.; Brennan, C.S. Effect of sugar replacement with stevianna and inulin on the texture and predictive glycaemic response of muffins. *Int. J. Food Sci. Technol.* **2016**, *51*, 1979–1987. [CrossRef]
31. Alencar, N.M.M.; de Morais, E.C.; Steel, C.J.; Bolini, H.M.A. Sensory characterisation of gluten-free bread with addition of quinoa, amaranth flour and sweeteners as an alternative for coeliac patients. *Int. J. Food Sci. Technol.* **2017**, *52*, 872–879. [CrossRef]
32. Abdel-Salam, A.M.; Ammar, A.S.; Galal, W.K. Evaluation and properties of formulated low calories functional yoghurt cake. *J. Food Agric. Environ.* **2009**, *7*, 218–221.
33. Edelstein, S.; Smith, K.; Worthington, A.; Gillis, N.; Bruen, D.; Kang, S.H.; Guiducci, G. Comparisons of Six New Artificial Sweetener Gradation Ratios with Sucrose in Conventional-Method Cupcakes Resulting in Best Percentage Substitution Ratios. *J. Culin. Sci. Technol.* **2007**, *5*, 61–74. [CrossRef]
34. Struck, S.; Jaros, D.; Brennan, C.S.; Rohm, H. Sugar replacement in sweetened bakery goods. *Int. J. Food Sci. Technol.* **2014**, *49*, 1963–1976. [CrossRef]
35. Röper, H.; Goossens, J. Erythritol, a new raw material for food and non-food applications. *Starch* **1993**, *45*, 400–405. [CrossRef]
36. Lin, S.D.; Hwang, C.F.; Yeh, C.H. Physical and Sensory Characteristics of Chiffon Cake Prepared with Erythritol as Replacement for Sucrose. *J. Food Sci.* **2003**, *68*, 2107–2110. [CrossRef]
37. Bornet, F.R. Undigestible sugars in food products. *Am. J. Clin. Nutr.* **1994**, *59*, 763S–769S. [CrossRef]
38. Lin, S.D.; Lee, C.C.; Mau, J.L.; Lin, L.Y.; Chiou, S.Y. Effect of Erythritol on Quality Characteristics of Reduced-Calorie Danish Cookies. *J. Food Qual.* **2010**, *33*, 14–26. [CrossRef]
39. Bornet, F.R.J.; Blayo, A.; Dauchy, F.; Slama, G. Plasma and Urine Kinetics of Erythritol after Oral Ingestion by Healthy Humans. *Regul. Toxicol. Pharm.* **1996**, *24*, S280–S285. [CrossRef]
40. Wang, Y.; Chen, L.; Li, Y.; Li, Y.; Yan, M.; Chen, K.; Xu, L. Efficient enzymatic production of rebaudioside A from stevioside. *Biosci. Biotech. Bioch.* **2016**, *80*, 67–73. [CrossRef]
41. Zahn, S.; Forker, A.; Krügel, L.; Rohm, H. Combined use of rebaudioside A and fibres for partial sucrose replacement in muffins. *LWT Food Sci. Technol.* **2013**, *50*, 695–701. [CrossRef]
42. AACC International. *Approved Methods of Analysis*, 9th ed.; AACC International: St. Paul, MN, USA, 1995; p. 76.
43. Martínez-Cervera, S.; Hera, E.; de la Sanz, T.; Gómez, M.; Salvador, A. Effect of using Erythritol as a Sucrose Replacer in Making Spanish Muffins Incorporating Xanthan Gum. *Food Bioprocess Tech.* **2012**, *5*, 3203–3216. [CrossRef]
44. Martínez-Cervera, S.; Sanz, T.; Salvador, A.; Fiszman, S.M. Rheological, textural and sensorial properties of low-sucrose muffins reformulated with sucralose/polydextrose. *LWT Food Sci. Technol.* **2012**, *45*, 213–220. [CrossRef]
45. Ghosh, S.; Sudha, M.L. A review on polyols: New frontiers for health-based bakery products. *Int. J. Food Sci. Nutr.* **2012**, *63*, 372–379. [CrossRef] [PubMed]
46. Morris, C.; Morris, G.A. The effect of inulin and fructo-oligosaccharide supplementation on the textural, rheological and sensory properties of bread and their role in weight management: A review. *Food Chem.* **2012**, *133*, 237–248. [CrossRef]

47. Rößle, C.; Ktenioudaki, A.; Gallagher, E. Inulin and oligofructose as fat and sugar substitutes in quick breads (scones): A mixture design approach. *Eur. Food Res. Technol.* **2011**, *233*, 167–181. [CrossRef]
48. Psimouli, V.; Oreopoulou, V. The Effect of Fat Replacers on Batter and Cake Properties. *J. Food Sci.* **2013**, *78*, C1495–C1502.
49. Ronda, F.; Gómez, M.; Blanco, C.A.; Caballero, P.A. Effects of polyols and nondigestible oligosaccharides on the quality of sugar-free sponge cakes. *Food Chem.* **2005**, *90*, 549–555. [CrossRef]
50. Alizadeh, M.; Azizi-Lalabadi, M.; Kheirouri, S. Impact of Using Stevia on Physicochemical, Sensory, Rheology and Glycemic Index of Soft Ice Cream. *FNS* **2014**, *5*, 390. [CrossRef]
51. Ishikawa, M.; Miyashita, M.; Kawashima, Y.; Nakamura, T.; Saitou, N.; Modderman, J. Effects of Oral Administration of Erythritol on Patients with Diabetes. *Regul. Toxicol. Pharm.* **1996**, *24*, S303–S308. [CrossRef]
52. Granfeldt, Y.; Eliasson, A.-C.; Björck, I. An Examination of the Possibility of Lowering the RGlycemic Index of Oat and Barley Flakes by Minimal Processing. *J. Nutr.* **2000**, *130*, 2207–2214. [CrossRef]
53. Anton, S.D.; Martin, C.K.; Han, H.; Coulon, S.; Cefalu, W.T.; Geiselman, P.; Williamson, D.A. Effects of stevia, aspartame, and sucrose on food intake, satiety, and postprandial glucose and insulin levels. *Appetite* **2010**, *55*, 37–43. [CrossRef] [PubMed]
54. Roberts, A.; Renwick, A.G. Comparative toxicokinetics and metabolism of rebaudioside A, stevioside, and steviol in rats. *Food Chem. Toxicol.* **2008**, *46*, S31–S39. [CrossRef] [PubMed]

4

The Effect of Astaxanthin-Rich Microalgae "Haematococcus pluvialis" and Wholemeal Flours Incorporation in Improving the Physical and Functional Properties of Cookies

A. K. M. Mofasser Hossain [1,2], Margaret A. Brennan [1], Susan L. Mason [1], Xinbo Guo [3], Xin An Zeng [3] and Charles S. Brennan [1,2,*]

1 Centre for Food Research and Innovation, Department of Wine, Food and Molecular Biosciences, Lincoln University, Lincoln 7647, New Zealand; AKMMofasser.Hossain@lincolnuni.ac.nz (A.K.M.M.H.); Margaret.Brennan@Lincoln.ac.nz (M.A.B.); Sue.mason@lincoln.ac.nz (S.L.M.)

2 Riddet Institute, Palmerston North 4442, New Zealand

3 School of Food Science and Engineering, South China University of Technology, Guangzhou 510640, China; xbg720@gmail.com (X.G.); xazeng@scut.edu.cn (X.A.Z.)

* Correspondence: charles.brennan@lincoln.ac.nz

Abstract: Marine-based food supplements can improve human nutrition. In an effort to modulate glycaemic response and enhance nutritional aspects, marine-derived algal food rich in astaxanthin was used in the formulation of a model food (wholemeal cookie). Astaxanthin substitution of cookies made from three flours (wheat, barley and oat) demonstrated a significant reduction in the rate of glucose released during in vitro digestion together with an increase in the total phenolic content (TPC) and antioxidant capacity of the food. The significantly ($p < 0.005$) lower free glucose release was observed from cookies with 15% astaxanthin, followed by 10% and then 5% astaxanthin in comparison with control cookies of each flour. Total phenolic content, DPPH radical scavenging and Oxygen Radical Absorbance Capacity (ORAC) value also notably increased with increase in astaxanthin content. The results evidence the potential use of microalgae to enhance the bioactive compounds and lower the glycaemic response of wholemeal flour cookie.

Keywords: microalgae; *Hematococcus pluvialis*; astaxanthin; bakery products; glycaemic response; antioxidant

---

1. Introduction

Whole-grains such as wheat, barley and oat make a substantial contribution to our diet. They contain a significant amount of bioactive compounds such as fibre, minerals, vitamins and phytochemicals [1,2] and as such mayplay a major role in enhancing human health by reducing the risk of diabetes [3,4] and cancer [5], while also regulating serum cholesterol [6] and stimulating beneficial gut microbiota [7]. In recent years there has been an increased interest in the utilisation of whole-grain food materials as well as fibre rich ingredients, in cereal products, including bread [8], extruded snack products [9,10], and pasta [11,12]. These pieces of research have investigated the impact of wholegrains and fibre on both the physicochemical characteristics of cereal food products as well as their nutritional quality. A recent review on this subject illustrated that the incorporation of fibre rich ingredients into cereal products often results in negative consumer acceptability [13]. There therefore remains a challenge to both utilise wholegrain cereal products as well as functional food ingredients such a fibre rich materials, into mainstay food products.

Recent research into functional food ingredients has shown an interest in the development of foods containing seaweed or algal materials [14,15]. These materials have been part of the human diet since 600 BC [16] and they have a role of diet in sustaining human due to their diverse range of nutrients and bioactive compounds; such as polysaccharides, proteins, polyunsaturated fatty acids, minerals and significant amounts of antioxidants [17,18]. One such material is *Haematococcus pluvialis*, a single-cell microalgal strain, which is rich source of astaxanthin (10,000–40,000 mg/kg) and associated bioactive ingredients including dietary fibre [19]. Several cell culture and animal studies have reported that astaxanthin has potent antioxidant activity 10 times higher than other carotenoids such as β-carotene, lutein, and zeaxanthin, and 500 times higher than vitamin E [20–22]. Carotenoids play a role in preventing or delaying degenerative diseases such as cancer and atherosclerosis diseases [23–25], and may be useful in the development of functional foods [15].

There is a paucity of information regarding combining the nutritional compounds of marine-based material and whole-grains. Therefore, the present study is the first to show the glycaemic glucose equivalents (GGE) as a predictor of glycaemic response, antioxidant capacities and physical properties of cereal and *Hematococcus pluvialis* in a model food.

2. Materials and Methods

2.1. Sample Collection and Preparation

Driedmicroalgae *Hematococcus pluvialis* was provided by Supreme Biotechnologies Ltd. (Nelson, New Zealand) and ground using a grinder (AutoGrinder, M-EM0415, Sunbeam Corp Ltd., Auckland, New Zealand). The ground material was sieved through a 0.5 mm screen to obtain flour. Wholemeal wheat (Champion Flour, Auckland, New Zealand), barley (Ceres Organics, Auckland, New Zealand) and oat flours (Ceres Organics, Auckland, New Zealand) were purchased locally.

2.2. Cookie Preparation

Cookies were prepared following the standard American Association of Cereal Chemistry (AACC) method 10–50D [26] with slight modification. Table 1 illustrates the dry ingredients used (sugar, salt and sodium bicarbonate). All dry ingredients (except flour) were mixed in an electric mixer (Breville, Melbourne, Australia) with vegetable shortening (Kremelta, Peerless foods, Braybook, Australia) for 3 min on speed 1. Dextrose solution (8.9 g dextrose anhydrous in 150 mL water) and distilled water were added to the mixer and mixed for a further 1 min on speed 2 with scraping down every 30 s. The flour was added and mixed for 2 min with scraping down every 30 s. The experimental samples were prepared by replacing the wholemeal flour with astaxanthin powder 5%, 10% and 15%. The cookie dough was rolled to a 6 mm thickness using measuring roller and cut with a 57 mm diameter cookie cutter. The cookies were placed on metal trays and baked in a preheated electric oven (BAKBAR turbofan convection oven, E3111, Moffat Pty Ltd., Rolleston, New Zealand) for 8 min at 180 °C. The cookies were cooled at room temperature, placed in air-tight plastic bags and stored at room temperature for 24 h prior to laboratory analysis.

Table 1. Model food formulation.

Sample	Wholemeal Flour (g)	Astaxanthin Powder (g)	Other Ingredients
Control	225.00	-	Vegetable shortening (64.0 g), sugar (130 g), salt (2.1 g), sodium bicarbonate (2.5 g), dextrose solution (33 g), water (16 g)
5% Astaxanthin powder	213.75	11.25	Vegetable shortening (64.0 g), sugar (130 g), salt (2.1 g), sodium bicarbonate (2.5 g), dextrose solution (33 g), water (16 g)
10% Astaxanthin powder	202.50	22.50	
15% Astaxanthin powder	191.25	33.75	

2.3. Physical Characteristics

Cookie diameter (mm) and thickness (mm) were measured using calipers (INSIZE digital caliper, series 1112, INSIZE Inc., Loganville, GA, USA). The colour of the cookie samples were measured in terms of Comission Internationale de l'Eclairage (CIE) L^*, a^* and b^* systems by using a colorimeter (Konica Minolta, Chroma Meters CR-210, Tokyo, Japan). The colour differences of the cookies were calculated by the following equation.

$$\Delta E = \sqrt{(\Delta L^*)^2 + (\Delta a^*)^2 + (\Delta b^*)^2}$$

2.4. Texture

The hardness of the cookies (fracture force) was measured by using a texture analyser (TA.XT plus Texture Analyser, Stable Micro Systems, Godalming, UK) with a 3-point bend rig. The analyser was set at a load cell 50 kg; pre-test speed 2 mm/s; test speed 5 mm/s; post-test speed 10 mm/s; return to start mode. The whole cookies were placed on the support ring and the probe moved downward until the samples were broken. The peak force (kg) was recorded as hardness. Measurements were made in triplicate.

2.5. Moisture

Moisture content of the cookie samples were measured after drying cookie ground samples (2 g) overnight in an oven at 105 °C.

2.6. Determination of Total Phenolic Content

The content of total phenolics of samples was measured by Folin-Ciocalteu reagent (mixture of phosphotungstic and phosphomolybdic acid; that is reduced by phenolics forming a blue complex) using the method described by Floegel et al., 2011 [27] with some modifications. The ground samples (1 g) were dispersed in 20 mL of 70% methanol (by placing on a stirrer overnight). The sample mixture was centrifuged at 700 g Relative centrifugal force (RCF) for 10 min and the supernatant collected to determine the total phenolics. Crude extracts (0.5 mL) were mixed thoroughly with freshly prepared 0.2 N Folin-Ciocalteu's reagent (2.5 mL), followed by 2.0 mL of 7.5% sodium carbonate (Na_2CO_3) and incubated in the dark for 2 hours. The absorbance reaction mixture was measured at 760 nm. Gallic acid (gallic acid, 97%, CAS: 149-91-7, Sigma-Aldrich, St. Louise, MO, USA) was used as a standard and results were expressed as mg gallic acid equivalent (GAE) per g sample.

2.7. Antioxidant Properties

The antioxidant capacity of the samples was measured by the DPPH (2,2-diphenyl-1-picrylhydrazyl) assay as described by Floegel et al., 2011 [27] with some modifications. Briefly, 0.5 mL of crude extract was mixed with freshly prepared 1 mL of 0.1 mM methanolic DPPH (CAS: 1898-66-4, Sigma-Aldrich, St. Louise, MO, USA) solution and incubated in the dark at room temperature for 30 min. The reaction mixture absorbance was measured at 517 nm. In order to calculate the DPPH radical scavenging capacity, trolox (CAS: 53188-07-1, ACROS Organics™, Morris, NJ, USA) was used as a standard and result were expressed as µmol trolox equivalent (TE) per g sample.

Oxygen radical absorbance capacity (ORAC) was determined as described by Floegel et al., 2011 with some modifications. Briefly, 25 µL diluted extract were mixed with 150 µL of 10 nM fluorescein into the microplate well and incubated for 30 min at 37 °C temperature. Twenty five microlitres AAPH (2,2-azobis (2-amidinopropane) dihydrochloride) (CAS: 2997-92-4, Cayman Chemical, Ann Arbor, MI, USA) solution was added to the pre-incubated reaction mixture. Fluorescence was measured (excitation 485 nm; emission 510 nm) from the bottom microplate every 60 s for a total of 60 min. Data analysed by using Omega MARS data analysis software (program version 3.02 R2, BMG Labtech, Mornington, Australia), in order to calculate antioxidant capacity, trolox was used as a standard and results were expressed as a mmol trolox equivalent (TE) per g sample.

2.8. InVitro Carbohydrate Digestion (Glycaemic Glucose Equivalent-GGE) Analysis

The in vitro digestion process was carried out with the method developed by Foschia, Peressini, Sensidoni, Brennan and Brennan, 2015 [28] and used by Gao, J.R. et al., 2016 [29]. The method estimates the glucose released from the cookie samples during enzymatic hydrolysis over 120 min to predict glycaemic response. In brief: digestions were held in 60 mL plastic pots placed on a controlled temperature stirring hot plate (IKA RT 15, IKA Werke GmbH & Co. KG, Mendelheim, Germany). The samples (0.5 g) were mixed with 30 mL of reverse osmosis water and kept at 37 °C for 10 min with constant stirring on a magnetic starrier. Pepsin solution (1 mL of 1 g pepsin in 10 mL 0.05 M hydrogen chloride (HCl) was added and incubated for 30 min at 37 °C. Aliquots (1 mL) were collected (time 0) from the digestion mixture and added to 4 mL alcohol to arrest enzyme reaction. Amyloglucosidase (0.1 mL) was added to the digestion mixture to prevent end product inhibition of pancreatic α-amylase. Then pancreatin solution (5 mL of 2.5% pancreatin in 0.1 M Malate buffer pH 6.0) was added to the mixture. Further 1 mL aliquots were collected at 20, 60 and 120 min and treated as before, then stored at 4 °C until reducing sugar analysis was carried out. The 3,5-dinitrosalicylic acid (DNS) method was followed to measure reducing sugar content of the samples during in vitro digestion. Glucose release was calculated in mg glucose/g sample and plotted against time and area under the curve (AUC) was calculated by dividing the graph into trapezoids.

2.9. Statistical Analysis

All data was analysed by using the data analysis software, Minitab (version 17, Minitab Inc., State College, PA, USA) to establish significant differences. Analysis of Variance (One-way) was employed with Tukey's test at 95% confidence interval ($p < 0.05$) in all cases. All values were presented as the mean of triplicate determinations ± standard deviation.

3. Results and Discussion

Cookies were prepared using astaxanthin powder and wholemeal flour. The effects of astaxanthin powder replacement on the physical properties and functional properties of wholemeal flour cookies were analysed.

3.1. Physical Properties of Cookies

The physical characteristics of the cookies are summarised in Table 2. The results showed a significant reduction ($p < 0.05$) in the height and diameter gain of the cookies containing astaxanthin and a significant reduction of ($p < 0.05$) weight loss of the wheat and oat flour cookies with 15% addition of astaxanthin. As the amount of astaxanthin powder increased the weight loss, height and diameter decreased. The largest height changes were observed in cookies made from wholemeal wheat flour, and the largest diameter changes were observed in cookies made from wholemeal oat flour. This observation could be attributed to the hydrophilic nature of the ingredients [30]. The spread factor of a cookie is affected by dough viscosity as well as the acid-base reaction of the ingredients (sodium bicarbonate and fat), causing bubbles in the dough to expand in volume [31]. Physical evaluation of the cookies reported by [32,33], suggested that the spread factor is affected by the water holding capacity of the ingredients. Cookies made with wholemeal barley had increased moisture content with increasing astaxanthin addition. The reason for this phenomenon is that the physical state of starch, protein and fibre are the key determinants of the water holding capacity of the flour as suggested in other papers [34–36]. The moisture content of wheat, oat and barley cookies increased significantly ($p < 0.05$) at all levels of astaxanthin addition (Table 2). This can be attributed to differences in water holding capacity of the ingredients especially different flours [37]. Correspondingly, the hardness of the cookies decreased with the addition of astaxanthin (Table 2). The study indicated that when astaxanthin was incorporated into wheat and oat cookies they were softer and barley cookies were harder in comparison to control cookies. This suggests that water holding capacity of astaxanthin is intermediary between oat and barley flour and it could be due to the nature of the starch and starch-protein interface of different flour. The [38] found that differences in swelling behaviour of the starch granules resulted in cookies with different textural properties, while [34] showed that increased protein content affected the interaction of starch and protein and their hydrogen bonding during dough development.

Table 2. Physical characteristics (after baking: changes in height (%), diameter (%) and weight loss (%); moisture content (%) and hardness (kg) of the model cookies).

Sample	Increase in Height (%)	Increase in Diameter (%)	Weight Loss (%)	Moisture Content (%)	Hardness (kg)
WCC	94.39 ± 3.06 ^{a}	3.93 ± 0.226	9.71 ± 0.04 ^{a}	7.50 ± 0.11 ^{c}	9.26 ± 0.13 ^{a}
W5A	71.44 ± 8.39 ^{b}	2.96 ± 1.139 ^{b}	9.63 ± 0.02 ^{a,b}	7.83 ± 0.01 ^{b}	7.79 ± 0.16 ^{b}
W10A	59.39 ± 3.06 ^{b,c}	2.27 ± 0.216 ^{b}	9.48 ± 0.12 ^{a,b}	7.91 ± 0.07 ^{b}	7.35 ± 0.58 ^{b}
W15A	52.94 ± 0.75 ^{c}	1.15 ± 0.925	9.44 ± 0.12 ^{b}	8.21 ± 0.03 ^{a}	7.06 ± 0.48 ^{b}
BCC	94.33 ± 6.78 ^{a}	5.23 ± 1.168	10.31 ± 0.11 ^{a}	7.74 ± 0.02 ^{d}	4.12 ± 0.12 ^{c}
B5A	83.50 ± 1.04 ^{a,b}	4.76 ± 0.444	10.41 ± 0.11 ^{a}	7.79 ± 0.02 ^{c}	4.98 ± 0.20 ^{b}
B10A	74.61 ± 2.91 ^{b,c}	3.67 ± 0.731 ^{b}	10.46 ± 0.20 ^{a}	7.90 ± 0.01 ^{b}	5.26 ± 0.22 ^{b}
B15A	65.50 ± 4.84 ^{c}	2.72 ± 0.314	10.67 ± 0.28 ^{a}	8.17 ± 0.02 ^{a}	6.21 ± 0.10 ^{a}
OCC	70.94 ± 0.91 ^{a}	23.20 ± 0.25 ^{a}	11.54 ± 0.17 ^{a}	5.55 ± 0.05 ^{d}	7.57 ± 0.05 ^{a}
O5A	67.94 ± 2.46 ^{a,b}	12.81 ± 0.49 ^{a}	11.14 ± 0.23 ^{a,b}	6.09 ± 0.04 ^{c}	7.23 ± 0.14 ^{a,b}
O10A	64.55 ± 0.25 ^{b}	7.80 ± 0.05 ^{c}	10.63 ± 0.22 ^{b,c}	6.66 ± 0.04 ^{b}	7.02 ± 0.12 ^{b}
O15A	55.55 ± 0.91 ^{c}	3.62 ± 0.14 ^{d}	10.23 ± 0.23 ^{c}	7.12 ± 0.09 ^{a}	6.16 ± 0.23 ^{c}

Data are presented as mean ± standard deviation, $n = 3$; (a–d): Means within same columns for same flour cookie group that do not share the same superscript are significantly different ($p < 0.05$). W, Wheat; B, Barley; O, Oat; CC, Cookie Control; A, Astaxanthin (5%, 10% or 15%).

3.2. Colour

The colour profile of the cookie samples (surface and ground) are summarised in Table 3. Both the surface colour and the total colour (represented by the ground sample) were measured to determine if there was any interaction in terms of food addition and colour enhancement. The addition of astaxanthin to three types of flour cookies significantly ($p < 0.05$) decreased the lightness (L^*), causing the cookies to became red (a^*) and decreased yellowness (b^*). There was a significant colour change as illustrated by the $\triangle E$ value of the three kind of flour cookies in the following order: control >5% astaxanthin >10% astaxanthin >15% astaxanthin cookies. The main factor causing the colour change of the cookies is due to the pigment of astaxanthin powder, as the level of substitution increased lightness of the cookies decreased and greenness increased. However, the reaction between reducing sugars and amino acids (maillard reaction; starch dextrinization and caramelization) which is induced by heating during baking time also enhances darkness the cookie colour [39] as reflected in colour change (Table 3; $\triangle E$ value).

3.3. Total Phenolic Content (TPC) and Antioxidant Activity of Cookies

The phenolic content, DPPH radical scavenging and ORAC activity of the cookies are summarised in Table 4. It can be seen that the phenolic content increased significantly ($p < 0.05$), and proportionately, with the replacement of astaxanthin powder. This phenomenon is likely to be due to the high amount of phenolic compounds present in astaxanthin (10,000–40,000 mg/kg). Spiller and Dewell (2003) [40] and Sharma and Gujral (2014) [41] have shown that wheat flour has less phenolic compounds compared to barley and oat flour. ORAC values were observed to increase as astaxanthin increased in the formulation (Table 4). Increasing the level of astaxanthin in cookies resulted in a significant increase ($p < 0.05$) of DPPH scavenging activity. These results are due to the addition of astaxanthin derived from microalgae. Previous research has illustrated that astaxanthin compounds are 10 times stronger than the other carotenoids [20] in terms of phenolic antioxidant activities.

Table 3. The CIE colour profiles of the cookies.

Sample	L^*	a^*	b^*	△E
Surface Cookie colour				
WCC	90.40 ± 0.42 ^{a}	−5.79 ± 0.35 ^{a}	33.05 ± 0.09 ^{a}	96.43 ± 0.44 ^{a}
W5A	84.14 ± 0.26 ^{b}	−7.37 ± 0.08 ^{b}	29.16 ± 0.23 ^{b}	89.36 ± 0.32 ^{b}
W10A	82.20 ± 0.10 ^{c}	−8.72 ± 0.20 ^{c}	27.42 ± 0.06 ^{c}	87.09 ± 0.13 ^{c}
W15A	81.42 ± 0.32 ^{c}	−8.27 ± 0.08 ^{c}	26.45 ± 0.34 ^{d}	86.01 ± 0.40 ^{d}
BCC	94.43 ± 0.45 ^{a}	−8.16 ± 0.76 ^{a}	34.55 ± 0.27 ^{a}	100.89 ± 0.58 ^{a}
B5A	86.97 ± 0.19 ^{b}	−9.25 ± 0.04 ^{b}	32.16 ± 0.07 ^{b}	93.19 ± 0.20 ^{b}
B10A	84.77 ± 0.23 ^{c}	−7.88 ± 0.25 ^{a}	30.06 ± 0.15 ^{c}	90.29 ± 0.27 ^{c}
B15A	83.10 ± 0.14 ^{d}	−7.83 ± 0.01 ^{a}	27.95 ± 0.14 ^{d}	88.02 ± 0.18 ^{d}
OCC	91.31 ± 0.69 ^{a}	−5.64 ± 0.34 ^{a}	35.24 ± 0.15 ^{a}	98.04 ± 0.71 ^{a}
O5A	84.19 ± 0.14 ^{b}	−7.63 ± 0.34 ^{b}	30.64 ± 0.15 ^{b}	89.91 ± 0.20 ^{b}
O10A	82.21 ± 0.13 ^{c}	−7.87 ± 0.13 ^{b}	28.26 ± 0.11 ^{c}	87.31 ± 0.17 ^{c}
O15A	80.77 ± 0.15 ^{d}	−8.17 ± 0.13 ^{b}	26.56 ± 0.19 ^{d}	85.39 ± 0.22 ^{d}
Ground Cookie colour				
WCC	87.20 ± 0.20 ^{a}	−0.32 ± 0.03 ^{a}	45.33 ± 0.10 ^{a}	97.55 ± 0.30 ^{a}
W5A	77.82 ± 0.06 ^{b}	−6.32 ± 0.04 ^{c}	43.72 ± 0.26 ^{b}	90.29 ± 0.01 ^{b}
W10A	75.42 ± 0.22 ^{c}	−6.98 ± 0.03 ^{d}	38.31 ± 0.15 ^{c}	84.88 ± 0.13 ^{c}
W15A	69.10 ± 0.30 ^{d}	−6.20 ± 0.02 ^{b}	34.13 ± 0.12 ^{d}	77.32 ± 0.22 ^{d}
BCC	95.13 ± 0.07 ^{a}	−13.41 ± 0.21 ^{c}	43.14 ± 0.41 ^{a}	105.32 ± 0.13 ^{a}
B5A	82.96 ± 0.62 ^{b}	−5.86 ± 0.23 ^{a}	43.95 ± 0.65 ^{a}	94.06 ± 0.30 ^{b}
B10A	74.46 ± 0.63 ^{c}	−6.56 ± 0.12 ^{b}	44.02 ± 0.09 ^{a}	86.74 ± 0.56 ^{c}
B15A	71.13 ± 0.77 ^{d}	−6.04 ± 0.38 ^{a,b}	39.85 ± 1.38 ^{b}	81.76 ± 0.24 ^{d}
OCC	93.15 ± 0.59 ^{a}	−9.32 ± 0.1.34 ^{b}	49.41 ± 1.35 ^{a}	105.86 ± 0.02 ^{a}
O5A	85.92 ± 0.27 ^{b}	−8.36 ± 0.09 ^{a,b}	39.58 ± 0.21 ^{b,c}	94.97 ± 0.16 ^{b}
O10A	73.24 ± 0.36 ^{c}	−7.33 ± 0.03 ^{a}	36.04 ± 0.07 ^{c}	81.96 ± 0.29 ^{c}
O15A	71.19 ± 0.47 ^{d}	−6.99 ± 0.57 ^{a}	41.34 ± 2.68 ^{b}	82.64 ± 0.97 ^{c}

L^*, lightness (0 = black, 100 = white); a^*, red (+) to green (-); b^*, yellow (+) to blue (-); △E, colour difference. Data are presented as mean ± standard deviation, n = 3; (a–d), Means within same columns for same flour cookie group that do not share the same superscript are significantly different ($p < 0.05$). W, Wheat; B, Barley; O, Oat; CC, Cookie Control; A, Astaxanthin (5%, 10% or 15%).

Table 4. Total phenolic content and antioxidant capacity.

Sample	TPC (mg GAE/g Sample)	DPPH (μmol TE/g Sample)	ORAC (mmol TE/g Sample)
WCC	0.59 ± 0.01 ^{d}	0.54 ± 0.01 ^{d}	0.09 ± 0.001 ^{b}
W5A	0.80 ± 0.01 ^{c}	0.95 ± 0.03 ^{c}	0.11 ± 0.001 ^{a}
W10A	0.95 ± 0.01 ^{b}	1.10 ± 0.01 ^{b}	0.12 ± 0.001 ^{a}
W15A	1.14 ± 0.01 ^{a}	1.26 ± 0.03 ^{a}	0.12 ± 0.004 ^{a}
BCC	0.63 ± 0.01 ^{c}	1.36 ± 0.01 ^{d}	0.08 ± 0.003 ^{b}
B5A	0.95 ± 0.02 ^{b}	1.69 ± 0.02 ^{c}	0.09 ± 0.002 ^{a}
B10A	1.15 ± 0.09 ^{a}	1.74 ± 0.01 ^{b}	0.09 ± 0.002 ^{a}
B15A	1.27 ± 0.01 ^{a}	1.79 ± 0.01 ^{a}	0.10 ± 0.002 ^{a}
OCC	0.87 ± 0.01 ^{d}	1.13 ± 0.01 ^{d}	0.08 ± 0.001 ^{c}
O5A	1.03 ± 0.01 ^{c}	1.22 ± 0.01 ^{c}	0.10 ± 0.002 ^{b}
O10A	1.28 ± 0.01 ^{b}	1.34 ± 0.01 ^{b}	0.10 ± 0.001 ^{a}
O15A	1.44 ± 0.01 ^{a}	1.46 ± 0.01 ^{a}	0.11 ± 0.001 ^{a}

Data are presented as mean ± standard deviation, n = 3; (a–d), Means within same columns for same flour cookie group do not share the same superscript are significantly different ($p < 0.05$). W, Wheat, B, Barley; O, Oat; CC, Cookie Control; A, Astaxanthin (5%, 10% or 15%).

3.4. *Glycaemic Glucose Equivalent (GGE) Analysis*

Figure 1 illustrates the in vitro digestion of cookies, calculated as the amount of reducing sugar released by digestive enzymes over 120 min. All the samples demonstrated the impact of the substitution of astaxanthin in the following order (5% > 10% > 15%) and significantly slowed the amount of reducing sugar released (calculated as mg glucose/g sample of incremental area under the curve (iAUC)) as compare with the control cookies.

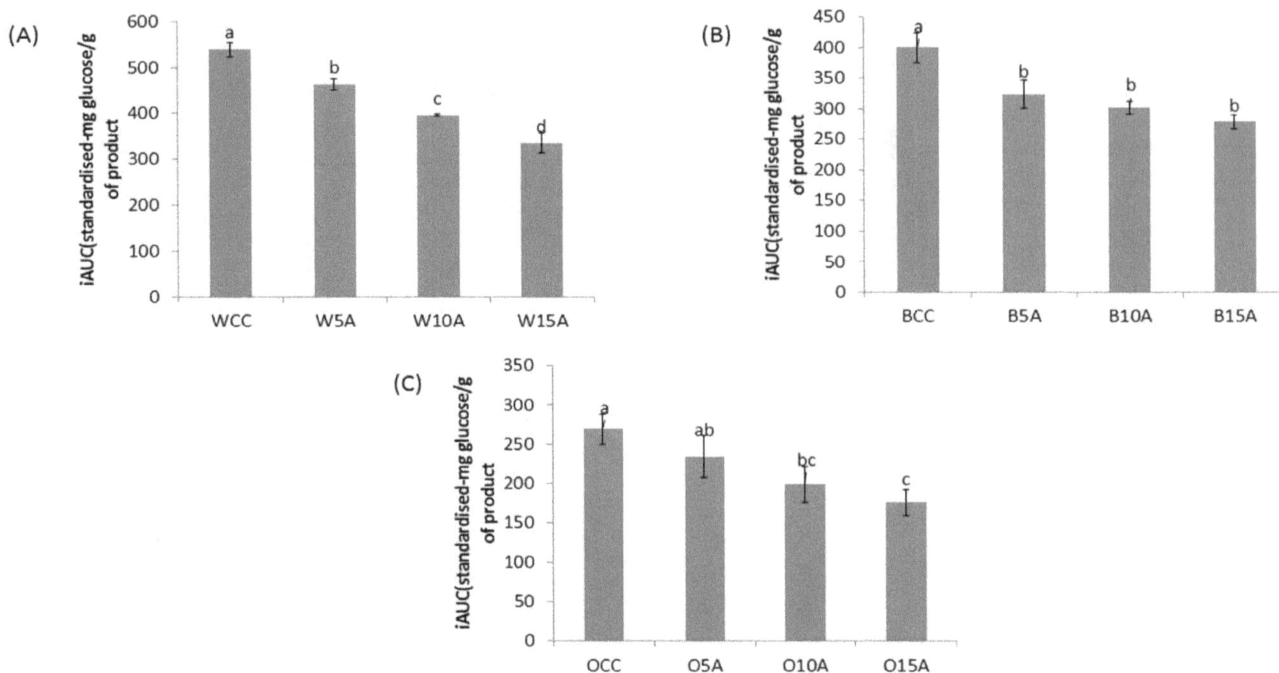

Figure 1. Reducing sugar released (mg/g sample) after 120 min digestion of (**A**) wheat, (**B**) barley and (**C**) oat wholemeal flour cookies with astaxanthin substitution. WCC, wheat cookie control; W5A, wheat + 5% astaxanthin cookie; W10A, wheat + 10% astaxanthin cookie; W15A, wheat + 5% astaxanthin cookie; BCC, barley cookie control; B5A, barley + 5% astaxanthin cookie; B10A, barley + 10% astaxanthin cookie; B15A, barley + 15% astaxanthin cookie; OCC, oat cookie control; O5A, oat + 5% astaxanthin cookie; O10A, oat + 10% astaxanthin cookie; O15A, oat + 15% astaxanthin cookie. (a–d), Means within same figure that do not share the same superscript are significantly different ($p < 0.05$).

It is possible that the high antioxidant activity of the astaxanthin powder could be related to the decreased rate of sugar released [21]. Researchers have shown that antioxidants can impair enzyme activity during the digestion [42]. The interaction between phenolic compounds and digestive enzymes [43] could affect the non-covalent starch-phenolic interactions thus impeding starch degradation [44,45]. Additionally, the rate of sugar release may also be decreased due to the non-starchy network of fibre and protein in the system which entraps starch granules and acts as a physical barrier thus limiting enzyme accessibility [28,46].

Figure 2 illustrates the rate of reaction of starch conversion to reducing sugar release over the 120 min in vitro digestion period. Form this figure it can be observed that the rate of reaction between 20–120 min appears to be greater for the control samples as compared with the samples containing astaxanthin. It can also be observed that the oat samples generally showed a lower sugar release profile than the barley and the wheat samples. It is possible that the in vitro digestion studies observed in Figures 1 and 2 are related to the total phenolic content/antioxidant activity of the samples (Table 4). Further work is required to determine whether this is an indirect relationship or if there is a mechanistic association between phenolic content of the cookies and reduced starch digestion.

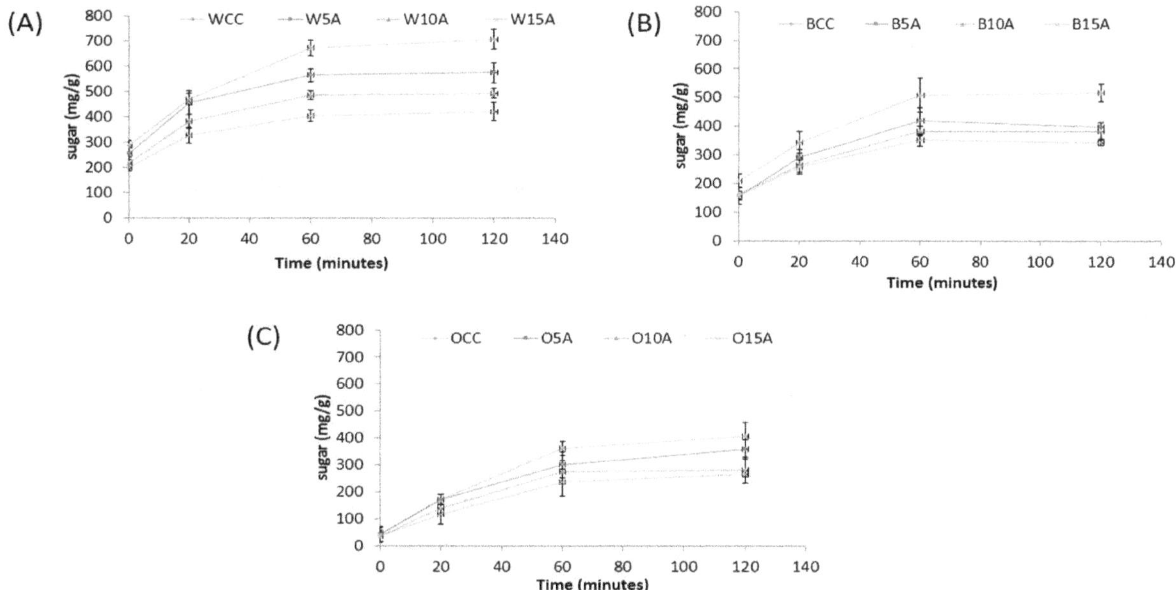

Figure 2. Reducing sugar released (mg/g sample) during the 120 min in vitro digestion process of (**A**) wheat, (**B**) barley and (**C**) oat wholemeal flour cookies with astaxanthin substitution. WCC, wheat cookie control; W5A, wheat + 5% astaxanthin cookie; W10A, wheat + 10% astaxanthin cookie; W15A, wheat + 5% astaxanthin cookie; BCC, barley cookie control; B5A, barley + 5% astaxanthin cookie; B10A, barley + 10% astaxanthin cookie; B15A, barley + 15% astaxanthin cookie; OCC, oat cookie control; O5A, oat + 5% astaxanthin cookie; O10A, oat + 10% astaxanthin cookie; O15A, oat + 15% astaxanthin cookie.

4. Conclusions

The research has illustrated the possible use of novel natural ingredients in alerting the functional quality and biological activity of simple foods. In particular, in vitro digestion (GGE analysis) of the cookies demonstrated significantly lower glucose release when astaxanthin increased in the formulation. The results also demonstrated that the combination of astaxanthin with wholemeal flour significantly improve the antioxidant properties of the cookies. Thus, the inclusion of astaxanthin illustrates a potential synergy between microalgae and wholemeal flour of the model food. As such this combination can contribute to the intake of natural bioactive compounds in the human diets for the potential health benefits.

Acknowledgments: The supply of microalgae by Supreme Biotechnologies Ltd., Nelson, New Zealand is kindly acknowledged. This research was funded by Lincoln University, New Zealand and National Science Challenge High Value Nutrition Award.

Author Contributions: A.K.M.M.H. and M.A.B. conducted the experiments. All authors were involved in the experimental design, data analysis, drafting, reading and approving the final manuscript.

References

1. Andersson, A.A.M.; Dimberg, L.; Aman, P.; Landberg, R. Recent findings on certain bioactive components in whole grain wheat and rye. *J. Cereal Sci.* **2014**, *59*, 294–311. [CrossRef]
2. Brennan, C.S.; Cleary, L.J. The potential use of cereal (1→3,1→4)-β-D-glucans as functional food ingredients. *J. Cereal Sci.* **2005**, *42*, 1–13. [CrossRef]
3. Brennan, C.S. Dietary fibre, glycaemic response, and diabetes. *Mol. Nutr. Food Res.* **2005**, *49*, 560–570. [CrossRef]
4. Ye, E.Q.; Chacko, S.A.; Chou, E.L.; Kugizaki, M.; Liu, S.M. Greater Whole-grain intake is associated with lower risk of type 2 diabetes, cardiovascular disease, and weight gain. *J. Nutr.* **2012**, *142*, 1304–1313. [CrossRef] [PubMed]

5. Knudsen, M.D.; Kyro, C.; Olsen, A.; Dragsted, L.O.; Skeie, G.; Lund, E.; Aringman, P.; Nilsson, L.M.; Bueno-de-Mesquita, H.B.; Tjonneland, A.; et al. Self-reported whole-grain intake and plasma alkylresorcinol concentrations in combination in relation to the incidence of colorectal cancer. *Am. J. Epidemiol.* **2014**, *179*, 1188–1196. [CrossRef] [PubMed]
6. Cho, S.S.; Qi, L.; Fahey, G.C.; Klurfeld, D.M. Consumption of cereal fiber, mixtures of whole grains and bran, and whole grains and risk reduction in type 2 diabetes, obesity, and cardiovascular disease. *Am. J. Clin. Nutr.* **2013**, *98*, 594–619. [CrossRef] [PubMed]
7. Zhou, A.L.; Hergert, N.; Rompato, G.; Lefevre, M. Whole grain oats improve insulin sensitivity and plasma cholesterol profile and modify gut microbiota composition in C57BL/6J mice. *J. Nutr.* **2015**, *145*, 222–230. [CrossRef] [PubMed]
8. Pasqualone, A.; Laddomada, B.; Centomani, I.; Paradiso, V.M.; Minervini, D.; Caponio, F.; Summo, C. Bread making aptitude of mixtures of re-milled semolina and selected durum wheat milling by-products. *LWT Food Sci. Technol.* **2017**, *78*, 151–159. [CrossRef]
9. Oliveira, L.C.; Rosell, C.M.; Steel, C.J. Effect of the addition of whole-grain wheat flour and of extrusion process parameters on dietary fibre content, starch transformation and mechanical properties of a ready-to-eat breakfast cereal. *Int. J. Food Sci. Technol.* **2015**, *50*, 1504–1514. [CrossRef]
10. Robin, F.; Theoduloz, C.; Srichuwong, S. Properties of extruded whole grain cereals and pseudocereals flours. *Int. J. Food Sci. Technol.* **2015**, *50*, 2152–2159. [CrossRef]
11. Lu, X.K.; Brennan, M.A.; Serventi, L.; Mason, S.; Brennan, C.S. How the inclusion of mushroom powder can affect the physicochemical characteristics of pasta. *Int. J. Food Sci. Technol.* **2016**, *51*, 2433–2439. [CrossRef]
12. Sobota, A.; Rzedzicki, Z.; Zarzycki, P.; Kuzawinska, E. Application of common wheat bran for the industrial production of high-fibre pasta. *Int. J. Food Sci. Technol.* **2015**, *50*, 111–119. [CrossRef]
13. Grigor, J.M.; Brennan, C.S.; Hutchings, S.C.; Rowlands, D.S. The sensory acceptance of fibre-enriched cereal foods: A meta-analysis. *Int. J. Food Sci. Technol.* **2016**, *51*, 3–13. [CrossRef]
14. Alves, C.; Pinteus, S.; Simoes, T.; Horta, A.; Silva, J.; Tecelao, C.; Pedrosa, R. *Bifurcaria bifurcata*: A key macro-alga as a source of bioactive compounds and functional ingredients. *Int. J. Food Sci. Technol.* **2016**, *51*, 1638–1646. [CrossRef]
15. Kadam, S.U.; Tiwari, B.K.; O'Donnell, C.P. Extraction, structure and biofunctional activities of laminarin from brown algae. *Int. J. Food Sci. Technol.* **2015**, *50*, 24–31. [CrossRef]
16. Aguilera-Morales, M.; Casas-Valdez, M.; Carrillo-Dominguez, B.; Gonzalez-Acosta, B.; Perez-Gil, F. Chemical composition and microbiological assays of marine algae *Enteromorpha* spp. as a potential food source. *J. Food Compost. Anal.* **2005**, *18*, 79–88. [CrossRef]
17. Lordan, S.; Ross, R.P.; Stanton, C. Marine bioactives as functional food ingredients: Potential to reduce the incidence of chronic diseases. *Mar. Drugs* **2011**, *9*, 1056–1100. [CrossRef] [PubMed]
18. Plaza, M.; Cifuentes, A.; Ibanez, E. In the search of new functional food ingredients from algae. *Trends Food Sci. Technol.* **2008**, *19*, 31–39. [CrossRef]
19. Wu, H.Y.; Hong, H.L.; Zhu, N.; Han, L.M.; Suo, Q.L. Two ethoxyquinoline metabolites from the alga *Heamatococcus pluvialis*. *Chem. Nat. Compd.* **2014**, *50*, 578–580. [CrossRef]
20. Miki, W. Biological functions and activities of animal carotenoids. *Pure Appl. Chem.* **1991**, *63*, 141–146. [CrossRef]
21. Naguib, Y.M.A. Antioxidant activities of astaxanthin and related carotenoids. *J. Agric. Food Chem.* **2000**, *48*, 1150–1154. [CrossRef] [PubMed]
22. Shimidzu, N.; Goto, M.; Miki, W. Carotenoids as singlet oxygen quenchers in marine organisms. *Fish. Sci.* **1996**, *62*, 134–137.
23. Barros, M.P.; Poppe, S.C.; Bondan, E.F. Neuroprotective properties of the marine carotenoid astaxanthin and omega-3 fatty acids, and perspectives for the natural combination of both in krill oil. *Nutrients* **2014**, *6*, 1293–1317. [CrossRef] [PubMed]
24. Raposo, M.F.D.; de Morais, A.; de Morais, R. Carotenoids from marine microalgae: A valuable natural source for the prevention of chronic diseases. *Mar. Drugs* **2015**, *13*, 5128–5155. [CrossRef] [PubMed]
25. Riccioni, G.; D'Orazio, N.; Franceschelli, S.; Speranza, L. Marine carotenoids and cardiovascular risk markers. *Mar. Drugs* **2011**, *9*, 1166–1175. [CrossRef] [PubMed]
26. American Association of Cereal Chemists. *Approved Methods of the American Association of Cereal Chemists*, 9th ed.; American Association of Cereal Chemists: St. Paul, MN, USA, 1995.

27. Floegel, A.; Kim, D.O.; Chung, S.J.; Koo, S.I.; Chun, O.K. Comparison of ABTS/DPPH assays to measure antioxidant capacity in popular antioxidant-rich US foods. *J. Food Compost. Anal.* **2011**, *24*, 1043–1048. [CrossRef]
28. Foschia, M.; Peressini, D.; Sensidoni, A.; Brennan, M.A.; Brennan, C.S. Synergistic effect of different dietary fibres in pasta on in vitro starch digestion? *Food Chem.* **2015**, *172*, 245–250. [CrossRef] [PubMed]
29. Gao, J.R.; Brennan, M.A.; Mason, S.L.; Brennan, C.S. Effect of sugar replacement with stevianna and inulin on the texture and predictive glycaemic response of muffins. *Int. J. Food Sci. Technol.* **2016**, *51*, 1979–1987. [CrossRef]
30. Okpala, L.; Okoli, E.; Udensi, E. Physico-chemical and sensory properties of cookies made from blends of germinated pigeon pea, fermented sorghum, and cocoyam flours. *Food Sci. Nutr.* **2013**, *1*, 8–14. [CrossRef] [PubMed]
31. Chung, H.J.; Cho, A.; Lim, S.T. Utilization of germinated and heat-moisture treated brown rices in sugar-snap cookies. *LWT Food Sci. Technol.* **2014**, *57*, 260–266. [CrossRef]
32. Brennan, C.S.; Samyue, E. Evaluation of starch degradation and textural characteristics of dietary fiber enriched biscuits. *Int. J. Food Prop.* **2004**, *7*, 647–657. [CrossRef]
33. Giami, S.Y.; Achinewhu, S.C.; Ibaakee, C. The quality and sensory attributes of cookies supplemented with fluted pumpkin (*Telfairia occidentalis* Hook) seed flour. *Int. J. Food Sci. Technol.* **2005**, *40*, 613–620. [CrossRef]
34. Mais, A.; Brennan, C.S. Characterisation of flour, starch and fibre obtained from sweet potato (kumara) tubers, and their utilisation in biscuit production. *Int. J. Food Sci. Technol.* **2008**, *43*, 373–379. [CrossRef]
35. Ragaee, S.; Abdel-Aal, E.S.M. Pasting properties of starch and protein in selected cereals and quality of their food products. *Food Chem.* **2006**, *95*, 9–18. [CrossRef]
36. Yamsaengsung, R.; Berghofer, E.; Schoenlechner, R. Physical properties and sensory acceptability of cookies made from chickpea addition to white wheat or whole wheat flour compared to gluten-free amaranth or buckwheat flour. *Int. J. Food Sci. Technol.* **2012**, *47*, 2221–2227. [CrossRef]
37. Inglett, G.E.; Chen, D.J.; Liu, S.X. Physical properties of gluten-free sugar cookies made from amaranth-oat composites. *LWT Food Sci. Technol.* **2015**, *63*, 214–220. [CrossRef]
38. Kweon, M.; Slade, L.; Levine, H. Solvent retention capacity (SRC) testing of wheat flour: Principles and value in predicting flour functionality in different wheat-based food processes and in wheat breeding—A review. *Cereal Chem.* **2011**, *88*, 537–552. [CrossRef]
39. Chevallier, S.; Colonna, P.; Lourdin, D. Contribution of major ingredients during baking of biscuit dough systems. *J. Cereal Sci.* **2000**, *31*, 241–252. [CrossRef]
40. Spiller, G.A.; Dewell, A. Safety of an astaxanthin-rich *Haematococcus pluvialis* algal extract: A randomized clinical trial. *J. Med. Food* **2003**, *6*, 51–56. [CrossRef] [PubMed]
41. Sharma, P.; Gujral, H.S. Cookie making behavior of wheat-barley flour blends and effects on antioxidant properties. *LWT Food Sci. Technol.* **2014**, *55*, 301–307. [CrossRef]
42. Matsiu, T.; Ebuchi, S.; Kobayashi, M.; Fukui, K.; Sugita, K.; Terahara, N.; Matsumoto, K. Anti-hyperglycemic effect of diacylated anthocyanin derived from Ipomoea batatas cultivar Ayamurasaki can be achieved through the alpha-glucosidase inhibitory action. *J. Agric. Food Chem.* **2002**, *50*, 7244–7248. [CrossRef]
43. Paliwal, C.; Ghosh, T.; Bhayani, K.; Maurya, R.; Mishra, S. Antioxidant, anti-nephrolithe activities and in vitro digestibility studies of three different cyanobacterial pigment extracts. *Mar. Drugs* **2015**, *13*, 5384–5401. [CrossRef] [PubMed]
44. Bordenave, N.; Hamaker, B.R.; Ferruzzi, M.G. Nature and consequences of non-covalent interactions between flavonoids and macronutrients in foods. *Food Funct.* **2014**, *5*, 18–34. [CrossRef] [PubMed]
45. Soong, Y.Y.; Tan, S.P.; Leong, L.P.; Henry, J.K. Total antioxidant capacity and starch digestibility of muffins baked with rice, wheat, oat, corn and barley flour. *Food Chem.* **2014**, *164*, 462–469. [CrossRef] [PubMed]
46. Wolter, A.; Hager, A.S.; Zannini, E.; Arendt, E.K. Influence of sourdough on in vitro starch digestibility and predicted glycemic indices of gluten-free breads. *Food Funct.* **2014**, *5*, 564–572. [CrossRef] [PubMed]

5

Lipids and Fatty Acids in Italian Durum Wheat (*Triticum durum* Desf.) Cultivars

Valentina Narducci, Enrico Finotti, Vincenzo Galli and Marina Carcea *

Research Centre for Food and Nutrition, Council for Agricultural Research and Economics (CREA), Via Ardeatina 546, 00178 Rome, Italy; valentina.narducci@crea.gov.it (V.N.); enrico.finotti@crea.gov.it (E.F.); vincenzo.galli@crea.gov.it (V.G.)

* Correspondence: marina.carcea@crea.gov.it

Abstract: The level of variation in lipids and their fatty acids was determined in the grains of 10 popular durum wheat cultivars commercially grown in Central and Southern Italy. Samples were harvested for two consecutive years to account for differences due to changes in climatic conditions. Total fat content was determined by means of the International Association of Cereal Science and Technology (ICC) Standard Method No. 136, whereas the fatty acid profile was determined by gas chromatography. Total lipid content ranged from 2.97% to 3.54% dry basis (d.b.) in the year 2010 and from 3.10% to 3.50% d.b. in the year 2011, and the average value was 3.22% d.b. considering both years together. Six main fatty acids were detected in all samples in order of decreasing amounts: linoleic (C18:2) > palmitic (C16:0) ≈ oleic (C18:1) > linolenic (C18:3) > stearic (C18:0) > palmitoleic (C16:1). Significant variations in the levels of single acids between two years were observed for three samples. These results will be very useful in the updating of food composition databases in general and will help authorities to set proper quality standards for wholegrain flours and products where the germ should be preserved, considering also the recent interest of industry and consumers for these kinds of products.

Keywords: durum wheat; fatty acids; grain; kernel; lipids

---

1. Introduction

Durum wheat (*Triticum durum* Desf.) kernels contain about 2.4–3.8% dry basis (d.b.) of lipids [1]. Roughly two thirds (66%) of them are contained in the germ, 15% are in the bran (particularly in the aleuronic layer), and about 20% are distributed in the endosperm, partly within the starch granules. From a chemical point of view, the most abundant fraction is composed by nonpolar lipids, which are mainly storage acylglycerols. Phospholipids, glycolipids and other classes are present in lesser amounts. The fatty acids of wheat lipids are mostly unsaturated (C18:2, C18:1, C18:3 and C16:1) and two of them are essential (linoleic and linolenic). This increases the value of wheat lipids for human nutrition, because essential fatty acids are precursors of important classes of biomolecules in the human body (like prostaglandins and membrane phospholipids) and are involved in metabolic processes like regulation of blood lipid levels, particularly cholesterol [1–3].

Lipid content, lipid classes and fatty acid levels in wheat kernels depend on a set of factors, some of which are genetic, such as species and variety [4], whereas others depend on the environment and are related to pedoclimatic conditions, agronomic practices and maturity level [1,4,5]. For example, durum wheat and hard red wheat generally have a higher lipid content than soft white wheat and the levels of fatty acids are different in durum and in soft wheat. In regard to climatic conditions, it has been seen that cold weather favors an increase of lipid content in wheat and a higher degree of unsaturation in fatty acids due to the need for membrane fluidification [6]. Other kinds of biotic and abiotic stresses can influence the level of saturated and unsaturated fatty acids in plants [7].

Moreover, different extraction and analytical methods can also account for the differences found in the literature [1,8]. Notwithstanding the number of samples analyzed, we can assume that data about fatty acid levels in durum wheat are abundant in the literature, but it is difficult to have a clear idea of their content and to make comparisons for a number of reasons: (i) different authors report fatty acids as percentage, alternatively referring to: (1) total lipids, (2) total fatty acids, or (3) kernel weight (in addition, some authors analyze germ oil and others analyze whole kernels); (ii) authors interested in statistic elaborations (e.g., in order to investigate variation factors or to look for discriminating parameters) often report charts and graphs rather than tables of data; (iii) cultivars are different in different countries and new ones are constantly bred; and (iv) databases do not always report the sample numerosity and the standard variation of the means.

In this work, the content and level of variation in lipids and of their fatty acids in the durum wheat kernels commercially grown in Italy (where durum wheat is an important cereal crop mainly used for pasta manufacturing) were assessed. For this reason, we selected 10 cultivars amongst the most commonly grown for pasta making. Samples were collected in several locations of Central and Southern Italy to account, at least partially, for differences due to different pedoclimatic environments; Southern Italy is characterized by milder winters and warmer springs and summers with respect to Central Italy, however both areas are considered highly suitable for durum wheat cultivation. Moreover, crops from two consecutive years were collected from the same fields.

The knowledge generated by this research will be very useful in the updating of food composition databases in general and will help authorities in setting proper quality standards for wholegrain flours and products where the germ should be preserved, considering also the recent interest of industry and consumers for these kinds of products and the lack, in several cases, of specific legislation.

2. Materials and Methods

2.1. Samples and Sample Preparation

Representative samples of durum wheat grains, belonging to 10 cultivars selected amongst the most frequently grown in Italy, were collected at harvest for two consecutive years (2010–2011) in 10 different locations of Central and Southern Italy (Table 1). Eight samples came from the Central regions of Italy (Tuscany and Marche) whereas twelve were from different locations in the Sicilian region, in the South. All locations belong to the area traditionally dedicated to durum wheat cultivation in Italy.

Table 1. Durum wheat sample specifications: cultivar, region and location.

Cultivar	Region	Location
Ancomarzio	Tuscany (Central Italy)	Siena (SI)
Creso	Tuscany (Central Italy)	Pisa (PI)
Dylan	Marche (Central Italy)	Macerata (MC)
Rusticano	Marche (Central Italy)	Ancona (AN)
Bronte	Sicily (Southern Italy)	Palermo (PA)
Ciccio	Sicily (Southern Italy)	Enna (EN)
Duilio	Sicily (Southern Italy)	Trapani (TP)
Iride	Sicily (Southern Italy)	Agrigento (AG)
K26	Sicily (Southern Italy)	Enna (EN)
Simeto	Sicily (Southern Italy)	Catania (CT)

Durum wheat in Italy is grown under rain-fed production: it is planted in late autumn or early winter and harvested in early summer, which often leads to limited rainfall and high temperatures, resulting in water stress during grain filling. Crop rotation and balanced nutrient management (mainly nitrogen and phosphorus, pre-sowing and topdressing fertilization) are practiced to ensure that the crop produces the greatest possible high-quality yield with the moisture that is available. The main climate factors influencing durum wheat crop quality are rainfall and temperature during the growing season. Data on these two factors of the years 2009–2011 in Central and Southern Italy can be found in the reports by the Italian High Institute for Environmental Protection and Research (ISPRA,) [9–11].

Fifty grams of each cleaned sample were milled by means of a Cyclotec laboratory mill (Foss-Tecator, Hillerød, Denmark) equipped with a 0.5 mm screen, to obtain wholemeal flours that were used for the subsequent analyses.

2.2. Chemicals

Chloroform, ethyl alcohol (96% *w/w*), methanol, *n*-hexane, formic acid (99% *w/w*) hydrochloric acid (37% *w/w*) and anhydrous sodium sulphate were of analytical grade and were purchased from Carlo Erba (Milan, Italy). Boron trifluoride (approximately 10% *w/w* in methanol for gas chromatography (GC) derivatization) was purchased from Sigma-Aldrich (St. Louis, MO, USA). Fatty acid standards (C16:0, C16:1, C17:0, C18:0, C18:1, C18:2, C18:3) were also purchased from Sigma-Aldrich.

2.3. Analyses

Moisture of wholemeal flours was determined by oven drying at 130 °C according to the ICC Standard No. 110/1 [12].

Total fat was determined by hydrolysis in formic acid and hydrochloric acid at 75 °C reflux for 20 min followed by extraction in hexane and evaporation, according to the ICC Standard No. 136 [12].

The fatty acid profile was determined by gas chromatography (GC). About 5 g of wholemeal flour (in duplicate) was introduced in a Corning tube and suspended in 10 mL of chloroform–methanol 2:1 acidulated with 6 N HCl. A magnetic bar was added, and the tube was left to extract overnight at room temperature on a magnetic stirrer. The mixture was filtered through Whatman Grade 1 (1–11 μm) filter paper into an oven dried flask, then the solvent was evaporated by nitrogen flux followed by oven drying at 30 °C. The contents of the flask were re-dissolved in chloroform–methanol 2:1 to a volume of exactly 10 mL, then an aliquot was derivatized according to Zweig and Sherma [13] as follows: 100 μL of this solution was introduced into a Corning tube containing 3 mL of methanol and a few boiling stones, then 0.5 mL of BF_3–methanol (10% *w/w*) was added and the tube caps were loosely screwed. The tubes were put onto a heating plate in a water bath and left to gently reflux at 72 °C for 30 min. Following this, the reaction was quenched with 2 mL of water, then the mixture was cooled to room temperature and extracted three times with 3 mL of *n*-hexane. The hexane extracts were reunited into a vial and finally the hexane was evaporated by nitrogen flux. The vial was stored under nitrogen at −18 °C for a few days. Immediately prior to GC analysis, the contents of the vial were re-dissolved in 300 μL of hexane and 2 μL were injected. The GC instrument was an HP 5890 equipped with a Supelco (Sigma-Aldrich, St. Louis, MO, USA) SPB®-PUFA (poly unsaturated fatty acids) column of 30 m length and a flame ionization detector (F.I.D.). The instrumental analysis was run according to Finotti et al. [14]: 50 °C for 1 min, ramp of 10 °C/min until 160 °C, stay at 160 °C for 1 min, ramp of 2 °C/min until 240 °C. The detected peaks were individuated by comparison with chromatograms of standards (C16:0, C16:1, C18:0, C18:1, C18:2, C18:3) and quantified by using C17:0 as an internal standard.

2.4. Statistics

The Shapiro–Wilks normality test, *F*-test for homogeneity of variance, Student's *t*-test and Friedman test followed by Wilcoxon pairwise comparisons were performed by means of the PAleontological STatistics (PAST) statistical package [15]. Two-way ANOVA followed by Tukey's test (only in cases with a normal variable and homogeneous variances) and box-plots were performed by means of StatSoft Statistica 8.0 (TIBCO Software, Palo Alto, CA, USA). Calculations were performed by means of Microsoft Excel (Redmond, Washington State, USA).

3. Results

3.1. Total Lipids

Total lipids ranged from 2.97% to 3.54% d.b. in the year 2010 and from 3.10% to 3.50% d.b. in the year 2011, and the average value was 3.22% d.b. considering both years together (Table 2). The moisture content of grains ranged between 10.5% and 12.3% and the average was 11.4% (Table 2). Total lipid content was strongly dependent on the combination of cultivar (cv)/growing site ($p < 0.01$) and to a minor extent on the growing year ($p < 0.05$), whereas the interaction cv/site × year was not a statistically significant factor of variation. In any case, differences were very small: up to 0.57 between samples of different cultivars and up to 0.18 between years for samples of a same cv/site (Table 2). Differences between years for samples of the same cv/site were not significant. The total lipid values found in this study are in line with those reported by the USDA National Nutrient Database (2.8 g/100 g d.b. for product N. 20076 "wheat, durum", mean of 18 samples, standard error 0.060) and by the Italian food composition tables (3.3 g/100 g d.b. for "durum wheat") compiled by the Italian National Institute for Research on Food and Nutrition (INRAN) [16,17]. If we take into account the geographical separation into Central and Southern Italy, we can say that the average total lipid values for all samples were 3.24% and 3.21% d.b. respectively, whereas the range of values was 2.97–3.54% for Central Italy and 3.09–3.41% d.b. for Southern Italy.

Table 2. Moisture and total lipids in the grains of 10 Italian durum wheat cultivars grown in different locations for two consecutive years.

Cultivar and Location		Moisture (g/100 g)		Total Lipids (g/100g d.b.)			
		2010	2011	2010	2011	Difference 2011–2010	
Central Italy	Ancomarzio SI	11.2	11.0	3.11 ^{ef}	3.25 ^{cde}	0.14	ns
	Creso PI	11.8	11.4	3.24 ^{cde}	3.25 ^{cde}	0.01	ns
	Dylan MC	11.7	11.7	3.54 ^{a}	3.50 ^{ab}	−0.04	ns
	Rusticano AN	12.3	12.0	2.97 ^{f}	3.10 ^{ef}	0.13	ns
Southern Italy	Bronte PA	11.3	11.1	3.09 ^{ef}	3.28 ^{bcde}	0.18	ns
	Ciccio EN	11.5	10.8	3.39 ^{abcd}	3.41 ^{abc}	0.02	ns
	Duilio TP	11.2	11.4	3.11 ^{ef}	3.15 ^{def}	0.05	ns
	Iride AG	11.0	10.5	3.31 ^{abcde}	3.24 ^{cde}	−0.07	ns
	K26 EN	11.3	11.0	3.10 ^{ef}	3.24 ^{cde}	0.14	ns
	Simeto CT	11.7	11.6	3.13 ^{ef}	3.10 ^{ef}	−0.02	ns

^{abcdef}: different letters correspond to significant differences ($p < 0.05$) according to 2-way ANOVA and Tukey's test. ns: not significant.

3.2. Fatty Acid Profile

Six main fatty acids were detected in all samples, as expected. In order of decreasing amounts, they are: linoleic (C18:2) > palmitic (C16:0) ≈ oleic (C18:1) > linolenic (C18:3) > stearic (C18:0) > palmitoleic (C16:1). This can be clearly seen from the box plot elaboration reported for each separate year and for the two years together (Figure 1). This distribution did not change whether considering both years separately or together. Detailed data of fatty acids in all samples are reported in Table 3.

Linoleic acid (C18:2) was present in amounts ranging from 0.50–1.14 g/100 g d.b. throughout all samples, with a mean of 0.68 and a standard deviation (SD) of 0.16 (Table 3). For comparison, the USDA National Nutrient Database reports 1.04 g/100 g d.b. for product N. 20076 "wheat, durum" and the INRAN food composition tables report 1.36 g/100 g d.b. for durum wheat. Neither database reports any information on standard errors for all acids.

Palmitic (C16:0) and oleic (C18:1) acids were detected in equal amounts. Palmitic acid ranged from 0.17–0.36 g/100 g d.b., mean 0.24 (SD 0.04) and oleic acid ranged from 0.17–0.43 g/100 g d.b., mean 0.24 (SD 0.07). The USDA reports 0.51 g/100 g d.b. for palmitic acid and 0.40 g/100 g d.b. for oleic acid, whereas the INRAN database reports 0.47 g/100 g d.b. and 0.38 g/100 g d.b., respectively (Table 3).

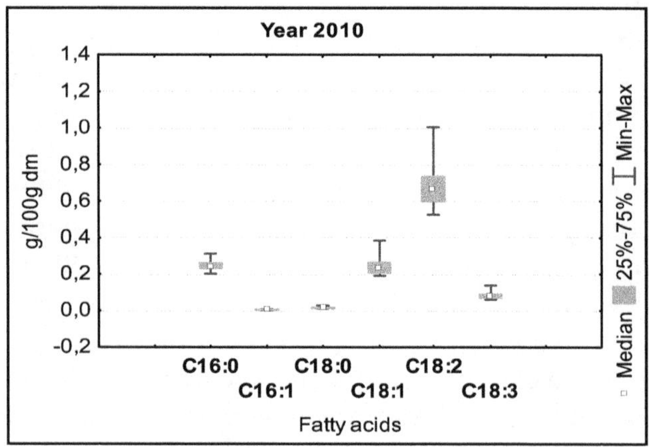

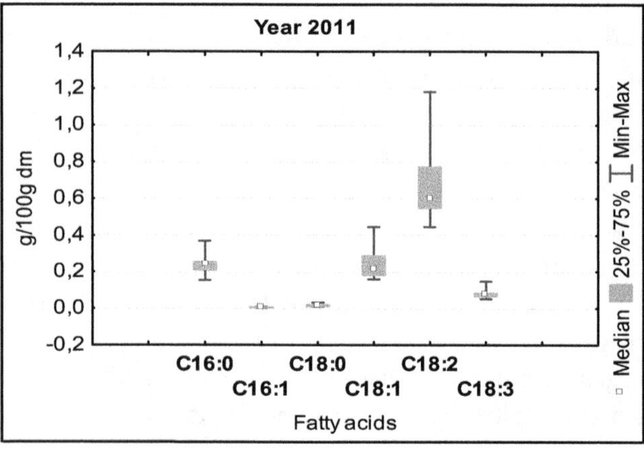

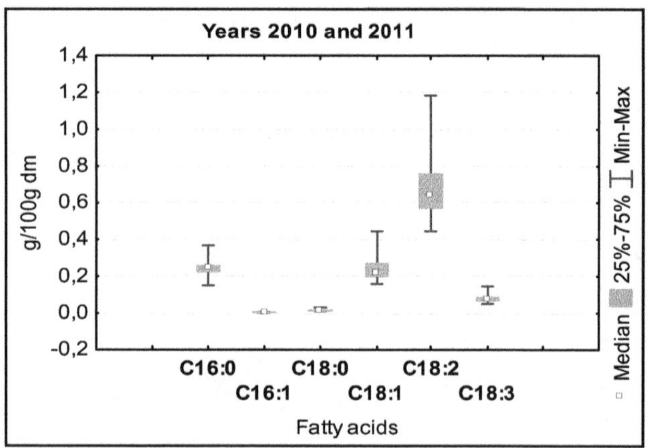

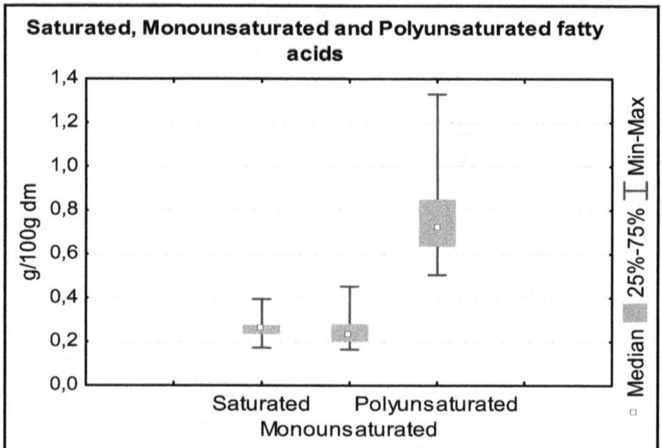

Figure 1. Box plot (percentiles) of fatty acids in samples of Italian durum wheat (10 cultivars, grown in the same location for two consecutive years).

Linolenic acid (C18:3) ranged from 0.06–0.14 g/100 g d.b., mean 0.08 (SD 0.02). The USDA and the INRAN databases report 0.05 g/100 g d.b. and 0.11 g/100 g d.b., respectively. Stearic acid (C18:0) ranged from 0.01–0.03 g/100 g d.b., mean 0.02 (SD 0.005). The USDA and the INRAN databases report, for this acid, 0.03 g/100 g d.b. and 0.02 g/100g d.b. respectively. Finally, palmitoleic acid (C16:1) was detected in very small amounts, ranging from 0.004–0.007 g/100 g d.b., mean 0.005 (SD 0.001). Both the USDA and INRAN databases report 0.01 g/100 g d.m. for this acid.

A series of *t*-tests, performed for each fatty acid on each pair of samples from the same cv/site between the two growing years, showed a significant difference between the years 2010 and 2011 in a few cases only, namely: all acids except C16:1 varied in Ancomarzio SI and Iride AG; only the acids C18:1, C18:2 and C18:3 varied in Ciccio EN (Table 3).

Table 3. Fatty acids in 10 Italian durum wheat cultivars, grown in different locations for two consecutive years (g/100 g sample, d.m.).

Sample	Total Lipids	C16:0	C16:1	C18:0	C18:1	C18:2	C18:3	Saturated	Monoun-Saturated	Polyun-Saturated	Ratio Unsaturated/ Saturated
Ancomarzio (SI) 2010	3.01	0.28	0.006	0.02	0.28	0.80	0.10	0.30	0.29	0.90	3.96
Ancomarzio (SI) 2011	3.03	0.23	0.004	0.01	0.18	0.54	0.06	0.24	0.18	0.60	3.24
		*			*	*	*				*
Creso (PI) 2010	3.02	0.23	0.004	0.02	0.24	0.68	0.07	0.25	0.24	0.75	3.97
Creso (PI) 2011	3.02	0.17	0.004	0.02	0.20	0.51	0.06	0.19	0.21	0.57	4.05
Dylan (MC) 2010	3.05	0.26	0.007	0.01	0.28	0.68	0.07	0.27	0.28	0.75	3.80
Dylan (MC) 2011	3.05	0.27	0.005	0.02	0.34	0.84	0.08	0.29	0.34	0.92	4.39
Rusticano (AN) 2010	3.00	0.23	0.005	0.02	0.22	0.65	0.08	0.25	0.23	0.72	3.87
Rusticano (AN) 2011	3.01	0.26	0.006	0.02	0.30	0.85	0.09	0.28	0.30	0.94	4.42
Bronte (PA) 2010	3.01	0.30	0.006	0.02	0.33	0.89	0.13	0.32	0.34	1.02	4.20
Bronte (PA) 2011	3.03	0.22	0.004	0.01	0.18	0.50	0.07	0.23	0.18	0.57	3.24
Ciccio (EN) 2010	3.04	0.24	0.004	0.02	0.25	0.73	0.09	0.26	0.25	0.83	4.11
Ciccio (EN) 2011	3.04	0.20	0.004	0.01	0.17	0.54	0.07	0.21	0.18	0.61	3.69
					*	**	**				
Duilio (TP) 2010	3.01	0.22	0.004	0.01	0.20	0.60	0.08	0.23	0.20	0.68	3.87
Duilio (TP) 2011	3.02	0.23	0.004	0.01	0.22	0.64	0.08	0.24	0.22	0.73	3.94
Iride (AG) 2010	3.03	0.23	0.007	0.01	0.22	0.59	0.07	0.24	0.22	0.66	3.62
Iride (AG) 2011	3.02	0.36	0.007	0.03	0.43	1.14	0.14	0.39	0.44	1.28	4.44
		**			**	**	**				*
K26 (EN) 2010	3.01	0.24	0.005	0.02	0.21	0.54	0.06	0.26	0.21	0.60	3.15
K26 (EN) 2011	3.02	0.24	0.005	0.01	0.22	0.59	0.07	0.26	0.23	0.66	3.48
							*				**
Simeto (CT) 2010	3.01	0.23	0.005	0.01	0.21	0.64	0.08	0.25	0.21	0.72	3.76
Simeto (CT) 2011	3.01	0.25	0.006	0.01	0.20	0.63	0.08	0.26	0.21	0.71	3.48
Max	3.00	0.36	0.007	0.03	0.43	1.14	0.14	0.39	0.44	1.28	4.44
Min	3.05	0.17	0.004	0.01	0.17	0.50	0.06	0.19	0.18	0.57	3.15
Mean	3.02	0.24	0.005	0.016	0.24	0.68	0.08	0.26	0.25	0.76	3.83
SD	0.014	0.04	0.001	0.005	0.07	0.16	0.02	0.04	0.07	0.18	0.38
Durum wheat USDA ‡	2.8	0.47	0.01	0.02	0.38	1.04	0.05	0.50	0.39	1.10	3.0
Durum wheat INRAN ‡	3.3	0.51	0.01	0.03	0.40	1.36	0.11	0.54	0.41	1.47	3.5

Asterisks indicate significant difference between the year 2010 and 2011, * $p < 0.05$, ** $p < 0.01$ (*t*-test). ‡: values on dry basis, calculated by the authors from original data in USDA and INRAN databases that are expressed on as-is basis.

3.3. Saturated and Unsaturated Fatty Acids

As expected, polyunsaturated fatty acids were preponderant over saturated and monounsaturated fatty acids in all samples ($p < 0.01$, Friedman test; see Figure 1), ranging from 0.57–1.28 g/100 g d.b. (Table 3). Total monounsaturated and total saturated, whose levels were roughly similar ($p < 0.01$), covered from 0.18–0.44 g/100 g d.b. and from 0.19–0.39 g/100 g d.b., respectively. The unsaturated/saturated ratio ranged from 3.15–4.44 g/100 g d.b. considering all samples, with a mean of 3.83 (SD 0.38). This mean is higher than that reported by USDA (3.0) and INRAN (3.5). A series of *t*-tests, performed on each pair of samples from the same cv/site grown in different years, showed a significant difference for the unsaturated/saturated ratio between years in only three cases (Ancomarzio SI, Iride AG and K26 EN) (Table 3).

4. Discussion

Total lipids were in line with the values reported by the USDA and the INRAN databases (nearer to the Italian value) and it was not possible to detect any difference between the geographical areas of Central and Northern Italy.

In regard to fatty acid composition, even if Bottari et al. in 1999 [18] observed the presence of more than 60 peaks by gas chromatography and mass spectrometry (GC-MS) and identified fatty acids with even numbers of carbon atoms from C12 to C30 as well as C15 and C17, the major fat components were saturated and unsaturated C16 and C18 and particularly C16:0, C18:1 and C18:2, which together represented around 90% of the total.

Actually, the USDA database (but not the INRAN one) and other works also report small amounts of C14:0 in durum wheat kernels (USDA 0.003 g/100 g fresh matter, corresponding to 0.0035 g/100 g d.b.). We did not detect this acid, as it was at the limit of detection of our method. There are publications reporting other fatty acids as well (i.e., C17, C20, C22 and C24), some in kernels (Beleggia et al. [5] who uses a GC-MS instrument) and others in germ oil [19,20]. However, only C16:0, C18:0, C18:1, C18:2 and C18:3 are constantly reported by all published works and are regarded as the most important ones in durum wheat, with others amounting to about 1–2% in total [1].

For all fatty acids except C18:3 and for total saturated, total monounsaturated and total polyunsaturated acids, the mean calculated for our samples was lower than the values reported by USDA and INRAN (roughly two thirds–half, $p < 0.01$ against a hypothetical value; see Table 3). However, the range of the detected values contained the reference values, except for C16:0 and for total saturated acids, for which the detected range extended entirely below the USDA and INRAN means. Neither database reports the standard deviations for fatty acids in durum wheat and only the USDA one reports sample numerosity (that is, 29); in this latter case, a certain width around the reported value can be supposed, but it is not quantified. On the contrary, for the unsaturated/saturated ratio, the range of the detected values extends entirely above the mean reported by USDA and contains that reported by INRAN. As a matter of fact, there are notable differences between the two references used. The INRAN values are equal to or higher than the USDA values for the considered variables, in particular for C18:0 (+50%), C18:2 (+31%), C18:3 (+120%), total polyunsaturated acids (+34%) and unsaturated/saturated ratio (+17%).

All the reported differences can be explained by the differences in genetic characteristics, pedoclimatic conditions, agronomical treatments and analytical procedure, as stated in the Introduction. In particular, Beleggia et al. [5] identified the interaction genotype × year × treatment as the main contributor to the variability of the fatty acid levels observed in 24 durum wheat samples, especially for linoleic, oleic and stearic acids. Armanino et al. [4] linked the fatty acid profile of 135 samples of durum wheat to the cultivar, the geographic origin and the harvest year. The variation in saturated and unsaturated fatty acids within the same variety is also associated with various kinds of biotic and abiotic stresses, like low or high temperature, salt, drought, pathogens and others [6,7].

Also, in our study, different conditions related to location and climatic factors can account for some of the observed variability in lipid parameters. In fact, from the ISPRA reports [9–11], we can briefly say that in both areas of Italy (Central and South), temperatures were similar in the first part of the two growing seasons (October–December 2009 and 2010), except the month of December which was warmer in 2009 than in 2010. In the second part of the growing season (January–June, particularly April–June), the Central area showed warmer temperatures in 2011 than in 2010. In regard to precipitation, the first growing season (2009) started with a lesser amount of rain in October–December with respect to the second one (2010) and continued with a higher amount of rain in the January–June period. This happened both in Central and Southern Italy.

5. Conclusions

This work contributes to the knowledge on the content and variability of total fats and of the main fatty acids in durum wheat kernels. The values obtained in this study are also compared with reference values from national and international databases. In this paper, the use of standard methods of analysis, statistical data (numerosity of samples, mean, standard errors) and the specification of all the elements that allow for conversion of results into different units of measure (g/100 g dry or wet sample, g/100 g fat matter) make this data very useful in the compilation of databases and easy to compare with other data. Moreover, updated data on lipids are needed to set proper quality standards for products such as wheat wholegrain flours and foods where the presence of germ is desirable.

Author Contributions: Conceptualization and supervision, M.C. and E.F.; investigation, E.F., V.N. and V.G.; data curation and writing—original draft preparation, V.N.; funding acquisition and writing—review and editing, M.C.

Acknowledgments: The authors wish to acknowledge Luigi Bartoli's technical assistance in sample preparation.

References

1. Lafiandra, D.; Masci, S.; Sissons, M.; Dornez, E.; Delcour, J.A.; Courtin, C.M.; Caboni, M.F. Kernel components of technological value. In *Durum Wheat Chemistry and Technology*, 2nd ed.; Sissons, M., Marchylo, B., Abecassis, J., et al., Eds.; AACC International Inc.: St. Paul, MN, USA, 2012; pp. 85–124.
2. Russo, G.L. Dietary *n*-6 and *n*-3 polyunsaturated fatty acids: From biochemistry to clinical implications in cardiovascular prevention. *Biochem. Pharmacol.* **2009**, *77*, 937–946. [CrossRef] [PubMed]
3. Mozaffarian, D.; Wu, J.H.Y. Omega 3 fatty acids and cardiovascular disease. *J. Am. Coll. Cardiol.* **2011**, *58*, 2047–2067. [CrossRef] [PubMed]
4. Armanino, C.; De Acutis, R.; Festa, M.R. Wheat lipids to discriminate species, varieties, geographical origins and crop years. *Anal. Chim. Acta* **2002**, *454*, 315–326. [CrossRef]
5. Beleggia, R.; Platani, C.; Nigro, F.; De Vita, P.; Cattivelli, L.; Papa, R. Effect of genotype, environment and genotype-by-environment interaction on metabolite profiling in durum wheat (*Triticum durum* Desf.) grain. *J. Cereal Sci.* **2013**, *57*, 183–192. [CrossRef]
6. Nejadsadeghi, L.; Maali-Amiri, R.; Zeinali, H.; Ramezanpour, S.; Sadeghzade, B. Membrane fatty acid compositions and cold-induced responses in tetraploid and hexaploid wheats. *Mol. Biol. Rep.* **2015**, *42*, 363–372. [CrossRef] [PubMed]
7. Upchurch, R.G. Fatty acid unsaturation, mobilization, and regulation in the response of plants to stress. *Biotechnol. Lett.* **2008**, *30*, 967–977. [CrossRef] [PubMed]
8. Rosicka-Kaczmarek, J.; Miśkiewicz, K.; Nebesny, E.; Makowski, B. Composition and functional properties of lipid components from selected cereal grains. In *Plant Lipids Science, Technology, Nutritional Value and Benefits to Human Health*; Budryn, G., Żyżelewicz, D., Eds.; Transworld Research Network: Kerala, India, 2015; pp. 119–145.
9. Istituto Superiore per la Protezione e la Ricerca Ambientale (ISPRA). Gli indicatori del clima in Italia nel 2009. Available online: http://www.isprambiente.gov.it/it/pubblicazioni/stato-dellambiente/gli-indicatori-del-clima-in-italia-nel-2009 (accessed on 14 June 2019).
10. Istituto Superiore per la Protezione e la Ricerca Ambientale (ISPRA). Gli indicatori del clima in Italia nel 2010. Available online: http://www.isprambiente.gov.it/it/pubblicazioni/stato-dellambiente/gli-indicatori-del-clima-in-italia-nel-2010-anno (accessed on 14 June 2019).
11. Istituto Superiore per la Protezione e la Ricerca Ambientale (ISPRA). Gli indicatori del clima in Italia nel 2011. Available online: http://www.isprambiente.gov.it/it/pubblicazioni/stato-dellambiente/gli-indicatori-del-clima-in-italia-nel-2011-anno-vii (accessed on 14 June 2019).
12. International Association for Cereal Science and Technology. *Standard Methods of the ICC*, The Association: Vienna, Austria, 2003.
13. Zweig, G.; Sherma, J. *Handbook of Chromatography*; CRC Press: New York, NY, USA, 1974; pp. 95–240.
14. Finotti, E.; Bersani, A.; Bersani, E. Total quality index for extra virgin olive oil. *J. Food Qual.* **2007**, *30*, 911–931. [CrossRef]
15. Hammer, Ų.; Harper, D.A.T.; Ryan, P.D. PAST: Paleontological statistics software package for education and data analysis. *Palaeontol. Electron.* **2001**, *4*, 1–9.
16. Istituto Nazionale di Ricerca per gli Alimenti e la Nutrizione (INRAN). Tabelle di composizione degli alimenti: 'frumento duro' (Food composition tables 'durum wheat'). Available online: http://nut.entecra.it/646/tabelle_di_composizione_degli_alimenti.html (accessed on 21 May 2019).
17. USDA National Nutrient Database for Standard Reference. Nutrient data for product 20076 'Wheat, durum'.

Available online: https://ndb.nal.usda.gov/ndb/foods/show/20076?n1=%7BQv%3D1%7D&fgcd=&man=&lfacet=&count=&max=25&sort=default&qlookup=WHEAT+DURUM&offset=&format=Full&new=&measureby=&Qv=1&ds=&qt=&qp=&qa=&qn=&q=&ing= (accessed on 21 May 2019).

18. Bottari, E.; De Acutis, R.; Festa, M.R. On the lipid constituents of wheat of different species, variety, origin and crop year. *Ann. Chim.* **1999**, *89*, 849–862.

19. Zarroug, Y.; Mejri, J.; Dhawefi, N.; Ali, S.B.S.; El Felah, M.; Hassouna, M. Comparison of chemical composition of two durum wheat (*Triticum durum* L.) and bread wheat (*Triticum aestivum* L.) germ oils. *EKIN J. Crop Breed. Genet.* **2015**, *1*, 69–76.

20. Güven, M.; Kara, H.H. Some chemical and physical properties, fatty acid composition and bioactive compounds of wheat germ oils extracted from different wheat cultivars. *J. Agric. Sci.* **2016**, *22*, 433–443.

6

The Content of Tocols in South African Wheat; Impact on Nutritional Benefits

Maryke Labuschagne [1], Nomcebo Mkhatywa [1], Eva Johansson [2,*], Barend Wentzel [3] and Angeline van Biljon [1]

1 Department of Plant Sciences, University of the Free State, Bloemfontein 9300, South Africa; LabuscM@ufs.ac.za (M.L.); 2006041384@ufs4life.ac.za (N.M.); avbiljon@ufs.ac.za (A.v.B.)
2 Department of Plant Breeding, The Swedish University of Agricultural Sciences, Box 101, SE-230 53 Alnarp, Sweden
3 Small Grains Institute, Bethlehem 9700, South Africa; wentzelb@arc.agric.za
* Correspondence: Eva.johansson@slu.se

Abstract: Wheat is a major component within human consumption, and due to the large intake of wheat, it has an impact on human nutritional health. This study aimed at an increased understanding of how the content and composition of tocols may be governed for increased nutritional benefit of wheat consumption. Therefore, ten South African wheat cultivars from three locations were fractionated into white and whole flour, the content and concentration of tocols were evaluated by high performance liquid chromatography (HPLC), and vitamin E activity was determined. The content and composition of tocols and vitamin E activity differed with fractionation, genotype, environment, and their interaction. The highest tocol content (59.8 mg kg^{-1}) was obtained in whole flour for the cultivar Elands grown in Ladybrand, while whole Caledon flour from Clarence resulted in the highest vitamin E activity (16.3 mg kg^{-1}). The lowest vitamin E activity (1.9 mg kg^{-1}) was found in the cultivar C1PAN3118 from Ladybrand. High values of tocotrienols were obtained in whole flour of the cultivars Caledon (30.5 mg kg^{-1} in Clarens), Elands (35.5 mg kg^{-1} in Ladybrand), and Limpopo (33.7 mg kg^{-1} in Bultfontein). The highest tocotrienol to tocopherol ratio was found in white flour (2.83) due to higher reduction of tocotrienols than of tocopherols at fractionation. The quantity and composition of tocols can be governed in wheat flour, primarily by the selection of fractionation method at flour production, but also complemented by selection of genetic material and the growing environment.

Keywords: *Triticum aestivum*; tocopherol; tocotrienol; vitamin E; genotype; environment

---

1. Introduction

Wheat is, together with rice, the major food crop in the world, supporting 20% of the daily energy for the human population [1]. In certain parts of the world, wheat is even the main staple food, contributing up to 70% of the daily energy and protein in the human diet [2]. Due to its high consumption, wheat provides a significant amount of energy, proteins, and selected micronutrients and vitamins to the consumer [3–5]. Thus, despite the fact that food from other origins might to a large extent have a higher relative content of certain compounds, wheat serves as a source of important nutritional components such as iron and zink, vitamin E, phenolics, and carotenoids [6]. The content of vitamin E and its activity is determined by the content of certain tocols [7]. The tocols are known as bioactive compounds with antioxidant traits, for e.g., they prevent oxidation of double bonds by reacting with peroxyl radicals and protecting lipids and membrane proteins against oxidative stress [8,9]. Tocols cannot be produced by humans and are, therefore, important components of any diet, and they are obtained from a large number of plant based foods [6]. Tocols consists of eight lipid-soluble compounds: α-, β-, γ-, δ-tocotrienol, and α-, β-, γ-, δ-tocopherol. Previous literature has accounted different vitamin E activity to the various tocopherols due to their chemical structures and physiological factors. However, recent opinion considers only α-tocopherol as the source of vitamin E activity [7]. For whole wheat flour, a mean vitamin E content of 0.71 mg/100 g has been reported by the U.S. Department of Agriculture (USDA) [10]. However, higher levels of vitamin E have been reported in whole wheat flour from certain genetic material, resulting in the presence of 20% of the daily requirement of vitamin E in 200 g of whole wheat flour [11]. Poor nutritional status together with a high prevalence of stressors, for e.g., malaria and HIV as may be the status of many in developing countries, are known to contribute towards vitamin E deficiency [12]. Thus, selection of suitable wheat material with high vitamin E content might contribute to solving the problems of vitamin E deficiency. Tocotrienols do not show vitamin E activity but are known to have higher antioxidant activity than the tocopherols and also have additional important health promoting effects [11,13]. Tocopherols are widely distributed in higher plants whereas tocotrienols occur mainly in some non-photosynthetic tissues such as seeds and endosperm of monocot grains [14]. In the wheat grain, α- and β-tocopherols are mainly found in the wheat germ, while tocotrienols are concentrated in the pericarp, testa, aleurone, and in the endosperm.

Fractionation of the crushed grain during milling is known to have a critical implication for the distribution of many nutrients [15]. The consumption of whole grain is a healthy alternative to white flour [16]. Previous studies have also shown genotype, environment, and cultivation practices to have an impact on tocol content and composition [6,11,14]. Increased understanding of the impact and interactions of genotype, environment, and processing on content of tocols and vitamin E activity in wheat flour will positively impact a healthy intake of these compounds from wheat.

Thus, the aim of this study was to evaluate the effects of genotype, environment, and fractionation through milling on the quantity and composition of tocol components in South African wheat flour. Interactions as well as importance of the various evaluated factors will be investigated and conclusions drawn as related to opportunities to govern these health components in wheat flour.

2. Materials and Methods

2.1. Plant Material

Ten South African bread wheat cultivars, Betta-DN, Caledon, Elands, Gariep, Komati, Limpopo, Matlabas, PAN3118, PAN3349, and PAN3377, grown in four replicates in each location, were used in the present study. The trials were conducted at three different locations in one season: Bultfontein (28°16′53.14″ S 26°27′02.77″ E, north western Free State with low rainfall, high temperatures, high evaporation requirements and deep, yellow sandy loam soils with a water table present), Ladybrand (29°14′30.75″ S 27°20′18.55″ E, central Free State, moderate rainfall, moderate temperatures, a lower evaporation requirement and relatively shallow duplex soils), and Clarens (28°24′26.63″ S 27°20′18.55″ E, eastern Free State, higher rainfall, lower temperatures, lower evaporation requirement with predominantly yellow soils of average effective depth). The trials were planted under dryland conditions in a randomized complete block design. Trial plots consisted of five rows of 5 m length and inter-row spacing of 5 cm. Fertilization was done after soil analysis and according to normal production practices for each location.

2.2. Extraction of Tocols

Milled grain samples were freeze dried for three days before tocol extraction. The extraction [17] was performed with modifications as suggested by Labuschagne et al. [18].

2.3. Analytical High Performance Liquid Chromatography (HPLC)

A normal phase-HPLC method [19] with modification [18] was used to separate the tocol compounds (Figure 1). A Phenomenex Luna Silica column (250 mm × 4.6 mm inner diameter (i.d.), 5 μm particle size) was used. The mobile phase was *n*-hexane/ethyl acetate/acetic acid (97.3:1.8:0.9 *v*/*v*/*v*) at a flow rate of 1.6 mL min^{-1}. All peaks were detected by fluorescence and the wavelength of detection was set to 290 nm and emission wavelength of 330 nm. HPLC injection volume was 10 μL per injection. A standard solution was used to carry out the linearity test over the different concentration ranges (ng μL^{-1}) close to the amount of tocols found in the samples: α-tocopherol 0.47–9.57 ng μL^{-1}; β-tocopherol 0.23–4.7 ng μL^{-1}; γ-tocopherol 0.65–13.1 ng μL^{-1}; δ-tocopherol 0.62–12.4 ng μL^{-1}; β-tocotrienol 0.54–10.82 ng μL^{-1}. Total tocols were the sum of α-tocopherol, β-tocopherol, α-tocotrienol, β-tocotrienol, and δ-tocotrienol.

2.4. Data Analysis

Statistical evaluation applying ANOVA followed by mean comparison with Duncan post-hoc test at $p < 0.05$, Spearman rank correlation analyses, and Principal component analyses (PCA) was carried out using the statistical package SAS (2004; SAS Institute Inc., Cary, NC, USA). In order to explain the proportion of the contribution of variation by the environments, genotypes, and flour fractionation on the tocol composition, regression analysis was applied [20,21]. Vitamin E activity was calculated based on α-tocopherol content according to the Scientific Opinion of an EFSA (European Food Safety Authority) Panel [7]. The Recommended Daily Intake (RDI) of vitamin E set by European Parliament and the Council in the Regulation No. 1169/2011 of 25 October 2011 is 12 mg/day [22].

3. Results

3.1. Importance of Genotype, Environment, and Fractionation on Tocols Content and Composition

The percentage recovery of tocols was more than 95%, and the different tocols were successfully separated by HPLC (Figure 1). The major tocols found were α- and β-tocopherol and α- and β-tocotrienol (Figure 1). Delta-tocopherols and especially γ-tocopherols were only found in small amounts and often only in traces. Flour type (white flour versus whole flour) was shown to explain by far the highest part of the variation in tocols content and composition except for δ-tocotrienol, where location was a significant parameter for the variation (Table 1). However, combination of flour type, cultivar, and location resulted in a higher degree of explanation as compared to each of the factors alone (Table 1), and analysis of variance (ANOVA) also showed significant interactions among the factors for content and composition of the tocols ($p < 0.01$). Similarly, the PCA analysis showed samples clearly clustering in two separate groups as related to flour type, although a number of whole flour samples from Ladybrand were also diverging into a separate group of whole flour samples based on lower values on the second principal component value (Figure 2).

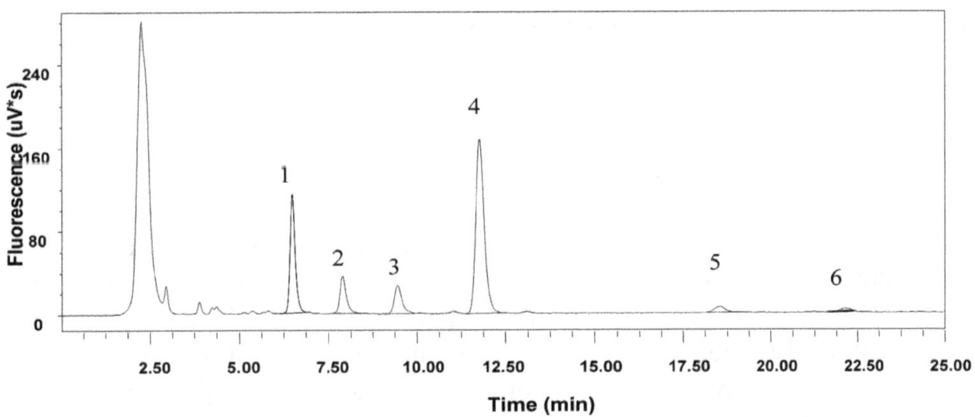

Figure 1. Example of separation of tocols by HPLC (High Performance Liquid Chromatography) from one wheat sample. Peak 1 = α-tocopherol, Peak 2 = α-tocotrienol, Peak 3 = β-tocopherol, Peak 4 = β-tocotrienol, Peak 5 = δ-tocopherol, and Peak 6 = δ-tocotrienol.

Table 1. Percentage of explanation (obtained through R-square from simple linear regression) of flour types (Flour; F), varieties (V), and growing locations (L) as well as their combinations on various tocols.

	α-TP	β-TP	α-TT	β-TT	δ-TT	TP	TT	Tot
Flour	89.0	89.6	87.8	83.5	11.2	89.9	85.8	90.3
Variety	1.06	1.45	3.53	1.46	4.29	1.18	2.06	1.64
Location	0.90	0.01	0.46	1.38	15.1	0.49	1.16	0.70
F, V, L	90.9	91.1	91.8	86.4	30.7	91.6	89.0	92.6

TP = tocopherols, TT = tocotrienols, Tot = total tocols.

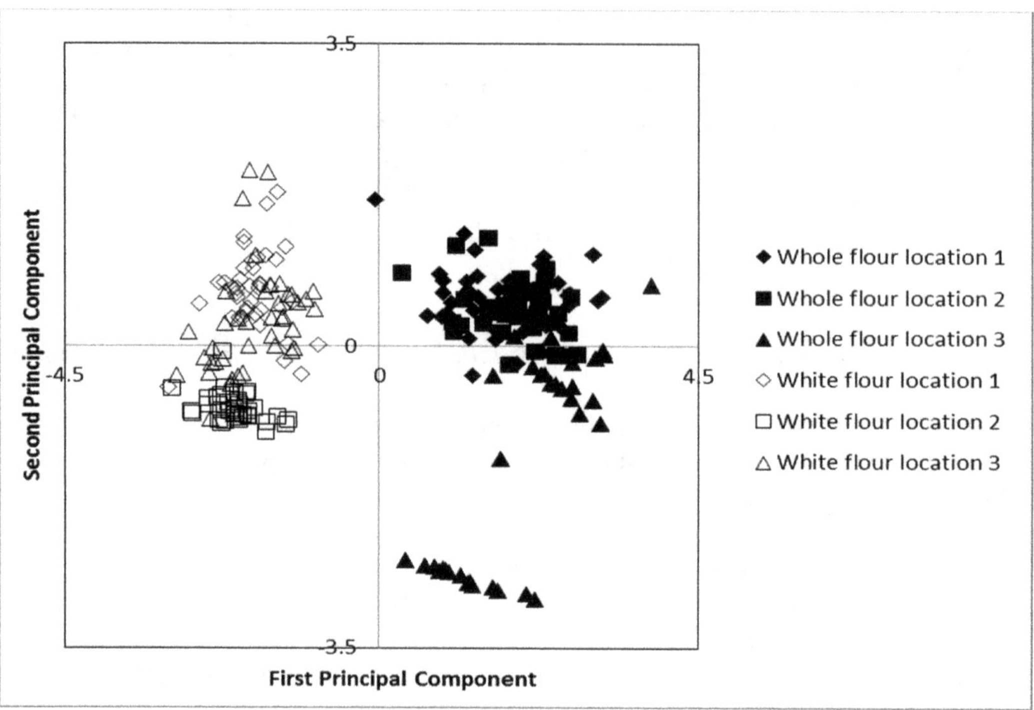

Figure 2. Loading plot from principal component analysis of tocopherols in two flour types of ten varieties grown at three locations in South Africa. Location 1 = Bultfontein, Location 2 = Clarens, Location 3 = Ladybrand. First principal component explained 79.3% of the variation while the second principal component explained 17.4% of the variation.

3.2. Effect of Flour Type on Content and Composition of Tocols

Whole flour had significantly ($p < 0.005$) higher tocol concentrations than white flour, the latter having on average 40% of the concentration of whole flour (Table 2). Concentration in white flour of α-tocopherol was 24% of that in whole flour and concentration in white flour of β-tocopherol was 31% of that in whole flour. Furthermore, white flour contained 25% of the α-tocotrienol concentration found in whole flour and 53% of the β-tocotrienols. The fact that the β-tocotrienols were retained to a higher degree than the other tocols from the whole to the white flour could also be seen as a higher tocotrienol to tocopherol quota (TT/TP) in the white flour as related to whole flour (Table 2). Tocol concentration in white flour as a percentage of that in whole flour varied in genotypes and locations, from 31% (PAN 3349 in Ladybrand) to 51% (Caledon at Bultfontein; Table 3).

Table 2. Mean values (mg kg^{-1}) of various tocols depending on flour type (white versus whole meal flour).

Flour	α-TP	β-TP	α-TT	β-TT	δ-TT	TT/TP	Tot
White	3.34 ^{b}	2.00 ^{b}	1.24 ^{b}	12.7 ^{b}	0.45 ^{b}	2.83 ^{a}	19.7 ^{b}
Whole	13.3 ^{a}	6.43 ^{a}	4.93 ^{a}	24.0 ^{a}	0.60 ^{a}	1.49 ^{b}	49.4 ^{a}

Average values followed by the same letters are not significantly different at $p < 0.05$ applying Duncan post-hoc test. TP = tocopherols, TT = tocotrienols, Tot = total tocols.

Table 3. Total tocol content (mg kg^{-1}) mean values of ten cultivars in three locations in white and whole flour.

Flour Type	Cultivar	Bultfontein	Clarens	Ladybrand	Average
White	Betta-DN	21.2	17.5	19.0	19.3 ^{cd}
	Caledon	26.4	24.1	25.9	25.5 ^{a}
	Elands	16.4	20.6	23.8	20.3 ^{bc}
	Gariep	20.1	20.0	24.7	21.6 ^{b}
	Komati	20.6	21.4	23.6	21.9 ^{b}
	Limpopo	17.9	20.7	17.4	18.6 ^{cde}
	Matlabas	18.8	18.7	18.3	18.6 ^{cde}
	C1PAN3118	17.1	17.0	15.3	16.5 ^{f}
	C2PAN3349	18.0	16.6	15.9	16.8 ^{f}
	C3PAN3377	18.2	17.8	17.8	18.1 ^{def}
	Average	19.5 ^{a}	19.4 ^{a}	20.2 ^{a}	
Whole	Betta-DN	48.0	51.2	52.8	50.6 ^{bc}
	Caledon	52.0	55.0	57.6	55.0 ^{a}
	Elands	49.9	51.4	59.8	53.7 ^{a}
	Gariep	40.9	48.6	49.6	46.3 ^{d}
	Komati	43.8	51.8	52.3	49.3 ^{bc}
	Limpopo	55.7	49.5	55.7	53.7 ^{a}
	Matlabas	39.4	52.8	52.0	48.2 ^{cd}
	C1PAN3118	43.5	42.9	45.4	43.9 ^{e}
	C2PAN3349	40.4	41.7	43.6	41.9 ^{e}
	C3PAN3377	50.2	47.7	54.5	51.0 ^{b}
	Average	46.5 ^{c}	49.2 ^{b}	52.3 ^{a}	

Average values followed by the same letters are not significantly different at $p < 0.05$ applying Duncan post-hoc test.

3.3. *Effect of Cultivar and Growing Location on Content and Composition of Tocols*

Tocol concentration in genotypes ranged between 16.49–25.49 mg kg^{-1} for white flour and 41.92–54.87 mg kg^{-1} for whole flour (Table 3). Thus, significant differences in tocol content and composition were found among certain of the evaluated cultivars (Table 3), despite the fact that only a limited amount of variation was explained by the differentiation in cultivars (Table 1 and Figure 2). Among the evaluated cultivars, Caledon was found to have a high concentration of tocols in whole flour and the highest concentration among the cultivars in white flour.

Cultivation of the cultivars in Ladybrand resulted in a higher tocol concentration in whole flour and a higher concentration in the white flour as compared to that of the other localities, with an average of 20.1 mg kg^{-1} for white flour and 52.3 mg kg^{-1} for whole flour (Table 3). In general, total tocol content in the samples differed significantly when grown at the different localities for whole flour but no such significant differences were found for white flour. Part of the explanation for this variation in the whole flour (Figure 2) might be the presence of δ-tocotrienol in samples grown in Ladybrand which were only found in trace amounts in samples from the other growing locations. However, a significant variation was found for the various tocol compound concentrations in both white and whole flour from the different locations. Samples from Clarens and Ladybrand had a significantly higher concentration of α-tocopherol in white and whole flour and β-tocopherol in white flour as compared to samples from Bultfontein, while samples from Clarence were higher than those from the other localities for β-tocopherol in whole flour. Significantly higher concentrations of α-tocotrienol and β-tocotrienol were found in whole flour samples from Ladybrand as compared to samples from the other locations, while for white flour, samples from Ladybrand and Bultfontein showed higher concentrations of α-tocotrienol than samples from Clarence (Table 4). In general, samples in Ladybrand showed a relatively high content of both tocopherols and tocotrienols in both white and whole flour, while samples from Clarence showed a relatively high tocotrienol concentration in both types of flours. Samples from Bultfontein showed a relatively high content of tocotrienols only in white flour. Due to differences in variations of concentrations of various tocol compounds by location, the tocotrienol to tocopherol quota (TT/TP) of the samples differed among locations; with significantly higher values in both white and whole flour samples from Ladybrand and Bultfontein as compared to those from Clarence (Table 4).

Table 4. Average content of each tocol compound (mg kg^{-1}) in three locations from white and whole wheat.

Flour Type	Characteristic	Bultfontein	Clarens	Ladybrand
White	α-Tocopherol	3.02 [b]	3.59 [a]	3.36 [a]
	β-Tocopherol	1.88 [b]	2.08 [a]	2.02 [a]
	α-Tocotrienol	1.32 [a]	1.12 [b]	1.28 [a]
	β-Tocotrienol	12.7 [a]	12.4 [a]	13.0 [a]
	TT/TP	3.07 [a]	2.51 [b]	2.92 [a]
Whole	α-Tocopherol	11.8 [b]	14.1 [a]	14.0 [a]
	β-Tocopherol	6.30 [b]	6.62 [a]	6.33 [b]
	α-Tocotrienol	4.80 [b]	4.45 [c]	5.52 [a]
	β-Tocotrienol	22.7 [c]	23.4 [b]	26.0 [a]
	TT/TP	1.53 [a]	1.36 [b]	1.57 [a]

TT = Tocotrienol, TP = Tocopherols; Average values of the different characteristics followed by the same letters are not significantly different at $p < 0.05$ applying Duncan post-hoc test.

4. Discussion

The present study clearly shows that the quantity and composition of tocols can be governed in South African wheat flour; fractionation through milling is the major determinant, but the effect was found to interact with the selection of genetic material and the growing environment. As can be seen from calculations of daily requirements of vitamin E, only 5% on average was obtained from white South African wheat flour while 22% was obtained from the corresponding whole flour (Table 5). However, by selecting whole flour of a high vitamin E cultivar (Caledon) grown on the locality (Clarence) contributing most to a high level of vitamin E activity, 27% of the daily requirement could be obtained by consumption of 200 g wheat flour per day (Table 5). Tocols are known to be destroyed when heated (25–94% reduction in vitamin E activity) [23,24]. A recent investigation showed a 40% reduction in tocopherols in bread as compared to their corresponding flour, although toasting of the bread resulted in an increase in tocopherol content so that the content reached 89% of the original content of the flour [25]. Today, most wheat is consumed after a heat treatment, thereby reducing the tocol content; consumption of wheat as whole and/or sprouted grain products is the best solution for wheat to be a tocol source [11]. However, the findings that toasting increases the amount of tocopherols as related to what is found in the bread calls for additional evaluations of how to best process wheat products in order to use these products as tocol sources [25]. To secure a high intake of tocols from the food, flour based products should be combined with other food items very high in tocols content [6,26,27].

Table 5. Vitamin E activity of wheat flour of different fractions, genotypes, and localities, calculated as tocopherol equivalents [7] and percentage of recommended intake [11,19] from the average flour consumption in the world of 200 g/person/day.

Flour Origin	Vitamin E Activity (mg kg^{-1})	Recommended Daily Intake (mg)	Percentage of Recommended Vitamin E from 200 g of Wheat Flour (%)
White	3.3	12	5.5
Whole	13.3	12	22.2
Whole flour at various locations			
Bultfontein	11.9	12	19.8
Clarence	14.1	12	23.5
Whole flour from Clarence in various cultivars			
Caledon	16.1	12	26.8
C1PAN3118	12.3	12	20.5

Vitamin E activity is primarily based on the presence of tocopherols in the food [24,28–30]. Besides variation in vitamin E activity, a large variation was also noted in the quantity and composition of tocotrienols in the present wheat material, and this related to variation in fractionation through milling, genotype, and location. Several investigations and results have indicated that tocotrienols are potentially as important for human health as are tocopherols. The tocotrienols have been found to have higher antioxidant capacity [31] and different health promoting properties than those of tocopherols [32–35]. Examples of biological tocotrienols-mediated activities not shared with the tocopherols are neuroprotection, radio-protection, anti-cancer, anti-inflammatory, and liquid lowering properties [36–39]. Similar to what was found for vitamin E activity, fractionation was by far the most important factor for the quantity of the tocotrienols found in the flour. However, tocotrienols content decreased less than tocols content with milling to white flour, resulting in a higher tocotrienols to tocols content in the white flour as compared to that of whole flour. Also, cultivation location resulting in the highest tocotrienols content varied for tocotrienols as compared to vitamin E activity. For tocotrienols, Ladybrand resulted in the highest amount among the locations with Caledon, Limpopo, and Elands showing the highest values among the cultivars. Scientifically based recommendations as to daily intake are only available for vitamin E [11] and not for the separate isoforms, although retailers are announcing that 34–43 mg per day of tocotrienols are beneficial [40]. If such a level should be recommended, the present white and whole flour samples would contribute to around 6%and 12%, respectively, of the daily requirements at a consumption of 200 g of flour per day. However, recent literature reports highly divergent bioavailability of tocotrienols based on the source of tocotrienols and on the target population [36]. Various sources of tocotrienols are rich to different degrees in different tocotrienol compounds, for e.g., tocotrienols from palm oil (the most common source of tocotrienol supplements) is particularly rich in δ-tocotrienol, while β-tocotrienol was the predominant compound in the present material, as also shown in previous studies on wheat [41,42]. The fact that the composition of tocotrienols varies with the source of tocotrienols may be one explanation for the difficulties of making recommendations for the daily intake requirements. Also, it is unclear what effect the relationship of the various tocotrienols and the ratio between tocotrienols and tocopherols is playing. Similar to previous studies [43], we were able in this study to show that cultivar and cultivation location affect composition of tocotrienols, for e.g., cultivation in Ladybrand did not only result in high levels of tocotrienols but also in higher levels of δ-tocotrienol in the whole flour than cultivation in the other locations. Ladybrand has a moderate rainfall and temperatures, resulting in lower evaporation and a relatively shallow duplex soil, growing parameters that might be the background for the content and composition of tocols. However, relationships among growing parameters and tocols content and composition have to be further evaluated before conclusions are made.

Scientific literature recommends not setting daily requirements of tocotrienols until more research based evidence is available [44]. However, from our study, we can conclude that fractionation, cultivation place, and cultivar need to be taken into consideration together with processing of the food in order to determine health effects of a certain food source of tocotrienols.

An increased understanding of how various tocol compounds can be governed through various production factors, including fractionation, genotype, and locality, opens up opportunities of producing specifically useful raw material for further food processing into nutritional beneficial food products with high bioavailability of wanted compounds. Fractionation was the factor effecting quantity of all tocols to the highest extent. In general, grain antioxidants are known to be concentrated in the bran and germ fractions, and thus these fractions are the major contributors to the total antioxidant activities of wheat [45,46]. A number of studies have also shown significantly more antioxidant activity in products manufactured with whole grains than products from refined wheat [47,48]. Previous studies have indicated that tocopherols are more concentrated in the germ fraction, while tocotrienols are found more in bran and are also observed in the endosperm [16,49]. This agrees with the findings in this study, which showed a higher content of all tocols in the whole flour compared to the white flour, but with the reduction to different extents depending on the compound. Fractionation procedures might, therefore, be a useful tool to effectively modulate tocol content and composition in wheat flour, although it can be complimented with genetic impact through the choice of cultivars and environmental impact through the choice of cultivation location.

5. Conclusions

The quantity and composition of tocols can be governed in wheat flour, primarily by the selection of the fractionation method at flour production, but also complemented by selection of genetic material and the growing environment. Total high content of tocopherols in the flour can best be obtained by the selection of whole flour from a high tocol producing cultivar cultivated in good conditions (not hot and dry). By doing so, 27% of the human daily requirement of vitamin E can be received by an average consumption of 200 g of wheat flour per day unless the tocols in the wheat flour are destroyed by harsh processing conditions.

Tocotrienols are possibly even more important than vitamin E in their contribution from wheat towards a healthy diet. Content and composition of these compounds can also be governed in wheat, as large variations are present due to fractionation, cultivar, and cultivation location. However, to do so, an increased knowledge on the requirements as to total amount, composition, and ratios of the different compounds is needed.

Acknowledgments: This study was supported by the Swedish University of Agricultural Sciences (SLU) and the UD-40 project (Ministry of Foreign Affairs in Sweden administered through the SLU). The National Research Foundation (project UID72056) is also acknowledged for financial support. Thanks to Maria Luisa Prieto-Linde for technical assistance with sample analyses at SLU.

Author Contributions: All authors planned the manuscript jointly and participated in discussions of the manuscripts as well as commented on the various drafted text versions of the manuscript. The first author (M.L.) came up with the idea of the manuscript and also completed the main part of the writing and compilation of various parts of the manuscript together with the third author (E.J.). The rest of the authors took the main responsibility for different parts of the experiments; N.M. carried out most of the lab work and a first compilation of the results of the data, B.W. took the main responsibility for the plant material in terms of its selection and cultivation, A.B. was responsible for analyses carried out in South Africa while E.J. was responsible for analyses (HPLC) carried out in Sweden.

References

1. Tilahun, D.; Shiferaw, E.; Johansson, E.; Hailu, F. Genetic variability of Ethiopian bread wheat genotypes (*Triticum aestivum* L.) using agro-morphological traits and their gliadin content. *Afr. J. Agric. Res.* **2016**, *11*, 330–339.
2. Husenov, B.; Makhkamov, M.; Garkava-Gustavsson, L.; Muminjanov, H.; Johansson, E. Breeding for wheat quality to assure food security of a staple crop: The case study of Tajikistan. *Agric. Food Secur.* **2015**, *4*, 9. [CrossRef]

3. Zielinski, H.; Kozlowska, H. Antioxidant activity and total phenolics in selected cereal grains and their different morphological fractions. *J. Agric. Food Chem.* **2000**, *48*, 2008–2016. [CrossRef] [PubMed]
4. Hussain, A.; Larsson, H.; Kuktaite, R.; Johansson, E. Mineral composition of organically grown wheat genotypes: contribution to daily merals intake. *Int. J. Environ. Res. Public Health* **2010**, *7*, 3442–3456. [CrossRef] [PubMed]
5. Hussain, A.; Larsson, H.; Kuktaite, R.; Olsson, M.E.; Johansson, E. Carotenoid content in organically produced wheat: Relevance for human nutritional health on consumption. *Int. J. Environ. Res. Public Health* **2015**, *12*, 14068–14083. [CrossRef]
6. Johansson, E.; Hussain, A.; Kuktaite, R.; Andersson, S.C.; Olsson, M. Contribution of organically grown crops to human health. *Int. J. Environ. Res. Public Health* **2014**, *11*, 3870–3898. [CrossRef] [PubMed]
7. European Food Safety Authority. Scientific opinion on dietary reference values for vitamin E as α-tocopherol. EFSA Panel on dietetic products, nutrition and allergies (NDA). *EFSA J.* **2015**, *13*, 4149.
8. Wolf, G. The discovery of the antioxidant function of vitamin E: The contribution of Henry A. Mattill. *J. Nutr.* **2005**, *135*, 363–366. [PubMed]
9. Dörmann, P. Functional diversity of tocochromanols in plants. *Planta* **2007**, *225*, 269–276.
10. United States Department of Agriculture. USDA National Nutrient Database for Standard Reference. Available online: https://ndb.nal.usda.gov/ndb/ (accessed on 1 August 2017).
11. Hussain, A.; Larsson, H.; Olsson, M.E.; Kuktaite, R.; Grausgruber, H.; Johansson, E. Is organically produced wheat a source of tocopherols and tocotrienols for health food? *Food Chem.* **2012**, *132*, 1789–1795. [CrossRef]
12. Dror, D.K.; Allen, L.H. Vitamin E deficiency in developing countries. *Food Nutr. Bull.* **2011**, *2*, 124–143. [CrossRef] [PubMed]
13. Piironen, V.; Lampi, A.; Ekholm, P.; Salmenkallio-Marttila, M.; Liukkonen, K. Micronutrients and phytochemicals in wheat grain. In *Wheat Chemistry and Technology*, 4th ed.; Khalil, K.K., Shewry, P.R., Eds.; American Association of Cereal Chemists, Inc.: Eagan, MN, USA, 2009; pp. 179–210.
14. Lampi, A.; Nurmi, T.; Piironen, V. Efects of the environment and genotype on tocopherols and tocotrienols in wheat in the HEALTHGRAIN diversity screen. *J. Agric. Food Chem.* **2010**, *58*, 9306–9313. [CrossRef] [PubMed]
15. Wrigley, C.W. Wheat: A unique grain for the world. In *Wheat Chemistry and Technology*, 4th ed.; Khalil, K.K., Shewry, P.R., Eds.; American Association of Cereal Chemists, Inc.: Eagan, MN, USA, 2009; pp. 1–15.
16. Bramley, P.M.; Elmadfa, I.; Kafatos, A.; Kelly, F.J.; Manios, Y.; Roxborough, H.E.; Schuch, W.; Sheehy, P.J.A.; Wagner, K.H. Vitamin E. *J. Sci. Food Agric.* **2000**, *80*, 913–938. [CrossRef]
17. Fratianni, A.; Caboni, M.F.; Irano, M.; Panfili, G. A critical comparison between traditional methods and supercritical carbon dioxide extraction for the determination of tocochromanols in cereals. *Eur. Food Res. Technol.* **2002**, *215*, 353–358. [CrossRef]
18. Labuschagne, M.T.; Mkhatywa, N.; Wentzel, B.; Johansson, E.; Van Biljon, A. Tocochromanol concentration, protein composition and baking quality of white flour of South African wheat cultivars. *J. Food Compos. Anal.* **2014**, *33*, 127–131. [CrossRef]
19. Panfili, G.; Fratianni, A.; Irano, M. Normal phase-high performance liquid chromatography method for the determination of tocopherols and tocotrienols in cereals. *J. Agric. Food Chem.* **2003**, *51*, 3940–3944. [CrossRef] [PubMed]
20. Malik, A.H.; Kuktaite, R.; Johansson, E. Combined effect of genetic and environmental factors on the accumulation of proteins in the wheat grain and their relationships to bread-making quality. *J. Cereal Sci.* **2013**, *57*, 170–174. [CrossRef]
21. Moreira-Ascarrunz, S.D.; Larsson, H.; Prieto-Linde, M.L.; Johansson, E. Mineral nutritional yield and nutrient density of locally adapted wheat genotypes under organic production. *Foods* **2016**, *5*, 89. [CrossRef] [PubMed]
22. European Parliament and Council. Regulation (EU) No 1169/2011 of the European Parliament and of the Council of 25 October 2011 on the Provision of Food Information to Consumers. *Off. J. Eur. Commun.* **2011**, *L304*, 18.
23. Hidalgo, A.; Brandolino, A. Tocol stability during bread, biscuit and pasta processing from wheat. *J. Cereal Sci.* **2010**, *52*, 254–259. [CrossRef]
24. Zielinski, H.; Ciska, E.; Kozlowska, H. The cereal grains: Focus on vitamin E. *Czech J. Food Sci.* **2001**, *19*, 182–188.

25. Nurit, E.; Lyan, B.; Pujos-Guillot, E.; Branlard, G.; Piquet, A. Change in B and E vitamin and lutein, β-sitosterol contents in industrial milling fractiona and during toasted bread production. *J. Cereal Sci.* **2016**, *69*, 290–296. [CrossRef]
26. Andersson, S.C.; Olsson, M.E.; Gustavsson, K.-E.; Johansson, E.; Rumpunen, K. Tocopherols in rose hips (*Rosa* spp.) during ripening. *J. Sci. Food Agric.* **2012**, *92*, 2116–2121. [CrossRef] [PubMed]
27. Andersson, S.C.; Rumpunen, K.; Johansson, E.; Olsson, M.E. Tocopherols and tocotrienols in Sea Buchthorn (*Hoppophae rhamnoides*) berries during ripening. *J. Agric. Food Chem.* **2008**, *56*, 6701–6706. [CrossRef] [PubMed]
28. Delgado-Zamarreno, M.M.; Bustamante-Rangel, M.; Sierra-Manzano, S.; Verdugo-Jara, M.; Carabias-Martinez, R. Simultaneous extraction of tocotrienols and tocopherols from cereals using pressurized liquid extraction prior to LC determination. *J. Sep. Sci.* **2009**, *32*, 1430–1436. [CrossRef] [PubMed]
29. Sramkova, Z.; Gregova, A.; Sturdik, E. Chemical composition and nutritional quality of wheat grain. *Acta Chim. Slovaca* **2009**, *2*, 115–138.
30. Tiwari, U.; Cummins, E. Nutritional importance and effect of processing on tocols in cereals. *Trends Food Sci. Technol.* **2009**, *20*, 511–520. [CrossRef]
31. Serbinova, E.; Kagan, V.; Han, D.; Packer, L. Free-radical recycling and intramembrane mobility in the antioxidant properties of alpha-tocopherol and alpha-tocotrienol. *Free Radic. Biol. Med.* **1991**, *10*, 263–275. [CrossRef]
32. Schaffer, S.; Müller, W.E.; Eckert, G.P. Tocotrienols: Constitutional effects in aging and disease. *J. Nutr.* **2005**, *135*, 151–154. [PubMed]
33. Shibata, A.; Kobayashi, T.; Asai, A.; Eitsuka, T.; Oikawa, S.; Miyazawa, T.; Nakagawa, K. High purity tocotrienols attenuate atherosclerotic lesion formation in apoE-KO mice. *J. Nutr. Biochem.* **2017**, *48*, 44–50. [CrossRef] [PubMed]
34. Alawin, O.A.; Ahmed, R.A.; Dronamraju, V.; Briski, K.; Sylvester, P.W. γ-Tocotrienol-indusced disruption of lipid rafts in human breast cancer cells in associated with a reduction in exosome heregulin content. *J. Nutr. Biochem.* **2017**, *48*, 83–93. [CrossRef] [PubMed]
35. Allen, L.; Ramlingam, L.; Menikdiwela, K.; Scoggin, S.; Shen, C.-L.; Tomison, M.D.; Kaur, G.; Dufour, J.M.; Chung, E.; Kalupahana, N.S.; et al. Effects of delta-tocotrienol on obesity-related adipocyte hypertrophy, inflammation and hepatic steatosis in high-fat-fed mice. *J. Nutr. Biochem.* **2017**, *48*, 128–137. [CrossRef] [PubMed]
36. Fu, J.-Y.; Che, H.-L.; Tan, D.M.-Y.; Teng, K.-T. Bioavailability to tocotrienols: Evidence in human studies. *Nutr. Metab.* **2014**, *11*, 5. [CrossRef] [PubMed]
37. Miyazawa, T.; Shibata, A.; Sookwong, P.; Kawakami, Y.; Eitsuka, T.; Asai, A.; Oikawa, S.; Nakagawa, K. Antiangiogenic and anticancer potential of unsaturated vitamin E (tocotrienol). *J. Nutr. Biochem.* **2009**, *20*, 79–86. [CrossRef] [PubMed]
38. Sen, C.K.; Khanna, S.; Roy, S.; Packer, L. Molecular basis of vitamin E action—Tocotrienol potently inhibits glutamate-induced pp60(c-Src) kinase activation and death of HT4 neuronal cells. *J. Biol. Chem.* **2000**, *275*, 13049–13055. [CrossRef] [PubMed]
39. Tonini, T.; Rossi, F.; Claudio, P.P. Molecular basis of angiogenesis and cancer. *Oncogene* **2003**, *22*, 6549–6556. [CrossRef] [PubMed]
40. Miscellaneous Nutrients. Available online: https://www.dcnutrition.com/miscellaneous-nutrients/tocotrienols/ (accessed on 1 August 2017).
41. Lampi, A.; Nurmi, T.; Ollilainen, V.; Piironen, V. Tocopherols and tocotrienols in wheat genotypes in the HEALTHGRAIN diversity screen. *J. Agric. Food Chem.* **2008**, *56*, 9716–9721. [CrossRef] [PubMed]
42. Okarter, N.; Liu, C.; Sorrells, M.; Liu, R.H. Phytaochemical content and antioxidant activity of six diverse varieties of whole wheat. *Food Chem.* **2010**, *119*, 249–257. [CrossRef]
43. Wong, R.S.; Radhakrishnan, A.K. Tocotrienol research: Past into present. *Nutr. Res.* **2012**, *70*, 483–490. [CrossRef] [PubMed]
44. Fardet, A.; Rock, E.; Remesy, C. Is the in vitro antioxidant potential of whole-grain cereals and cereal products well reflected in vivo? *J. Cereal Sci.* **2008**, *48*, 258–276. [CrossRef]
45. Shewry, P.R.; Piironen, V.; Lampi, A.-M.; Edelmann, M.; Kariluoto, S.; Nurmi, T.; Fernandez-Orozco, R.; Ravel, C.; Charmet, G.; Andersson, A.A.M.; et al. The HEALTHGRAIN wheat diversity screen: Effects of genotype and environment on phytochemicals and dietary fiber components. *J. Agric. Food Chem.* **2010**, *58*, 9291–9298. [CrossRef] [PubMed]

46. Miller, H.E.; Rigelhof, F.; Marquart, L.; Prakash, A.; Kanter, M. Antioxidant content of whole grain beakfast cereals, fruits and vegetables. *J. Am. Coll. Nutr.* **2000**, *19*, 312–319. [CrossRef]
47. Baublis, A.J.; Lu, C.; Clydesdale, F.M.; Decker, E.A. Potential of wheat-based breakfast cereals as a source of dietary antioxidants. *J. Am. Coll. Nutr.* **2000**, *19*, 308–311. [CrossRef]
48. Perez-Jimenez, J.; Saura-Calixto, F. Literature data may underestimate the actual antioxidant capacity of cerreals. *J. Agric. Food Chem.* **2005**, *53*, 5036–5040. [CrossRef] [PubMed]
49. Hidalgo, A.; Brandolino, A. Protein, ash, lutein and tocols distribution in einkorn (*Triticum monococcum* L. subsp. *monococcum*) seed fractions. *Food Chem.* **2008**, *107*, 444–448. [CrossRef]

7

Micronutrient Analysis of Gluten-Free Products: Their Low Content is not Involved in Gluten-Free Diet Imbalance in a Cohort of Celiac Children and Adolescent

Idoia Larretxi [1,2], Itziar Txurruka [1,2], Virginia Navarro [1,2], Arrate Lasa [1,2], María Ángeles Bustamante [1,*], María del Pilar Fernández-Gil [1], Edurne Simón [1,2] and Jonatan Miranda [1,2]

1 Gluten Analysis Laboratory of the University of the Basque Country, Department of Nutrition and Food Science, University of the Basque Country, UPV/EHU, 01006 Vitoria, Spain
2 GLUTEN3S research group, Department of Nutrition and Food Science, University of the Basque Country, UPV/EHU, 01006 Vitoria, Spain
* Correspondence: marian.bustamante@ehu.eus

Abstract: Data about the nutritional composition of gluten-free products (GFP) are still limited. Most studies are based on ingredient and nutrition information described on the food label. However, analytical determination is considered the gold standard for compositional analysis of food. Micronutrient analytical content differences were observed in a selection of GF breads, flakes and pasta, when compared with their respective gluten-containing counterparts. In general terms, lower iron, piridoxin, riboflavin, thiamin, niacin, folate, manganese and vitamin B5 can be underlined. Variations in biotin and vitamin E content differed among groups. In order to clarify the potential contribution of the GFP to the gluten-free diet's (GFD) micronutrient shortages, analytical data were used to evaluate GFD in a cohort of celiac children and adolescent. Participants did not reach recommendations for vitamin A, vitamin E, folic acid, vitamin D, biotin, iodine, and copper. It does not seem that the lower micronutrient content of the analyzed GFP groups contributed to the micronutrient deficits detected in GFD in this cohort, whose diet was not balanced. Nevertheless, GFP fortification for folate and biotin is proposed to prevent the deficiencies observed in GFD, at least in the case of pediatric celiac disease.

Keywords: celiac disease; gluten-free diet; gluten-free product; micronutrient; vitamin and minerals; dietary recommendation

---

1. Introduction

Celiac disease (CD) is a chronic immune-mediated inflammatory pathology triggered by the gluten in the diet of genetically predisposed individuals. The need to avoid this protein in the diet of celiac people brought about some years ago the development of specific cereal-based gluten-free products (GFP). Despite the fact that these GFP allowed them to include a wide variety of foods in their diets, in recent years researchers have highlighted differences in the nutrient composition of GFP with respect to gluten containing counterparts [1,2], leading to a minor health rating in some food-groups [3,4].

It is important to note that most of the studies about the nutrient composition of the GFP are based on ingredients and the nutrition information described on the food label [2–4]. To improve these data, some works, such as that carried out by Mazzeo et al. (2015) [5], take advantage of the retention factors for each nutrient, including losses due to heating or other food preparation steps. However, analytical determination is considered the gold standard for composition analysis of food. Accurate analysis could also provide detailed information about vitamins and minerals, which is not totally or commonly available on label [6]. Therefore, access to micronutrient data is already restricted to hardly any research [7–9].

Furthermore, a gluten-free diet (GFD) often implies some nutritional imbalances, as recognized in the literature [10,11]. Not only have inadequate fat, protein, sugar and fiber consumption been observed in GFD, but also a poor intake of micronutrients such as iron, zinc, magnesium, calcium, folate, vitamin D and B_{12} [12]. Similarly, celiac people seem to have lower blood values for hemoglobin, ferritin, vitamin D, and copper than the rest of the population [13,14]. There has been speculation about whether the characteristic composition of GFP is responsible for GFD inadequacy. A potential correlation between both facts has been proposed by others [15].

In the case of GFP, the use of raw material such as unenriched rice or maize refined flours, gums or enzymes in their formulation could lead to a different composition compared to their gluten containing homologues [16]. Moreover, as the micronutrient content of gluten-free pseudocereals and legumes is higher than that of the gluten free cereals [15,17], some authors proposed to promote their use in GFP formulation [12,18,19].

In view of the above, the aim of this study was to assess analytically the macronutrient and micronutrient content of a selection of GF breads, flakes and pasta, and to compare it with their respective gluten-containing counterparts. Additionally, in order to clarify the potential contribution of the GFP to the GFD's micronutrient shortages, vitamin and mineral analytical data were used to evaluate GFD in a cohort of celiac children and adolescents.

2. Materials and Methods

2.1. Analytical Nutrient Content of GF Bread, Breakfast Cereals and Pasta

The measured samples were thirty-seven selected GFP signed with the Crossed Grain symbol: 13 breakfast cereals, 12 breads and 12 pasta products (Supplementary Table S1). All the food items were purchased from the local market (Vitoria, Spain) and they were stored frozen (−20 °C) until analyzed. The analytically determined composition of GF foodstuffs was compared with the data of equivalent gluten-containing breads ($n = 19$), breakfast cereals ($n = 18$), and pasta products ($n = 8$), analyzed in the same way and at the same time for macronutrients, and with micronutrient data obtained from the Spanish Food Composition Database—BEDCA database [20]. These results were also compared with the data described in the food label of GFPs.

Analysis of the nutrient content of foodstuff has been carried out using official methods. Crude protein content was determined by the Kjeldahl method (AOAC, 960.52A) [21] in a Foss Kjeltec™ distillation unit (Höganäs, Sweden). Fat content was analyzed by the Soxhlet extraction method based on the official method (AOAC, 2003.05) [21], using a Soxtherm extraction system (Gerhardt, Bonn, Germany). Determinations were performed in duplicate.

For mineral determination, microwave-assisted digestion was carried out in a closed microwave device Mars 5 (CEM, Vertex, Barcelona, Spain) equipped with 8–24 teflon vessels and temperature controllers. The quantitative analysis of selenium, manganese and cooper was performed by using ICP-MS (7700x, Agilent Technologies, Palo Alto, CA, USA) and MicroMist micro-uptake glass concentric nebulizer (Glass Expansion, West Melbourne, Victoria, Australia). ICP-OES (Horiba Jobin Yvon Activa, Kyoto, Japan) was used with a quartz Meinhard concentric nebulizer, a Scott-type spray chamber and a standard quartz sheath connection between the spray chamber and the torch in the case of calcium, sodium, zinc and iron quantification. Working standard solutions of Ca, Na (0–20 mg/L), Fe, Zn and Se (0–100 μg/L) were prepared immediately prior to their use, by stepwise dilution of certified standard multi-element solution (100 mg/L) (Merck, Darmstadt, Germany) with HNO3 1.0 % *v*/*v* (Merck, Darmstadt, Germany). Additionally, a 10 mg/L multi-element standard solution (Y, Rh) from Inorganic Ventures (Equilab, Madrid, Spain) was also used as the internal standard in direct ICP-MS analysis.

As a step prior to vitamin quantification, samples were extracted by liquid-liquid extraction using an aqueous acidic mixture, centrifuged and filtrated, except for vitamin E. Biotin, Folate, Niacin, Pyridoxine, Riboflavin, Thiamine, vitamin B_5 and B_{12} were measured by liquid chromatography (LC) with triple quadrupole mass spectrometry detection. High purity (>95%) standards (Merck, Darmstadt, Germany) were used for the identification of each vitamin by positive ionization of the electrospray and multiple reaction monitoring. Quantification was developed using the standard addition method. Vitamin E determination was carried out by previous saponification of the samples, followed by a liquid-liquid extraction and purification of the extracts. Afterwards, high performance LC with the fluorescence detector method was used to analyze vitamin E in each extract. Quantification was performed by an external calibration method using the calibration curve of the tocopherol standard (Merck, Darmstadt, Germany). Analytical determinations of micronutrients were carried out once in each sample, but it was verified before the analysis that the reproducibility of the methods was less than 5%.

As mentioned, the micronutrient content of GF foodstuffs was compared with that of gluten-containing counterparts, obtained from the Spanish Food Composition Database—BEDCA database- [20]. Data for biotin in all studied food groups and copper in cereals were obtained from McCance and Widdowson's "composition of foods integrated dataset" from the United Kingdom [22]. No available data were found with regard to the manganese content of cereal flakes in food composition databases from the UK, Australia, the USA or Spain [20,22–24].

2.2. *Dietary Assessment: Participants and Procedure*

Eighty-three minor celiac (age: 3 to 18 years; 53 girls and 30 boys) from the Basque Country took part in the study. The age of the participants was selected due to their higher consumption of GFP compared to adults [25,26]. All participants received oral and written information about the nature and purpose of the survey, and all of them gave written consent for involvement in the study. This study was approved by the Ethical Committee in University of Basque Country (CEISH/76/2011 and CEISH/194M/2013).

The dietary assessment followed in the research was described elsewhere [26]: three days food records (two weekdays and one weekend day) were selected for each patient, 24-h food recalls (24HRs) were filled in by each celiac patient. Micronutrient intake was calculated by a computerized nutrition program system (AyS, Software, Tandem Innova, Inc., Huesca, Spain). The analytically measured vitamin and mineral content of tested GF products was added into the food composition database of the program before calculations. Dietary reference intakes (DRI) for the Spanish population issued by the Spanish Societies of Nutrition, Feeding and Dietetics (FESNAD) in 2010 were taken as references for the interpretation of the 24HRs [27].

2.3. *Statistical Analysis*

Results are presented as mean ± standard deviation (SD) of the mean. Statistical analysis was performed using SPSS 24.0 (SPSS Inc., Chicago, IL, USA). After confirming the normal distribution of lipid and protein content variables using Shapiro-Wilks normality, paired-samples student's t test was used for comparison. Due to their skewed distribution, micronutrients variables for analytical and database information were analyzed by Mann–Whitney U. The level of significance was set to $p < 0.05$.

3. Results and Discussion

3.1. *Macronutrient Content of GF Rendered Foods*

With the aim of assessing representative products of a GFD, GFP from the three main cereal food-types contributing to a balanced diet, such as flakes, pasta and bread, were selected. Protein and lipid contents of the three GFP groups analyzed are shown in Table 1. Results were compared to the nutritional composition of their gluten-containing counterparts. With regard to breads, lipid content was higher and the protein content was lower than that of gluten containing products. Similarly, GF bread has been described as poor in proteins and rich in fat content by others [28]. GF pasta provided a lower protein amount, although the comparison to gluten containing pasta did not reach statistical significance. In general terms, lower protein content in GFP than in their counterpart has been proposed by previous research [2–4]. Nevertheless, and in good accordance with our data, Missbach et al. did not observe this pattern in flakes [2].

Table 1. Analytical protein and lipid content in gluten-free rendered foodstuffs divided by food groups, compared to gluten-containing products, expressed by 100 g of foodstuffs.

	Cereal Flakes			Bread			Pasta		
	GFP	GCP	*P*	GFP	GCP	*p*	GFP	GCP	*p*
Lipids	3.9 ± 5.3	2.6 ± 2.0	NS	5.6 ± 4.2	3.5 ± 4.1	0.05	3.2 ± 4.5	2.2 ± 1.1	NS
Proteins	7.4 ± 0.7	7.8 ± 3.1	NS	2.4 ± 2.0	9.0 ± 1.5	<0.001	6.5 ± 1.4	9.8 ± 4.2	NS

Values are means ± SD. SD, standard deviation; GFP, gluten-free product; GCP, gluten-containing product; *p*, statistical significance; NS, not significant.

Some clues for justifying the results could be extracted from the list of ingredients of GFP (Supplementary Table S1). Rice and maize flours are extensively used in GFP, especially in breads, and according to composition databases, their protein content is lower than that of wheat. Moreover, maize and rice starches, usually added as a substitute, are especially poor in this macronutrient. For pasta and flakes, other ingredients could hinder the protein deficit, such as cocoa or eggs, soy protein or meat from the filled pasta. For lipids, the use of additives like mono and diglycerides of fatty acids (E-471) in GFP, especially in breads, could affect the final composition. However, this study did not consider the label information of ingredients of GCP, thus making conclusive statements is not possible.

It is important to point out that the comparative study between GFP and their homologues with gluten in the present work was performed as suggested by Staudacher and Gibson [6], by direct analytical methods and in paired form. As stated in the introduction, most of the studies evaluating the differences between both foodstuffs are based on nutrition information taken from the food label. For this reason, the analytical results obtained were compared to those reported in the nutritional panel information and some interesting data were collected. With regard to bread, experimental data reported a lower lipid (23%, $p = 0.07$) and higher protein (37%; $p = 0.03$) content than that supplied by the label. Similarly, in the case of cereal flakes, the measured protein amount was higher (19%; $p = 0.04$). No differences were observed between analyzed and labelled data in GF pasta.

In view of Regulation (EU) No 1169/2011 [29], the declared values on labels shall be average values based on (a) the manufacturer's analysis of the food; (b) a calculation from the known or actual average values of the ingredients used; (c) a calculation from generally established and accepted data. It is not possible for us to determine how each manufacturer calculated label information. However, it must be highlighted that nutrient variations observed in bread types are not within the tolerance ranges between label information and our direct food analysis (tolerance ranges: ±1.5 g for lipids and ±2 g for proteins, when its content in food is <10 g per 100 g). This information brings to light that previous studies about bread described in the literature could be reconsidered, and additionally, it validates, in part, others about pasta and cereals.

3.2. Micronutrient Content of GFP, Compared to Gluten-Containing Products

Despite the growing market of the GFP [30], data about their vitamin and mineral contribution remain scarce. Moreover, the data found in the literature are usually calculated from ingredients and their composition databases, which has been proposed to lead to overestimation [5]. Table 2 shows analytical micronutrient content of GF bread, flakes and pasta, compared to that of their gluten-containing counterparts. Lower iron, piridoxin, riboflavin and thiamin content was found in the three GFP groups analyzed. Niacin reduction was observed in GF flakes and breads. With regard to iron, similar results were found by Rybicka [8], who described that 273 of 408 GFP analyzed fulfilled less than 10% of recommended nutrient intake per portion and only 23 products were major contributors to daily intake (over 25% of recommendation intake per portion). In a study performed with 368 GFP, including flours, breads, pasta and cold cereals, overall it was observed that these kinds of products contained lower amounts of thiamin, riboflavin and niacin than the wheat product they were intended to replace [31]. These results are in line with the results obtained in the present study.

Folate content was lower in GF flakes and pasta types; manganese amount was lower only in GF pasta, and that of vitamin B_5 in GF flakes. As stated before, commonly used ingredients for GFP are maize and rice flours as well as a variety of starches (potato, corn), among others. It seems that removal of protein-rich fractions from flours may result in dramatic depletion of folates. Additionally, rice flours are not very rich in this vitamin [9]. In fact, we calculated a reduction of almost 80% of folate content in rice flour with respect to wheat flour ($p = 0.05$) comparing the nutrient composition of both flours obtained from food composition databases from the UK, Australia, the USA or Spain [20,22–24].

Several studies have claimed lower zinc and copper and higher sodium content for GFP [4,32]. However, no significant differences in those minerals were found in our data.

Finally, biotin content differed widely among groups, being higher in cereal flakes and lower in pasta GFP than in their counterparts. Moreover, we found that some GF cereals were fortified with biotin, thus explaining its higher content in this GF food group. Similarly, although vitamin E contribution from GFP was lower in flakes, no differences were observed in pasta and bread. Moreover, it is worth mentioning that half of the analyzed bread types showed a formulation with sunflower oil (Supplementary Table S1), which led to higher vitamin E content in those specific stuffs.

It is important to point out that food technology interventions to improve the shelf life and rheological properties of GFP have influenced their nutritional profile [12]. In order to avoid the absence of the mentioned micronutrients without fortifying foodstuffs, different strategies can be proposed: avoiding starch as a major ingredient, sourdough fermentation, and using less popular grain GF flour such as that from pseudocereals (buckwheat, quinoa, amaranth and teff) or legumes, including wholemeal forms of gluten-free cereals [18,19,33,34]. In our samples, only one out of twelve foodstuffs analyzed in each group contained pseudocereals in their ingredients list (4 to 5 g in 100 g), reflecting the need of more research on the properties and technological characteristics of these raw materials, and promotion of their use.

3.3. Micronutrient Intake in Celiac Children and Adolescents

It is known that GFD can lead to imbalanced macronutrient distribution. Our previous work [26] reported that celiac children and adolescents consumed more fat and less carbohydrate than recommended and pointed at GF rendered foods as one of the culprits. Thus, taking into account directly analyzed micronutrient content, their intake on that pediatric cohort was calculated considering their age group and gender, and compared to FESNAD recommendations (Supplementary Figure S1).

More than 1/4 of participants did not reach recommendations for vitamin A and vitamin E. Four out of ten children and adolescents with CD showed low intake of folic acid, which was even less than 66% of the recommendation for 25% of participants. Sixty percent of participants did not get that for vitamin D, and moreover, about 40% of them did not reach 25% of the recommendation. Most participants showed very low intakes of biotin, iodine and copper. Slightly over half the participants did not fulfil 50% of iodine recommendation and more than 40% were not able to achieve 25% of that of biotine. The intake of the rest of micronutrient was appropriate. With the exception of vitamin D, the results obtained differ from those obtained in similar pediatric research on celiac children, where low intake of iron, calcium, selenium and magnesium was observed [10,35,36].

Table 2. Analytical [4] micronutrient content in gluten-free rendered foodstuffs divided by food groups, compared to gluten-containing products, expressed by 100 g of foodstuffs.

Micronutients/Products	Cereal Flakes					Breads					Pasta				
	GCP		GFP		*p*	GCP		GFP		*p*	GCP		GFP		*p*
	Mean	SD	Mean	SD		Mean	SD	Mean	SD		Mean	SD	Mean	SD	
Calcium (mg)	141	183	22.3	16.8	NS	60.5	34.4	90.8	57.5	NS	22.9	10.0	27.3	27.3	NS
Iron (mg)	9.87	5.19	1.8	1.8	<0.001	6.75	19.99	1.1	0.9	0.009	1.83	0.88	0.7	0.5	0.002
Sodium (mg)	332	332	357.1	313.6	NS	423	280	570.8	248.1	NS	61.0	155	34.8	65.6	NS
Zinc (mg)	5.94	12.9	0.9	0.5	NS	0.84	0.48	0.5	0.4	NS	1.45	1.10	1.1	0.5	NS
Copper (mg)	0.2	0.2	0.3	0.3	NS	0.14	0.11	0.1	0.1	NS	0.31	0.20	0.1	0.1	NS
Manganese (mg)			0.4	0.4		0.58	0.51	0.2	0.3	NS	2.22	1.18	0.5	0.8	0.042
Biotin (ug)	2.3	2.9	40.7	95.7	0.001	12.7	13.6	9.74	21.6	NS	15.8	14.8	1.10	1.00	0.002
Folate (ug)	275	35.4	55.4	88.9	0.062	32.55	14.79	32.8	56.8	NS	19.4	10.3	3.14	3.42	0.003
Niacin (mg)	16.2	8.25	3.02	2.41	<0.001	3.49	2.15	1.02	1.46	0.004	3.75	3.46	3.62	10.58	NS
Piridoxin (mg)	1.80	0.90	1.19	4.15	0.001	0.12	0.10	0.02	0.02	<0.001	0.12	0.07	0.01	0.01	<0.001
Riboflavin (mg)	1.45	0.72	0.12	0.17	<0.001	0.13	0.11	0.04	0.09	0.001	0.07	0.04	0.01	0.02	0.002
Tiamin (mg)	1.32	0.70	0.19	0.28	<0.001	0.20	0.12	0.01	0.01	<0.001	0.19	0.15	0.03	0.04	0.001
B_5 (mg)	7.55	3.46	1.03	1.81	0.045	0.39	0.07	0.42	0.57	NS	0.70	0.40	0.29	0.36	0.067
B_{12} (ug)	0.85	0.52	3.68	4.18	0.03	0.02	0.05	88.2	236	0.026	0.04	0.08	0.73	1.37	NS
Vitamin E (mg)	3.00	6.22	0.14	0.47	0.01	0.30	0.33	1.04	1.2	NS	0.09	0.12	0.2	0.1	NS

Values are means ± SD. SD, standard deviation; GFP, gluten-free product; GCP, gluten-containing product; *p*, statistical significance; NS, not significant.

Considering all the above mentioned, it does not seem that the GFP groups analyzed contribute to the micronutrient deficits detected in young celiac people's diets. In fact, cereals have only a modest role as source of these micronutrients. It is important to highlight that in our previous study [26] we reported unhealthy dietary habits in these celiac children and adolescents: very low cereal and vegetable consumption, low fruit and nut intake and excessive meat consumption. Thus, general recommendations to promote healthy GFD should be given to amend the observed wrong habits. It is worth mentioning that this conclusion refers to our cohort, and that in other dietary patterns, GFPs role could be different.

It must be pointed out that, in the case of folic acid, we observed a lower content of this vitamin in GFP than in their gluten containing equivalents. In this regard, in Canada and USA [37,38] the fortification of wheat flour with folic acid is mandatory, but not for other alternative flours, such as the ones used in GFP. Taking into account the folate deficiency observed in GFD, its fortification in GFP or ingredients could be of interest for celiac children. Folate fortification measures could also be extended to biotin, whose widespread diet-deficiency in celiac population was alarming. In fact, some of the GF cereals analyzed were supplemented with this vitamin (Supplementary Table S1).

It is of interest to point out that some deficiency diseases found in celiac people, such as anemia, low bone density or zinc depletion [39] are not only justified by nutritional shortages. Other pathological situations such as systemic inflammation or intestinal microbiota alteration appear to contribute to the persistence of those deficiencies in some celiac individuals [12,40,41].

It has to be highlighted that this paper presents wide-ranging high-quality nutritional information about GF bread, pasta and cereal micronutrient content. This remains limited in the literature and even more so in food panels or in databases used for GFD design and evaluation, where it is crucial. Moreover, it has assessed not only GFP composition but also its dietetic role, discussing, in general terms, its involvement in micronutrient deficiencies of the GFD of children and adolescents. Nevertheless, extrapolation to celiac adults is limited and needs further research. Moreover, as proposed elsewhere [42], the bioavailability of GFP is a matter of concern that should also be taken into account in further studies. Finally, it is also of great interest to analyze the nutritional composition of GFPs considering their ingredients list to define the role of ingredients such as gluten free cereals or pseudocereals, starches and additives in the final composition of the product.

The practical outcomes of the present study are relevant in improving the universal guidelines for food fortification in CD [43,44]. Some individualized supplementation is usually proposed for celiac people based on micronutrient related blood monitoring. Nevertheless, GFP fortification for folate and biotin could contribute to preventing the deficiencies observed in GFD, at least in the case of celiac children and youngsters.

4. Conclusions

Even if lower micronutrient content was found in the analyzed GFP groups, this fact was not related with the micronutrient deficits detected in GFD in a cohort of celiac children and adolescent. Nevertheless, according to the obtained results, GFP fortification for folate and biotin seems to be a suitable proposal in order to prevent the deficiencies observed in GFD.

Author Contributions: E.S. carried out the experimental design. I.L. and I.T. analyzed lipid, protein and micronutrient content. V.N. and A.L. performed the analysis of diet. M.Á.B., M.d.P.F.-G. and J.M. analyzed all data and contributed to statistical analysis. I.L., I.T., V.N. and J.M. wrote the manuscript.

References

1. do Nascimento, A.B.; Fiates, G.M.; Dos Anjos, A.; Teixeira, E. Analysis of ingredient lists of commercially available gluten-free and gluten-containing food products using the text mining technique. *Int. J. Food Sci. Nutr.* **2013**, *64*, 217–222. [CrossRef] [PubMed]
2. Missbach, B.; Schwingshackl, L.; Billmann, A.; Mystek, A.; Hickelsberger, M.; Bauer, G.; König, J. Gluten-free food database: The nutritional quality and cost of packaged gluten-free foods. *PeerJ* **2015**, *3*, e1337. [CrossRef] [PubMed]
3. Wu, J.H.; Neal, B.; Trevena, H.; Crino, M.; Stuart-Smith, W.; Faulkner-Hogg, K.; Yu Louie, J.C.; Dunford, E. Are gluten-free foods healthier than non-gluten-free foods? An evaluation of supermarket products in Australia. *Br. J. Nutr.* **2015**, *114*, 448–454. [CrossRef] [PubMed]
4. Miranda, J.; Lasa, A.; Bustamante, M.A.; Churruca, I.; Simon, E. Nutritional differences between a gluten-free diet and a diet containing equivalent products with gluten. *Plant Foods Hum. Nutr.* **2014**, *69*, 182–187. [CrossRef] [PubMed]
5. Mazzeo, T.; Cauzzi, S.; Brighenti, F.; Pellegrini, N. The development of a composition database of gluten-free products. *Public Health Nutr.* **2015**, *18*, 1353–1357. [CrossRef] [PubMed]
6. Staudacher, H.M.; Gibson, P.R. How healthy is a gluten-free diet? *Br. J. Nutr.* **2015**, *114*, 1539–1541. [CrossRef]
7. Gliszczyńska-Świgło, A.; Klimczak, I.; Rybicka, I. Chemometric analysis of minerals in gluten-free products. *J. Sci. Food Agric.* **2018**, *98*, 3041–3048. [CrossRef]
8. Rybicka, I. The Handbook of Minerals on a Gluten-Free Diet. *Nutrients* **2018**, *10*, 1683. [CrossRef]
9. Yazynina, E.; Johansson, M.; Jägerstad, M.; Jastrebova, J. Low folate content in gluten-free cereal products and their main ingredients. *Food Chem.* **2008**, *111*, 236–242. [CrossRef]
10. Babio, N.; Alcázar, M.; Castillejo, G.; Recasens, M.; Martínez-Cerezo, F.; Gutiérrez-Pensado, V.; Masip, G.; Vaqué, C.; Vila-Martí, A.; Torres-Moreno, M.; et al. Patients with Celiac Disease Reported Higher Consumption of Added Sugar and Total Fat Than Healthy Individuals. *J. Pediatr. Gastroenterol. Nutr.* **2017**, *64*, 63–69. [CrossRef]
11. Barone, M.; Della Valle, N.; Rosania, R.; Facciorusso, A.; Trotta, A.; Cantatore, F.P.; Falco, S.; Pignatiello, S.; Viggiani, M.T.; Amoruso, A.; et al. A comparison of the nutritional status between adult celiac patients on a long-term, strictly gluten-free diet and healthy subjects. *Eur. J. Clin. Nutr.* **2016**, *70*, 23–27. [CrossRef]
12. Gobbetti, M.; Pontonio, E.; Filannino, P.; Rizzello, C.G.; De Angelis, M.; Di Cagno, R. How to improve the gluten-free diet: The state of the art from a food science perspective. *Food Res. Int.* **2018**, *110*, 22–32. [CrossRef]
13. Salazar Quero, J.C.; Espin Jaime, B.; Rodriguez Martinez, A.; Arguelles Martin, F.; Garcia Jimenez, R.; Rubio Murillo, M.; Pizarro Martin, A. Nutritional assessment of gluten-free diet. Is gluten-free diet deficient in some nutrient? *An. Pediatr.* **2015**, *83*, 33–39. [CrossRef]
14. Botero-López, J.E.; Araya, M.; Parada, A.; Méndez, M.A.; Pizarro, F.; Espinosa, N.; Canales, P.; Alarcón, T. Micronutrient deficiencies in patients with typical and atypical celiac disease. *J. Pediatr. Gastroenterol. Nutr.* **2011**, *53*, 265–270. [CrossRef]
15. Pellegrini, N.; Agostoni, C. Nutritional aspects of gluten-free products. *J. Sci. Food Agric.* **2015**, *95*, 2380–2385. [CrossRef]
16. Matos Segura, M.E.; Rosell, C.M. Chemical Composition and Starch Digestibility of Different Gluten-free Breads. *Plant Foods Hum. Nutr.* **2011**, *66*, 224. [CrossRef]
17. Schoenlechner, R.; Drausinger, J.; Ottenschlaeger, V.; Jurackova, K.; Berghofer, E. Functional Properties of Gluten-Free Pasta Produced from Amaranth, Quinoa and Buckwheat. *Plant Foods Hum. Nutr.* **2010**, *65*, 339–349. [CrossRef]
18. Hager, A.S.; Wolter, A.; Jacob, F.; Zannini, E.; Arendt, E.K. Nutritional properties and ultra-structure of commercial gluten free flours from different botanical sources compared to wheat flours. *J. Cereal Sci.* **2012**, *56*, 239–247. [CrossRef]
19. Alvarez-Jubete, L.; Arendt, E.K.; Gallagher, E. Nutritive value and chemical composition of pseudocereals as gluten-free ingredients. *Int. J. Food Sci. Nutr.* **2009**, *60*, 240–257. [CrossRef]

20. AESAN. Base de Datos Española de Composición De Alimentos (BEDCA) v 1.0. Available online: http://www.bedca.net/ (accessed on 30 July 2019).
21. Horwitz, W.; Latimer, G.W. *AOAC International. Official Methods of Analysis of AOAC International*, 18th ed.; (Revision 3, 2005); AOAC International: Gaithersburg, MD, USA, 2010.
22. Roe, M.; Pinchen, H.; Church, S.; Finglas, P. McCance and Widdowson's the Composition of Foods Seventh Summary Edition and updated Composition of Foods Integrated Dataset. *Nutr. Bull.* **2015**, *40*, 36–39. [CrossRef]
23. AUSNUT 2011-13 Food Nutrient Database. Available online: http://www.foodstandards.gov.au/science/monitoringnutrients/ausnut/ausnutdatafiles/Pages/foodnutrient.aspx (accessed on 30 July 2019).
24. USDA Food Composition Databases. Available online: https://ndb.nal.usda.gov/ndb/ (accessed on 30 July 2019).
25. Zuccotti, G.; Fabiano, V.; Dilillo, D.; Picca, M.; Cravidi, C.; Brambilla, P. Intakes of nutrients in Italian children with celiac disease and the role of commercially available gluten-free products. *J. Hum. Nutr. Diet.* **2013**, *26*, 436–444. [CrossRef]
26. Larretxi, I.; Simon, E.; Benjumea, L.; Miranda, J.; Bustamante, M.A.; Lasa, A.; Eizaguirre, F.J.; Churruca, I. Gluten-free-rendered products contribute to imbalanced diets in children and adolescents with celiac disease. *Eur. J. Nutr.* **2019**, *58*, 775–783. [CrossRef]
27. FESNAD. Dietary reference intakes (DRI) for spanish population, 2010. *Act. Diet.* **2010**, *14*, 196–197. [CrossRef]
28. Matos, M.E.; Rosell, C.M. Understanding gluten-free dough for reaching breads with physical quality and nutritional balance. *J. Sci. Food Agric.* **2015**, *95*, 653–661. [CrossRef]
29. Regulation (EU) No 1169/2011 of the European Parliament and of the Council of 25 October 2011 on the provision of food information to consumers, amending Regulations (EC) No 1924/2006 and (EC) No 1925/2006 of the European Parliament and of the Council, and repealing Commission Directive 87/250/EEC, Council Directive 90/496/EEC, Commission Directive 1999/10/EC, Directive 2000/13/EC of the European Parliament and of the Council, Commission Directives 2002/67/EC and 2008/5/EC and Commission Regulation (EC) No 608/2004 (Text with EEA relevance). Available online: http://data.europa.eu/eli/reg/2011/1169/2018-01-01 (accessed on 30 July 2019).
30. Lee, A.R.; Wolf, R.L.; Lebwohl, B.; Ciaccio, E.J.; Green, P.H.R. Persistent Economic Burden of the Gluten Free Diet. *Nutrients* **2019**, *11*, 399. [CrossRef]
31. Thompson, T. Thiamin, riboflavin, and niacin contents of the gluten-free diet: Is there cause for concern? *J. Am. Diet. Assoc.* **1999**, *99*, 858–862. [CrossRef]
32. Krupa-Kozak, U.; Wronkowska, M.; Soral-ŚMietaNa, M. Effect of Buckwheat Flour on Microelements and Proteins Contents in Gluten-Free Bread. *Czech J. Food Sci.* **2011**, *2*, 103–108. [CrossRef]
33. Rybicka, I.; Gliszczyńska-Świgło, A. Minerals in grain gluten-free products. The content of calcium, potassium, magnesium, sodium, copper, iron, manganese, and zinc. *J. Food Compos. Anal.* **2017**, *59*, 61–67. [CrossRef]
34. Rybicka, I.; Gliszczynska-Swiglo, A. Gluten-Free Flours from Different Raw Materials as the Source of Vitamin B. *J. Nutr. Sci. Vitaminol* **2017**, *63*, 125–132. [CrossRef]
35. Mariani, P.; Viti, M.G.; Montuori, M.; La Vecchia, A.; Cipolletta, E.; Calvani, L.; Bonamico, M. The gluten-free diet: A nutritional risk factor for adolescents with celiac disease? *J. Pediatr. Gastroenterol. Nutr.* **1998**, *27*, 519–523. [CrossRef]
36. Ohlund, K.; Olsson, C.; Hernell, O.; Ohlund, I. Dietary shortcomings in children on a gluten-free diet. *J. Hum. Nutr. Diet.* **2010**, *23*, 294–300. [CrossRef]
37. Food and Drug Regulations, Government of Canada. 2019. Available online: https://laws-lois.justice.gc.ca/eng/regulations/C.R.C.,_c._870/ (accessed on 30 July 2019).
38. Questions and Answers on FDA's Fortification Policy-Guidance for Industry. Available online: https://www.fda.gov/media/94563/download (accessed on 15 July 2019).
39. Melini, V.; Melini, F. Gluten-Free Diet: Gaps and Needs for a Healthier Diet. *Nutrients* **2019**, *11*, 170. [CrossRef]
40. Harper, J.W.; Holleran, S.F.; Ramakrishnan, R.; Bhagat, G.; Green, P.H. Anemia in celiac disease is multifactorial in etiology. *Am. J. Hematol.* **2007**, *82*, 996–1000. [CrossRef]

41. Olechnowicz, J.; Tinkov, A.; Skalny, A.; Suliburska, J. Zinc status is associated with inflammation, oxidative stress, lipid, and glucose metabolism. *J. Physiol. Sci.* **2018**, *68*, 19–31. [CrossRef]
42. Suliburska, J.; Krejpcio, Z.; Reguła, J.; Grochowicz, A. Evaluation of the content and the potential bioavailability of minerals from gluten-free products. *Acta Sci. Pol. Technol. Aliment.* **2013**, *12*, 75–79.
43. Caruso, R.; Pallone, F.; Stasi, E.; Romeo, S.; Monteleone, G. Appropriate nutrient supplementation in celiac disease. *Ann. Med.* **2013**, *45*, 522–531. [CrossRef]
44. Dennis, M.; Lee, A.R.; McCarthy, T. Nutritional Considerations of the Gluten-Free Diet. *Gastroenterol. Clin. N. Am.* **2019**, *48*, 53–72. [CrossRef]

Recent Advances in Physical Post-Harvest Treatments for Shelf-Life Extension of Cereal Crops

Marcus Schmidt [1], Emanuele Zannini [1] and Elke K. Arendt [1,2,*]

[1] School of Food and Nutritional Sciences, University College Cork, Western Road, T12 Y337 Cork, Ireland; marcus.schmidt@ucc.ie (M.S.); e.zannini@ucc.ie (E.Z.)

[2] Alimentary Pharmabotic Centre Microbiome Institute, University College Cork, T12 Y337 Cork, Ireland

* Correspondence: e.arendt@ucc.ie

Abstract: As a result of the rapidly growing global population and limited agricultural area, sufficient supply of cereals for food and animal feed has become increasingly challenging. Consequently, it is essential to reduce pre- and post-harvest crop losses. Extensive research, featuring several physical treatments, has been conducted to improve cereal post-harvest preservation, leading to increased food safety and sustainability. Various pests can lead to post-harvest losses and grain quality deterioration. Microbial spoilage due to filamentous fungi and bacteria is one of the main reasons for post-harvest crop losses and mycotoxins can induce additional consumer health hazards. In particular, physical treatments have gained popularity making chemical additives unnecessary. Therefore, this review focuses on recent advances in physical treatments with potential applications for microbial post-harvest decontamination of cereals. The treatments discussed in this article were evaluated for their ability to inhibit spoilage microorganisms and degrade mycotoxins without compromising the grain quality. All treatments evaluated in this review have the potential to inhibit grain spoilage microorganisms. However, each method has some drawbacks, making industrial application difficult. Even under optimal processing conditions, it is unlikely that cereals can be decontaminated of all naturally occurring spoilage organisms with a single treatment. Therefore, future research should aim for the development of a combination of treatments to harness their synergistic properties and avoid grain quality deterioration. For the degradation of mycotoxins the same conclusion can be drawn. In addition, future research must investigate the fate of degraded toxins, to assess the toxicity of their respective degradation products.

Keywords: cereal grains; shelf life; spoilage microorganisms; mycotoxins; physical decontamination

---

1. Introduction

At a time of rapid growth in global populations, sufficient nutritional supply to humanity has become increasingly challenging. On the basis of their long tradition as global staples of the human diet and livestock feed, agricultural crops such as cereals will have a key role in satisfying this growing nutritional need. However, global agricultural area is limited, making it difficult to expand cereal production. Considering that approximately 15% of all cereals worldwide are lost due to microbial pests [1], the most sensible approach to combat this issue is to increase both food safety and sustainability to reduce economic losses. Pre- and post-harvest microbial spoilage counts as one of the predominant factors in crop loss all over the world. Various strategies to prevent microbial contamination in the field have been investigated and reviewed by Oerke [2]. However, even the best management practices cannot completely eliminate the risk of contamination. Because of the permanent and ubiquitous presence of microorganisms and fungal spores in the environment, cereals always carry a certain microbial load when harvested. Additionally, climatic conditions, such as temperature and humidity, that are not under human control may be crucial for contamination with moulds [3]. Therefore, appropriate post-harvest crop treatment, before and during storage, is as important as pre-harvest strategies in the prevention of microbial spoilage. Thus, this review is focused exclusively on research regarding post-harvest treatments.

Depending on climatic conditions during growth, grains carry a microbial load with a high diversity of potential spoilage organisms when harvested. In addition, post-harvest contamination during transport is possible. This microbial load consists of bacteria, yeasts, and filamentous fungi belonging to many different genera. The activity of these micro-organisms during storage and, accordingly, the shelf life of the crop is dependent on a range of factors, as illustrated in Figure 1. Amongst the most influential parameters are moisture content and water availability during storage. As a result, grains are usually stored at low moisture contents of 12–13% and a water activity of <0.70 [4]. However, cereals are usually traded as wet weight and thus inefficient drying systems can lead to microbial spoilage during storage. Furthermore, even if dried properly, some xenerophilic species of *Aspergillus* can still develop during storage, resulting in quality deterioration and mycotoxin accumulation [5].

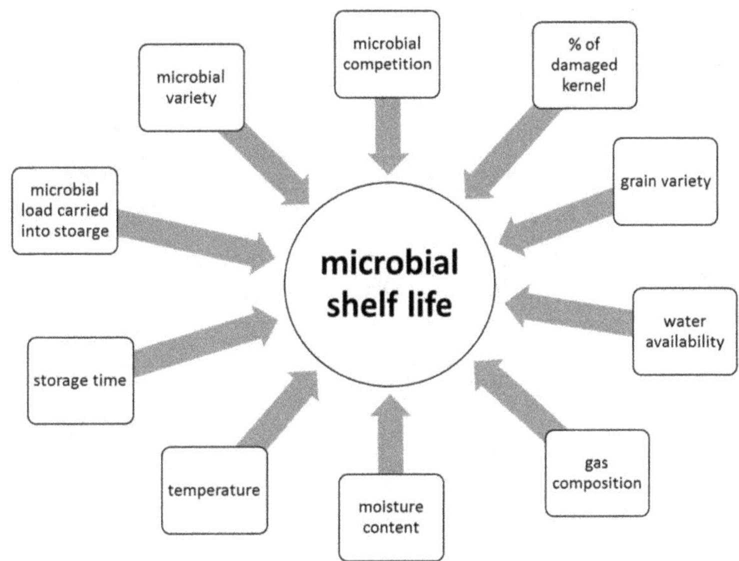

Figure 1. Biotic and abiotic factors influencing the microbial shelf-life of cereal grains during storage.

In addition, conventional storage systems, such as silos, are often cost intensive and inflexible as to volume. In these rigid systems, due to the inappropriate size for the amount of grains stored, the environmental conditions in the headspace cannot be controlled. Thus, it is likely that suitable conditions arise which promote microbial growth and the production of toxic metabolites [6]. As shown in a recent study conducted by Schmidt et al. [7], if the conditions during storage are suitable, a minimal fungal field contamination can rapidly evolve into a serious consumer health hazard.

The biggest microbial threat during storage is displayed by filamentous fungi, mostly belonging to the genera *Aspergillus* and *Penicillium*. This is largely a result of their relative tolerance to low water activities and the production of mycotoxins, which are secondary fungal metabolites with toxic effects on humans and animals. In addition, these fungi induce a loss of nutritional value in grain, produce off-odours, and result in reduced baking and milling quality [4]. Although *Fusarium* spp. are typical field pathogens and unlikely to develop during storage, previously produced and accumulated mycotoxins remain a serious issue during cereal storage and processing [8]. Hence, in addition to the living organisms, a broad variety of mycotoxins must be countered during post-harvest treatments, as the prevention of their production is not always possible. Table 1 shows the most commonly reported mycotoxins of cereal crops and the producing fungal genera. It has been reported that approximately 25% of the global cereal crops, equivalent to over 500 million tons per annum, are contaminated with mycotoxins and thus present a potential consumer health hazard [9]. In contrast to fungal mycelia, mycotoxin-contaminated grains often do not vary visually from clean grains and are therefore difficult to identify and eliminate.

Table 1. Chemical structures of mycotoxins commonly found on cereal grains sorted by the producing fungal species.

Aspergillus spp.	*Aspergillus* spp./*Penicillium* spp.	*Fusarium* spp.
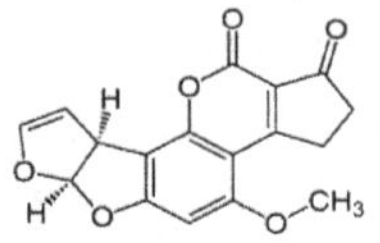 Aflatoxin B_1		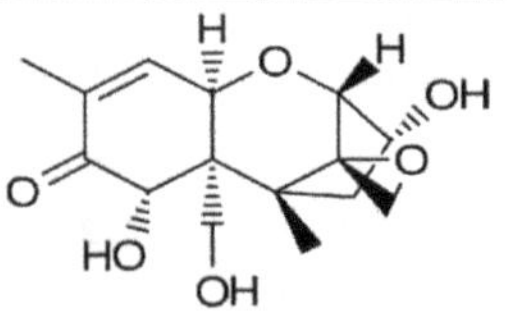 Deoxynivalenol
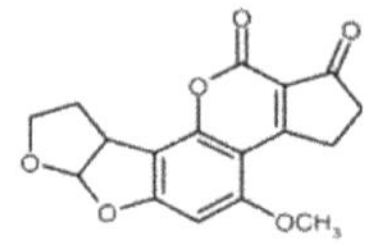 Aflatoxin B_2	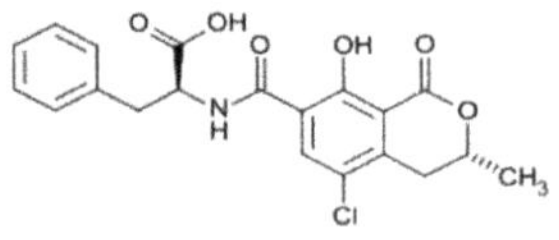 Ochratoxin A	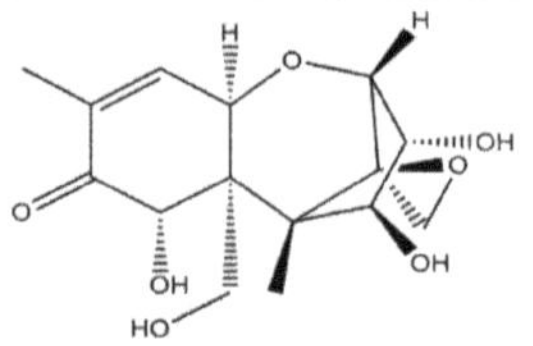 Nivalenol
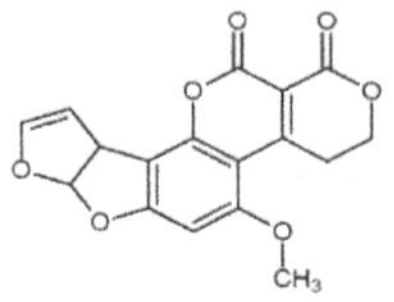 Aflatoxin G_1	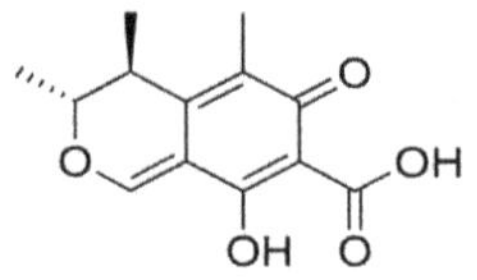 Citrinin	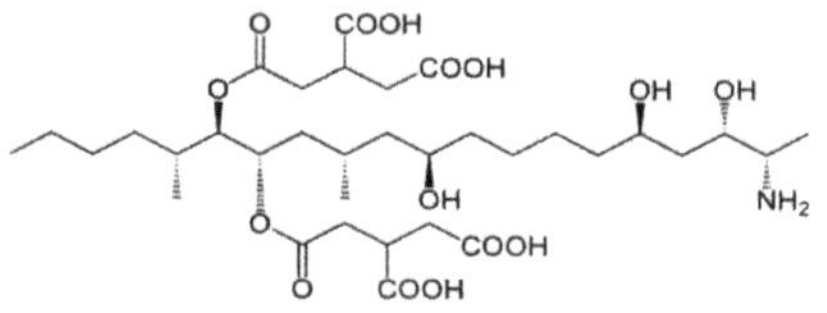 Fumonisin B_1
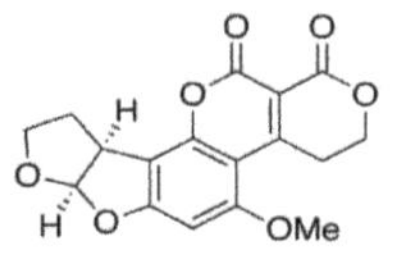 Aflatoxin G_2		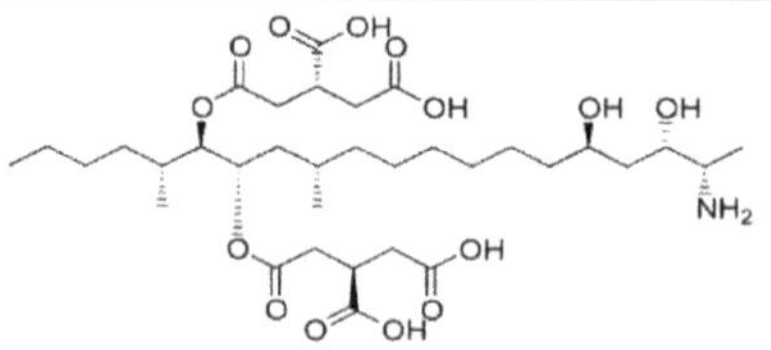 Fumonisin B_2
		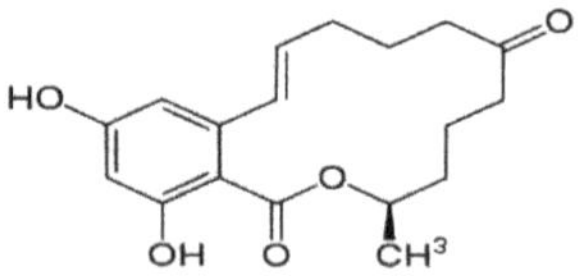 Zearalenone

Previous studies have established that mycotoxins are primarily located in the husk layers of grains. A study conducted by Vidal et al. [10] showed that wheat bran obtained from a Spanish market contained substantial amounts of various mycotoxins, mainly deoxynivalenol (DON) and zearalenone (ZEA). The authors concluded that the production of whole grain products from these wheat samples would constitute a substantial consumer health hazard. However, since wheat bran is rich in dietary fibre, there is a high interest in exploiting its application in food and feed products because of its potential health-promoting properties. In addition to these *Fusarium* toxins, different toxins produced by storage fungi, namely aflatoxins (AFs), ochratoxin A (OTA), and citrinin are commonly found as contaminants in cereals (Table 1). Finally, bacterial spoilage organisms must also be considered to ensure sufficient grain shelf life. Although most bacteria are unlikely to grow under conditions commonly applied to grain storage, their presence can result in significant quality deterioration during subsequent processing or in the final product [11].

In recent years, the consumer desire for more natural, less processed foods with fewer or no chemical additives has increased enormously; however, the requirement for the maintenance of the highest safety standards remains. This increases the emphasis on physical and microbiological treatments to control post-harvest microbial spoilage in cereals [12]. In addition, the application of both physical and microbiological decontamination methods into necessary food processing procedures while simultaneously enabling a "clean label" has attracted increasing interest from both the industry and researchers. Various approaches for bio-preservation, particularly the use of antifungal LAB (lactic acid bacteria), have been investigated and reviewed elsewhere [5,13,14]. In contrast, this article focuses on the recent advances in novel physical decontamination methods.

Physical grain treatments, including dry and wet heat, ionizing and non-ionizing irradiation, high hydrostatic pressure and modified atmosphere packaging, were critically reviewed as to their suitability to eliminate viable forms and spores of both food spoilage bacteria and fungi commonly found on cereals. Furthermore, the treatments' potential to remove previously produced mycotoxins as well as the impact on grain quality, viability and technological performance were evaluated based on the existing literature. This allowed for the identification of future research needs as well as possibilities for industrial application of the treatments discussed. It should be mentioned that classical physical treatments, such as milling, sorting, and hulling are not covered in this review, as these methods are well established and industrially applied. Therefore, they largely have not been the subject of recent research.

2. Modified Atmosphere Packaging (MAP)

Modified atmospheres have been investigated for the storage of cereals intended for food and feed. While fungi responsible for grain deterioration during storage often are considered obligate aerobes, many are microaerophilic. Hence, they can develop in niches where other species cannot grow and therefore can dominate in grain ecosystems. In many cases, the oxygen level must be <0.14% and the carbon dioxide level >50% to achieve significant growth inhibition [15,16]. Certain species, such as *P. roqueforti* Thom and some *Aspergillus* spp., can grow and infect grains even at >80% carbon dioxide, if at least 4% oxygen is present. In addition, post-harvest systems also use (oxygen-free) nitrogen to prevent grain deterioration [17]. However, it must be noted that results obtained in different sample systems are very difficult to compare, as the tolerance to low oxygen and high carbon dioxide levels is highly dependent on the sample matrix and water availability. Accordingly, low water availability has been reported to increase the sensitivity of microorganisms to the modified atmosphere. While MAP is used to control microbial spoilage and insect pests in moist grains during storage, different threats require different treatment conditions.

Exposure of various toxigenic fungi to ozone gas (60 μmol/mol) for up to 120 min resulted in significantly reduced growth and spore germination for *Fusarium graminearum*, *F. verticillioides* (Sacc.) Nirenberg, *Penicillium citrinum* Thom, C., *Aspergillus parasiticus* Speare, and *A. flavus* Link. However, the efficiency of the treatment was strongly dependent on the specific strain. *F. graminearum* was found to be particularly sensitive, as its growth was totally inhibited after exposure for 40 min, whereas *F. verticillioides* growth after 120 min of exposure was only slightly reduced [18].

However, very little research on modified atmosphere packaging has been conducted in recent years. This can be attributed to various reasons. Firstly, storage conditions under high carbon dioxide and low oxygen levels are difficult to apply to a conventional silo storage system. Additionally, environmental conditions, such as temperature, moisture content, and water availability determine the gas composition required to achieve sufficient microbial inhibition. The biggest potential drawback of this technology is that the microorganisms are not killed and therefore can induce product spoilage during subsequent processing. In addition, the removal of mycotoxins produced in field or the inactivation of microbial enzymes is not possible. In addition, microbial inhibition is substantially dependent on the fungal or bacterial strain. As cereals after harvest carry a wide range of microorganisms, it also appears very difficult to predict the success on a specific crop. Therefore, recent research to prevent post-harvest microbial spoilage has shifted towards novel and more flexible methods for application.

3. Thermal Treatments

Thermal treatments, including pasteurisation and sterilisation techniques, are the most regularly used treatment for the inactivation of microorganisms and enzymes in the food industry [19]. For post-harvest application of heat treatments various approaches, such as hot water dips, hot dry air, or superheated steam, are possible using different time-temperature combinations [20]. Table 2 summarises heat treatments reported to have been successful for microbial inactivation or toxin degradation and the side effects on the sample.

Table 2. The effects of different heat (wet and dry) treatments on microbial load and mycotoxin content in various sample matrices.

Target Organism/Toxin	Treatment	Sample Matrix	Technological Impact	References
Natural microbial load	Dry air 9 day/100 °C	Various cereals	No impact	[21,22]
Natural microbial load	Steam 60 min/82 °C	corn	No impact	[23]
Natural microbial load	Steam 210–250 °C/15 s	Wheat, barley, rye	Not investigated	[24]
F. graminearum	dry air 15 day/60 °C; 5 day/70 °C; 2 day/80 °C	Wheat	No impact	[25]
F. graminearum	Dry air 5 day/90 °C	Wheat	Reduced seed viability	[25]
F. graminearum	Dry air 21 day/60 °C; 9 day/70 °C; 5 day/80 °C	Barley	Reduced viability for 9 day/70 deg; 5 day/80 deg	[25]
Aspergillus spp., *Penicillium* spp., *Fusarium* spp., *E. coli*, *L. Monocytogenes*, *Salmonella* spp.	Steam 170–200 °C/<60 s	Various cereals	No impact	[26–28]
Geobacillus stearothermophilus spores	Steam 20 min/160 °C	Dried spore pellet-sand mixture	Not investigated	[29]
DON (50% reduction)	Steam 6 min/185 °C	wheat	Not investigated	[29]

3.1. Dry Heat Treatments

Described as an alternative to chemical grain disinfection, several applications of dry heat in the form of hot air treatments were studied for the ability to control fungal spoilage without compromising the kernels' viability [25]. Contradictory results have been reported as to the effects of dry heat treatments on the cereal's sensory quality and nutritional value. Several authors reported no impact on technological performance and enzymatic activities after nine days at up to 100 °C [21,22]. In contrast, Gilbert et al. [25] found a significant loss in seed viability after treatment for five days at 90 °C.

For inhibition of various fungal strains on wheat grains, time-temperature combinations of 15 day/60 °C, 5 day/70 °C and 2 day/80 °C, respectively, were found to inhibit fungal growth and spore germination completely without compromising the grain's viability [25,30]. When treating barley at the same temperatures, the fungi were completely inhibited after 21 days, 9 days, and 5 days, respectively. In contrast to wheat, after nine days at 70 °C, the germination capacity of barley was substantially reduced.

Although bacterial spoilage organisms, such as *Bacillus* spp., are unlikely to cause grain quality deterioration during storage, they have to be inactivated prior to grain processing to avoid subsequent product spoilage [11]. However, no studies specifically investigating the heat inactivation of grain spoilage bacteria post-harvest are available to date. In general, bacteria are reported to be less heat stable than fungal mycelia and it can therefore be assumed that they are also inactivated with the abovementioned antifungal treatments [31].

Thus, dry heat treatment prior to grain storage shows potential for the prevention of post-harvest microbial spoilage based on the heat inactivation of the microbes and the reduction of the grain's moisture content and water availability, which further supports microbial inhibition [32].

Depending on the processing conditions and sample matrix (i.e., the presence or absence of yeast), reports suggest a substantial reduction in the occurrence of mycotoxins during heating. However, cereal flours currently are not always heat treated during processing and this approach is very inconsistent. Therefore, an efficient pre-storage treatment to degrade mycotoxins is essential [33]. In general, conventional heat treatment is not suitable for detoxifying crops contaminated with mycotoxins. Commonly found mycotoxins, such as aflatoxins, trichothecenes, OTA, and others reportedly possess great heat stability (>300 °C) and thus cannot be degraded by dry heat without seriously damaging the treated cereal. To date, no studies reporting the total removal of mycotoxins by dry heat treatments in vitro or in situ are available. In addition, the reported partial degradation of different toxins by dry heat was always found to compromise the grain quality and viability. This indicates that dry heat can serve as a sufficient tool for the degradation of mycotoxins only in combination with other treatments [34]. In addition, the thermal degradation of mycotoxin into intermediate constituent products of unknown identity and toxicity must also be considered [35,36].

Available literature suggests that, depending on the target microorganism and cereal substrate, dry heat treatments have the potential to decrease the microbial load without compromising the grain quality. However, such treatments consume considerable energy and time, lasting up to several days. Furthermore, the conditions must be adjusted carefully to achieve satisfying results for both microbial decontamination and grain quality. In addition, the sole use of dry heat is unsuitable for killing spores of heat-resistant bacteria, as the applicable temperatures are too low and do not kill the grains. Hence, bacterial spores enter a dormant state and can germinate once suitable conditions return, particularly during cereal processing [26]. In terms of mycotoxin degradation, dry heat cannot serve as a sole treatment to efficiently remove mycotoxins produced in-field. The temperatures required are not feasible to maintain the grain's technological performance; decomposition is always incomplete and the resulting degradation products could display a health risk of yet unknown potential. Finally, the efficiency of hot air treatments is further compromised by the particle size of the treated sample. Thus, it is less efficient for the treatment of whole grains than for treating the milled product.

3.2. Wet Heat Treatments

Compared to conventional hot air treatments, the use of hot steam appears to be a more efficient approach in terms of both time and energy for microbial decontamination and mycotoxin degradation (Table 2). In addition, food spoilage bacteria and fungi were found to be less heat resistant when in conditions with high water availability [37]. Apart from the classic saturated water steam (up to 100 °C), superheated steam (SS, up to 250 °C) has recently gained considerable interest as a rapid, non-destructive, and safe decontamination method [38]. Hence, recent advances and novel applications of SS will be the focus of this section. SS, having higher enthalpy than saturated steam, can quickly transfer heat to the material being processed, resulting in rapid temperature increase in the sample. In addition, SS is reported to contribute to better product quality. The major advantages of using SS for food processing include better product quality (colour, shrinkage, and rehydration characteristics), reduced oxidation losses, and higher energy efficiency [39].

Researchers using SS achieved microbial decontamination from vegetative forms of food spoilage fungi (*Aspergillus* spp., *Penicillium* spp., *Fusarium* spp.) and bacteria, such as *Escherichia coli* O157:H7, *Salmonella Typhimurium*, *Salmonella enteritidis* phage type 30, and *Listeria monocytogenes*, on different cereals. Treatment times of less than 60 s with water steam temperatures of 170 °C–200 °C were reported to be sufficient to reduce the microbial load below the respective limit of detection [26–28]. However, none of those treatments resulted in a significant reduction of sensory or nutritional quality. In contrast, corn treated with conventional steam at 82 °C had to be exposed for 60 min in order to achieve a significant reduction of the microbial load by 4-log units [23]. No results regarding the impact of the treatment on the grain quality were reported. As a result, despite the ability of both approaches to decontaminate cereals, the use of superheated steam is a much more time efficient solution.

Compared to their vegetative forms, fungal and bacterial spore inhibition presents a much bigger challenge. As mentioned above, bacterial endospores can lay dormant and germinate when conditions are favourable during downstream processing. Nonetheless, SS was found to be efficient at permanently killing spores of *Geobacillus stearothermophilus*. However, exposure times of up to 20 min are required to kill spores. This is significantly longer than the inactivation of vegetative microbes. Thus, the biggest reduction in spore viability was detected during the first 5 min of treatment, independent from the processing temperature [29].

In addition, SS was also investigated for the removal of mycotoxins from different cereal matrices. Partial degradation of DON upon SS treatment was reported by Cenkowski et al. [29]. The authors found that increases in steam temperature and exposure time correlated with higher degradation rates for DON. Thus, the highest treatment temperature (185 °C), combined with the longest treatment time (6 min), resulted in the highest reduction of DON, by 50%, which was found to be independent of the steam velocity. Furthermore, the reduction was found to be exclusively due to thermal degradation, rather than solubilisation and water extraction with the steam. However, no investigation of the treatment's impact on the grain's technological performance were undertaken in the study of Cenkowski et al. [29]. Likewise, the dry decomposition temperature of aflatoxins (approximately 270 °C) is known to be significantly reduced under moist conditions [40]. Consequently, SS treatments present a much more efficient and promising approach for AF (aflatoxins) degradation than conventional dry heating.

In conclusion, the application of wet heat and superheated steam were found to be very effective in the decontamination of cereals without compromising the grain's technological quality and performance. However, despite extensive research, future work is still required to optimise the processing parameters which is dependent on the matrix present. The technological impact of treatments long enough to kill spores and degrade mycotoxins requires further investigation. Additionally, the fate of mycotoxins thermally degraded by the SS remains unclear. Thus, the degree of actual detoxification is still in question. Similarly, the possibility of degrading other toxins, such as patulin or bacterial toxins, requires closer investigation.

Finally, it is noteworthy that ultra-superheated steam (USS) has recently attracted considerable research interest. This technique employs temperatures of 400–500 °C. Exposure of different cereals, namely wheat, barley, and rye for 15 s to USS (actual contact temperature 210–250 °C) resulted in total inhibition of spoilage fungi and grain shelf-life extension without notable quality deterioration [24]. However, few studies have investigated the application of USS for the microbial decontamination of food commodities. Thus, the optimal conditions of use and the full potential of this method remain unclear. Further research is needed to clarify the suitability of USS treatments to decontaminate and potentially detoxify cereal grains post-harvest.

4. Ionizing Irradiation

Ionizing irradiation approaches largely are based on short waves of electromagnetic energy that travel at the speed of light. All treatments discussed in this section share the basic properties of electromagnetic radiation. Ionizing radiation treatment using either gamma rays or an electron beam (e-beam) is well established as a rapid, efficient, safe, and environmentally friendly technique for the reduction of food-borne diseases by destroying pathogenic and toxigenic microorganisms [41]. Their biggest advantage is their great penetrating power (inversely related to the frequency [42]), their high efficiency against various food spoilage organisms, and the absence of a rise in temperature in the treated sample [1]. In addition, irradiation treatments for food processing purposes are unconditionally regarded as safe for dosages of up to 10 kGy (1 Gy = 1 Joule of irradiation energy/kg sample matter, with 1 Joule = 1 $\frac{kg \cdot m^2}{s^2}$) [43]. Due to the unit of irradiation dosage containing the ratio of energy per time and sample matter, treatments are commonly compared by means of dose and form of application only. Successful treatments with ionizing irradiation against various food spoilage organisms and toxins are summarised in Table 3.

Table 3. The effects of different ionizing irradiation treatments (gamma- and e-beam irradiation) on microbial load and mycotoxin content in various sample matrices.

Target Organism/Toxin	Treatment	Sample Matrix	Technological Impact	References
Natural fungal population	0.75 kGy gamma	millet	none	[44]
Natural microbial load	6 kGy e-beam	chestnuts	No effect on nutritional value	[45,46]
L. monocytogenes	3.3 kGy e-beam (soft electrons)	Alfalfa sprouts	No quality deterioration	[47]
Aspergillus spp., *Alternaria* spp., *Fusarium* spp., *Curvularia* spp., *Helminthosporium* spp.	1.5–3.5 kGy gamma	wheat	Reduced quality for doses >2.5 kGy	[48]
Fusarium spp.	4 kGy gamma	Barley	Reduced quality	[49]
Fusarium spp.	6 kGy gamma	Wheat and maize	Reduced quality	[49]
Aspergillus spp., *Penicillium* spp.	10–15 kGy e-beam	Dry split beans	No quality deterioration (10 kGy)	[50]
Penicillium spp., *Fusarium* spp., *Aspergillus* spp.	1.7–4.8 kGy e-beam	corn	Not investigated	[41]
Fusarium spp. and DON	6–10 kGy e-beam	Barley, malt	Not investigated	[51]
OTA and aflatoxins	15 kGy gamma	Wheat and sesame	Not investigated	[52–54]
OTA	2 kGy gamma	Aqueous solution	-	[55]
DON, ZEN, T-2, FB_1	10 kGy gamma	Soy beans, corn, wheat	Not investigated	[56]
FB_1	7 kGy gamma	Barley, wheat, maize	Not investigated	[49]
aflatoxins	1.5 kGy e-beam	Ground almond flour	Not investigated	[57]

DON: Desoxynivalenol; OTA: Ochratoxin A; ZEN: Zearalenone; T-2: Fusariotoxin T 2; FB_1: Fumonisin B1; -: none.

4.1. Gamma Irradiation

This section discusses the application of irradiation to decontaminate cereals using gamma rays. These electromagnetic waves are usually produced by radioactive cobalt isotopes (^{60}Co). The use of gamma rays for irradiation treatments is characterised by their high penetration energy and short treatment times.

For millet grains exposed to gamma radiation, no significant decrease in fungal incidence or spore germination was reported for radiation doses up to 0.5 kGy. However, at doses of 0.75 kGy or higher, the rate of fungal incidences and spore germination sharply decreased by over 80% and 2-log units, respectively [44]. Salem et al. [48] applied gamma irradiation ranging from 0.5–3.5 kGy to wheat grains prior to storage. A dosage of 1.5 kGy was found to be sufficient for at least a 90% reduction of *Aspergillus* spp., *Alternaria* spp., *Fusarium* spp., *Curvularia* spp., and *Helminthosporium* spp. immediately after the treatment. However, after six months of subsequent storage, the degree of inhibition (compared to the untreated control) was significantly reduced for all species apart from *Fusarium* spp. The authors also reported that higher irradiation doses resulted in higher inhibition rates. In particular, 3.5 kGy, resulting in total inhibition directly after the treatment, also showed total inhibition after six months against all fungi apart from *Aspergillus* spp. (96.4%). In contrast, Aziz et al. [49] reported higher irradiation doses, 4 kGy for barley and 6 kGy for wheat and maize, necessary for total inhibition of *Fusarium* spp. However, analysis of selected physical, chemical, and rheological properties of these grains prior to and after storage showed that, from a technological performance point of view, irradiation dosages higher than 1.5–2.5 kGy were not feasible. This also correlates with findings reported by other researchers [58,59].

Available literature suggests that the radio sensitivity of different fungal species appears to differ significantly depending on the reference consulted. These discrepancies likely result from countless influencing factors which require further research. These factors include the form of fungal contamination (mycelium or spores) and the moisture contents of spores or commodities. Although moist conditions promote fungal growth and spore germination, dry spores are considered more irradiation resistant. Furthermore, the age of spores and the nature of the matrix irradiated can have a significant influence on the radio sensitivity. In addition, the fungal strain and the temperature before, during, and after irradiation influence the treatment's efficiency for each sample.

However, the most recent research on the application of gamma irradiation on cereals has focused on the degradation of mycotoxins in food and feed commodities. Several studies have investigated the degradation of aflatoxins (AFs) and ochratoxin A (OTA) in particular. Deberghes et al. [60] previously reported on the degradation of OTA in an aqueous solution due to gamma irradiation with 2–5 kGy. However, in situ degradation of mycotoxins such as OTA was found to be much more difficult. After gamma irradiation of wheat and sesame seeds using 15 kGy, degradation of OTA, AFB_1 (Aflatoxin B1), AFB_2, AFG_1 (Aflatoxin G1), and AFG_2 with reduction rates of 23.9%, 18.2%, 11.0%, 21.1%, and 13.6%, respectively, were found [52,61]. However, in both studies the application of lower irradiation doses showed no substantial reduction of AFs and OTA. Several other authors also reported similar results on various cereal matrices intended for food or feed use [53,54,62–64]. However, it must be noted that none of these studies took the moisture content of the seeds into consideration, which appears to have a critical impact on the radio stability of the toxins. Therefore, the meaningfulness of the results is limited. In another study, soybeans, corn, and wheat, with respective moisture levels of 9, 13, and 17%, showed no substantial reduction in AFs or OTA after irradiation dosages of up to 20 kGy [56]. Therefore, the success of AF degradation due to gamma rays is not dependent solely on the dose; the moisture content of the sample has a major impact on AF degradation. It is proposed that this is primarily due to the radiolysis of water, producing highly active radicals which can degrade AFs to compounds with lower biological activity [40,65]. Similar results were reported for the degradation of OTA in vitro and in situ. OTA showed great radiostability as a dry substance because irradiation with 8 kGy resulted in no noteworthy reduction. In contrast, when in an aqueous solution (50 ng/mL), significant reduction was achieved with just 2 kGy. Similarly, the degradation in moist wheat kernels (16% moisture) was substantially higher than in dry ones (11% moisture) when irradiated with 8 kGy [55].

On the basis of consulted literature, typical *Fusarium* toxins, such as DON, ZEN (Zearalenone), T-2 (Fusariotoxin T 2), and FB_1 (Fumonisin B1) appear to be more radio sensitive than AFs and OTA. DON, ZEN, and T-2 toxin in soybeans, corn, and wheat were significantly reduced by irradiation with 10 kGy [56]. Irradiation of barley, wheat, and maize naturally contaminated with FB_1 which resulted in a significant reduction (>85%) and total destruction of the toxin after exposure to 5 kGy and 7 kGy, respectively [49].

Nevertheless, irradiation results in degradation products of unknown identity and toxicity must be considered. Wang et al. [65] detected 20 radiolytic products of AFB_1 after irradiation in a water/methanol mixture. To date, just seven of these products have been identified and six are considered less toxic than AFB_1 due to the missing double bond on the terminal furan ring (Table 1). Given these results, it remains unclear if degradation of mycotoxins is responsible for the detoxification of the sample or if the resulting products are equally as toxic as the original substance. Furthermore, as the irradiation efficiency is highly dependent on water availability, the application in dry food matrices appears to be limited. Although AFs and OTA belong to the most commonly found toxins in cereal crops, the fate of other contaminants, such as DON, NIV (nivalenol), and ZEN requires further research.

In conclusion, gamma irradiation can reduce and potentially fully inhibit fungal and bacterial spoilage of grains during storage thus avoiding the production of mycotoxins. However, the irradiation dosages required for total inhibition of common storage fungi, such as *Aspergillus parasiticus*, are highly dependent on the sample matrix and fungal load. Necessary doses reported a range between 5 and 10 kGy. Unfortunately, such high irradiation dosages cause severe damage to the treated grains and are therefore not feasible from a technological point of view. On the other hand, a simple reduction of the microbial load is not sufficient either, as even minimal fungal contamination can lead to growth during storage. This ultimately results in huge economic losses and a potential consumer health hazard, as demonstrated by the authors in a previous study [7]. Therefore, gamma irradiation alone cannot serve as an efficient tool for cereal grain preservation during storage but could potentially be applied in combination with other treatments. However, for treatment of cereals purposed for animal feed, higher irradiation dosages are allowed. Thus, gamma irradiation may be a promising approach in the decontamination of animal feed.

4.2. Electron Beam Irradiation

The use of e-beam irradiation has several advantages over the use of conventional gamma irradiation. Table 4 summarises the comparison between gamma and e-beam irradiation. The main advantages include faster operation, lower irradiation dosages, and the use of electricity rather than radioactive materials to generate the electron, making the technology more flexible and easier to use. Unfortunately, its penetration power is lower, largely rendering it a tool for surface disinfection [1]. The general use of e-beam irradiation in the food industry, including the technological background and mode of action, was recently reviewed by Freita-Silva et al. [1]. Accordingly, this section will focus exclusively on recent advances in microbial decontamination using e-beam irradiation. With the exception of Europe, e-beam irradiation has been accepted and is widely applied towards the treatments of various food products worldwide, such as fruits and grains. Approximately 81,593 t are treated annually, out of which only 11 t are from Europe [66].

Table 4. Comparison of gamma (^{60}Co) and e-beam irradiation, adopted from Freita-Silva et al. [1].

Parameters	Gamma Irradiation	E-Beam Irradiation
Irradiation Time	Slow	Fast
Doses (kGy)	Higher doses	Lower doses
Source	Radioactive material	Electricity to generate electrons
Flexibility	Inflexible (cannot be turned off)	More flexible (can be turned off)
Penetration	Good penetration	Lower penetration power

Microbial decontamination and mycotoxin degradation in vitro with the potential of application in situ has been previously reported [67]. The irradiation dose necessary for sufficient decontamination depends on the type and species of grains to be treated [68].

When dry split beans were subjected to e-beam irradiation (0, 2.5, 5, 10, 15 kGy) to control storage moulds, irradiation resulted in a dose-dependent decrease in fungal contaminants. High irradiation doses (10 and 15 kGy) resulted in a complete absence of fungi and undetectable levels of aflatoxins B_1 and B_2. In contrast, un-irradiated beans carried *Aspergillus niger* van Tieghem at the highest level (33–50%), followed by *A. flavus* (14–20%), and *Penicillium chrysogenum* Thom (7–13%). For total inhibition of fungal incidence, irradiation doses of 10 and 15 kGy were necessary. Irradiated split beans (10 kGy) also showed improved shelf life of up to six months without quality deterioration [50]. In contrast, on raw corn under comparable conditions, doses as low as 1.7, 2.5, and 4.8 kGy were found to be sufficient to fully inhibit the growth of *Penicillium* spp., *Fusarium* spp., and *Aspergillus* spp., respectively [41]. Researchers concluded that, with sufficient optimisation of the processing parameters, e-beam irradiation has considerable potential in the microbial decontamination of cereals. For the reduction of the natural microbial load in chestnuts, 6 kGy were found sufficient for decontamination while nutritionally valuable constituents remained unaffected [45,46,69]. Interestingly, e-beam irradiation of *Fusarium* spp.-infected barley with 6–10 kGy showed no significant reduction in fungal incidence and DON contents in the fresh barley. However, the resulting barley malt was reported to have significantly reduced DON content and fungal occurrence [51]. In another study conducted by Stepanik et al. [70], wheat grains and dried distillers grain were irradiated with up to 55 kGy, which resulted in a maximum DON reduction of 17%.

To date, no studies investigating the fate of mycotoxins exposed to e-beam irradiation are available. This is likely due to the lower energy value of this irradiation compared to gamma irradiation (Table 4). Thus, e-beam irradiation is unlikely to create enough energy for mycotoxin degradation. This applies in particular if the toxins are not exclusively located on the grain surface but also in the inner layers. Therefore, the application on ground almond flour with a dose as low as 1.5 kGy was found to be sufficient for total degradation of aflatoxins [57].

In conclusion, e-beam treatment shows potential to reduce the microbial load and content of mycotoxins produced in-field. However, depending on the sample matrix, microbial load, and target organism, the irradiation dose necessary is likely to exceed that generally permitted, i.e., 10 kGy [43], leading to legislative difficulties. Furthermore, the impact of various e-beam treatments on the grain's sensory and nutritional properties have to be investigated further. Finally, difficulties such as the even treatment of the sample surface and the low penetration energy of the e-beam must be considered before any industrial application.

A variation of conventional e-beam irradiation is the use of so-called "soft electrons". The term "soft" refers to the low energy of the electrons fired at the sample. This results in less impact on the sample in terms of sensory and nutritional value. However, this approach only can serve as a surface treatment, as the e-beam does not have sufficient energy to penetrate the deeper layers of the sample. The use of 3.3 kGy applied at soft electrons was reported to successfully eliminate *L. monocytogenes* from alfalfa sprouts [47]. However, due to the low penetration power, a small particle size and an even sample surface are crucial to ensure uniform treatment. Consequently, the irradiation treatment of soybeans was found to be more difficult, as 17 kGy was insufficient to eliminate the natural microbes present on the surface [71]. Thus, because of the difficult applicability, soft electrons show very little potential for industrial post-harvest decontamination of cereal crops but could have potential for flour treatment after milling.

5. Non-Ionizing Irradiation

This section reviews recent advances in non-ionizing irradiation treatments for microbial decontamination and detoxification with possible applications for cereals. Treatments that were successfully applied for the various target organisms or toxins are summarised in Table 5. Because of the non-ionizing character of the treatments discussed here, the impact on the grain quality is likely to be negligible. In addition, consumer acceptance for ionizing irradiation is relatively low due to misinformation [72]. Use of non-ionizing irradiation should increase consumer acceptance of the final products.

Table 5. The effects of different non-ionizing (light, microwave, ultrasound) treatments on microbial load and mycotoxin content in various sample matrices.

Target Organism/Toxin	Treatment	Sample Matrix	Technological Impact	References
Different food spoilage bacteria and fungi	US (ultrasound) > 60 W/cm^2	Aqueous solution	-	[73]
A. parasiticus	Microwave: 900 W, 2.45 GHz, 1–5 min	Aqueous solution	-	[74]
Aspergillus spp. and *Penicillium* spp.	US: 6 min, 60 °C, 20–39 W/cm^2	Culture medium	-	[75]
Aspergillus spp.	51.2 J/g pulsed white light	wheat	15% reduced seed viability	[76]
Aspergillus spp.	Microwave: 120 s, 2450 MHz, 1.25 kW	Cereals and nuts	Not investigated	[77,78]
Bacillus subtilis	1.0 J/cm^2 * 10 pulses light with 200–1100 nm	spices	No quality deterioration	[79]
OTA, OTB (Ochratoxin B), citrinin	Light: 455 nm/470 nm for 5 day	Aqueous solution	-	[80]
Aflatoxins	UV (Ultraviolet)-light: 265 nm for 15–45 min	nuts	Not investigated	[81]
trichothecenes	US > 200 W/cm^2	corn	No quality deterioration	[82]

* Times (sign for multiplication), -: none.

5.1. Ultraviolet (UV) Light

The antimicrobial properties of UV light are well investigated and, taking surface disinfection as an example, long established. However, the conventional application of UV light in the form of continuous exposure has numerous disadvantages. As the sanitizing effect is primarily attributed to the high ionizing energy of vacuum-UV (wavelength < 180 nm), the consumer acceptance is very low. The induced DNA damage, responsible for the microbial inhibition, also occurs in the sample which results in a substantial loss of quality. In addition, depending on the water content, substantial internal heating of the sample can occur. To avoid these unwanted side effects, recent research has focused on the application of pulsed UV light. In these studies, the treatment was carried out with numerous short flashes of light with a broad wavelength spectrum. Although the inhibitory effect was still attributed to the UV spectrum of light (wavelength 200–400 nm), microbial inhibition could be achieved with non-ionizing UV (>180 nm). At the same time, the undesired side effects were substantially reduced. Thus, pulsed UV light presents a novel, non-thermal, antimicrobial treatment with potential applications for food preservation. Therefore, this section is focused exclusively on the application of non-ionizing UV light. Microbial inactivation as a result of exposure to pulsed light, in vitro and in situ, has been reported by several studies and comprehensively reviewed by Oms-Oliu et al. [83].

Oms-Oliu et al. [83] demonstrated the successful inhibition of food spoilage fungi and bacteria with pulsed light when applied to various food matrices, including milk, honey, and fruits. However, only one available study investigated the application of pulsed light for pre-storage decontamination of cereals. Maftei et al. [76] reported up to a 4-log unit reduction for naturally occurring *Aspergillus* spp. in wheat grains. Treatment was carried out with 40 flashes of broad spectrum white light (180–1100 nm) with an overall energy release of 51.2 J/g. In addition, the authors reported that the same treatment with light of a narrower wavelength spectrum (305–1100 nm and 400–1100 nm, respectively) resulted in significantly less fungal inhibition.

Although pulsed UV light causes less damage to the sample than continuous UV irradiation, significantly reduced seed viability was reported nonetheless. Alongside the reduction of *Aspergillus* spp. from 10^5 to 10 cfu/g, the seed viability was significantly reduced by 15% [76]. Consequently, despite showing the potential for microbial decontamination, further optimisation of the processing conditions is required to improve efficiency and make the treatment potentially suitable for industrial application.

However, inhibition of common food spoilage bacteria was generally found to be more difficult, as reductions of no more than 1-log unit could be achieved without substantial impact on the sample quality [83]. Furthermore, no studies investigating the inhibition of bacteria commonly found on cereals or in cereal matrices are available. However, Nicorescu et al. [79] achieved up to a 1-log unit reduction of *Bacillus subtilis* in a liquid medium and artificially contaminated spices. After the treatment, approximately 10^4 cfu/g remained on the samples, despite an equivalent 90% reduction in the bacterial population. Thus, further research is needed to improve the antibacterial properties of pulsed UV light.

Several studies have also investigated the possibility of photodegradation of mycotoxins in vitro and in situ using UV and visible light. Treatment of different mycotoxins (OTA, OTB, and citrinin) in aqueous solution with light of various wavelengths (455, 470, 530, 590, and 627 nm) for five days resulted in significant degradation of all three toxins after exposure to the 455 nm and the 470 nm light [80]. In particular, light of wavelength 455 nm was found to be very efficient in terms of mycotoxin degradation. Subsequently, 455 nm light was applied in situ on artificially fungal-infected wheat kernels. After five days of exposure, the OTA and OTB levels were reduced by >90% compared to the untreated control [80].

In addition, the total aflatoxin content of various nuts could be substantially reduced by treatment with UV light (265 nm) for 15–45 min [81]. However, numerous factors were found to have a significant impact on the level of aflatoxin reduction. The most influential factors included the moisture content of the nuts, the toxin targeted, the exposure time, and the type of nut. The authors also reported higher resistance of AFB_1 and AFG_1 to the UV light compared to AFG_2. For all toxins, increasing sensitivity towards the treatment could be attributed to increasing moisture levels and exposure time.

To evaluate the potential use of photodegradation for the detoxification of cereals, the fate of the degraded mycotoxins also must be considered. Liu et al. [84] proposed a pathway for the UV light-induced photodegradation of AFB_1 after identification of the three main degradation products using UPLC-MS (ultra performance liquid chromatography-tandem mass spectrometer). Identification of the degradation products revealed that, from the two most important parts of the molecule in terms of toxicity, namely the terminal furan ring and the lactone ring (Table 1), only the latter was affected by photodegradation. In addition, the authors reported first order reaction kinetics and found the process to be independent of the initial toxin concentration (within 0.2–5 ppm) but directly related to the irradiation intensity. On the basis of these results, a subsequent study investigated the cytotoxicity of UV light degraded AFB_1 in an aqueous solution [85]. The authors assessed the toxicity of the three previously identified degradation products using the Ames test. Interestingly, the cytotoxicity was reduced by 40% compared to native AFB_1 but not fully eliminated. This leads to the question as to whether photodegradation can serve as a suitable tool for mycotoxin detoxification. Given that 60% of the initial cytotoxicity remained even after complete degradation of the toxin, alternative treatments are likely to be more suitable.

In conclusion, despite some potential for microbial decontamination and mycotoxin degradation, UV light appears to be difficult to apply without affecting sample quality. Although the use of pulsed light rather than continuous irradiation reduces the negative effects, no complete inhibition without quality loss has been reported. This applies in particular to the decontamination of food spoilage bacteria. For application on cereal grains, the uneven sample surface makes a reliable application even more challenging as a result of the shadow spots on the grains. In terms of mycotoxin degradation, it was shown that UV light was capable of total degradation of toxins such as AFB_1, but the degradation products were found to remain cytotoxic. Therefore, it appears an unsuitable method for mycotoxin detoxification.

5.2. Microwave Treatments

Microwave technology is widely used in the food industry and offers several advantages, including safety, high efficiency, and environmental protection, but often affects food quality [74]. Microwaves are defined as electromagnetic waves with frequencies ranging from 300 MHz to 300 GHz. The mechanism of microbial inhibition is primarily based on the internal heating of the sample resulting from molecular movement in the pulsing electromagnetic field. This leads to the denaturation of proteins, enzymes, and nucleic acids. This implies the risk of losing enzymatic activities in the grain, activities which are essential for downstream processing steps [74]. However, with optimised processing conditions, microwave treatment has the ability to fully inhibit microbial growth on cereal grains without compromising the grain's germination quality [86]. Therefore, the impact of various factors, such as moisture content, microbial load, or sample matrix, need to be investigated further to determine the optimal processing conditions for each cereal matrix.

Available literature suggests a microwave treatment for up to 10 min with an energy output of 1.45 kW with 2450 MHz results in a very minor reduction of total AFs, including AFB_1 [53]. However, the possibility of inhibiting the growth and spore germination of *Aspergillus* spp. in cereals and nuts by 3-log units, without significant quality deterioration, was reported by different authors [77,78]. A treatment time of 120 s with 2450 MHz and 1.25 kW was found to be sufficient. Consequently, due to the fungal inhibition, the amount of mycotoxins produced was also significantly lower.

Furthermore, non-thermal inactivation of microorganisms resulting from repeated exposure to sub-lethal doses of high frequency microwaves has been reported [74]. The lethal effect of low-dose microwave radiation (LDMR) on spoilage microorganisms was a result of a disruption of the cell membrane and induced DNA damage rather than protein denaturation. Thus, the mechanism by which LDMR causes fungal death is different from a conventional heating treatment [74]. However, in a study conducted on *A. parasiticus*, the severity of DNA injury was found to increase with rising temperatures. Thus, the inactivation effect is still partially related to the processing temperature. However, few available studies have investigated this topic. Thus, future research is needed to exploit this technology through the establishment of non-thermal, microwave-based, microbial hurdle processes that do not compromise the grain quality.

Overall, microwave treatment, because of internal heating, shows little potential for the microbial decontamination of cereals. This is primarily a result of heat-induced damage to the sample. The same conclusion must be drawn for the microwave-induced degradation of mycotoxins which possess high heat stability. However, the concept of non-thermal microbial inactivation appears much more promising. However, as research on this approach is in its infancy, it is not yet possible to predict the full potential and applicability to industrial grain decontamination process until more extensive research has been conducted.

5.3. Ultrasonication

The term 'ultrasound' (US) describes sonic waves with frequencies above the human audible range and are generally divided into two categories: high frequency ultrasound and power ultrasound. The former uses high frequencies of 2–20 MHz with low sound intensity (0.1–1 W/cm^2) and is predominantly used in food quality analysis and medical imaging. In contrast, power ultrasound, or high-intensity ultrasound, is characterised by low frequencies (20–100 kHz) but high sound intensity (10–1000 W/cm^2). Research on the inactivation of enzymes and microorganisms has predominantly focused on the application of high power ultrasound, considered a promising, novel, and non-thermal approach for microbial disinfection of various surfaces and food matrices [87]. In contrast, high frequency US shows much less potential for microbial decontamination. Therefore, this review focuses on power ultrasound exclusively.

Only a few studies have investigated the sole application of US e for microbial decontamination with contradictory results. Butz and Tauscher [88] demonstrated that US alone does not sufficiently inactivate food spoilage microorganisms, as the inactivating effects are not severe enough. In contrast, Chemat et al. [73] reported that, if the acoustic power applied is sufficiently high (>60 W/cm^2), even US alone can induce cell rupture and thus microbial inactivation. Successful decontamination using US was only achieved under laboratory conditions and would be difficult to apply on an industrial scale. Most data available suggests that US alone is a very inefficient and energy consuming treatment for microbial disinfection and therefore must be used in combination with other treatments, such as sanitizing chemicals or heat [89]. Furthermore, the generation of such high-power US requires an immense energy input and is relatively inefficient compared to other techniques. This is further supported by O'Donnell et al. [19] who described the challenges encountered by the industrial scale-up of US technology. In addition, the application of this technology to cereal grains could prove difficult, as the treatment has to be carried out in a liquid medium. Therefore, it would be crucial that the cavitation of the liquid around the grains is evenly distributed.

In general, the biggest potential of US is in combination with mild heat or sanitizing agents, which have been shown to have a synergistic effect by several authors [90,91]. Herceg et al. [75] achieved total inhibition of *Aspergillus* and *Penicillium* spp., after exposure to ultrasound for at least 6 min at 60 °C when the applied power was ranging between 20 and 39 W/cm^2. However, these results were achieved in liquid sample matrices in which the US waves can easily travel, resulting in an evenly distributed cavitation effect. But for possible application on cereal crops, it remains unclear if enough cavitation throughout the whole sample can be generated for a noteworthy disinfection effect. Thus, a small sample size appears necessary to provide uniform cavitation. Furthermore, the grains would be required to be in a "washing solution", which produces a further challenge to the industrial use of this technology.

No available studies have investigated the application of US to decontaminate solid foods. Chemat et al. [73] recently reviewed the application of US in the food industry and its advances for decontamination of liquid food systems. However, chemical disinfection supported by US is likely to result in synergistic effects. Thus, it is apparently a promising improvement over conventional chemical disinfection (reduction of treatment time and unpleasant side effects) and therefore should be considered for further investigations. Ultrasound could be used to provide the energy necessary to form free radicals as reactive species and so support the disinfection efficiency of commonly used surface sanitizers. In particular, hydrogen peroxide- or sodium hypochlorite-based disinfection of food or food contact materials can be efficiently supported by US, creating more hydroxyl- and hypochlorite radicals, respectively. Furthermore, the use of US can substantially increase the speed and efficacy of conventional food preservation methods such as sterilisation and pasteurisation. This would allow a reduction in the processing time and temperature and therefore reduce undesirable side effects, such as changes in taste, colour, and nutritional value [73].

Few studies have investigated the impact of ultrasonication on mycotoxins. Lindner and Hasenhuti [82] reported the successful degradation of trichothecenes in contaminated corn while the technological performance of the treated samples remained unchanged. However, as discussed earlier, for the combination of gamma irradiation with chemical sanitizers, the production of hydroxyl radicals can lead to chemical degradation of aflatoxins. Theoretically it should be possible to produce such radicals using US. However, to the best of the authors' knowledge, no studies have been conducted on this topic.

On the basis of published research, clearly only a combination of US with heat or chemical sanitizers can sufficiently inactivate vegetative cells, spores, and enzymes simultaneously. Only then can consistent and high product quality be ensured, as the microbial enzymes can cause great damage to proteins and carbohydrates of the grains, even after killing of the vegetative cells [7].

6. High Hydrostatic Pressure (HHP)

Another emergent approach for the decontamination of food and feed products from spoilage microbes is treatment with high hydrostatic pressure (HHP). Well-established applications include the preservation of meat products, oysters, fruit juices, and many ready-to-eat foods. HHP may inactivate vegetative microorganisms and fungal spores at relatively low temperatures without compromising sensory and nutritional properties [92,93]. Thus, it has potential use in the expansion of the production of value-added foods.

Microbial inactivation is reported for processing pressures ranging from 100 to 800 MPa and relatively short times (a few seconds to several minutes). Combined treatment with mild temperatures between 20 and 50 °C to inactivate enzymes also have been reported. The treatment conditions depend fundamentally on the food matrix as well as the microorganisms and enzymes targeted. However, it is noteworthy that this technology cannot inactivate bacterial endospores with the application of the processing parameters commonly used in the food industry [94]. Pressures of at least 600 MPa with mild temperatures (60 °C) are required for the killing of spores of most food spoilage bacteria. Certain strains of *Clostridium botulinum* and *Bacillus species* are reported to withstand hydrostatic pressures of up to 1000 MPa [92]. Therefore, they present a much bigger challenge and cannot be inhibited by HHP alone, but which may be possible in combination with more severe heat treatment [95].

For the inactivation of *Escherichia coli* K-12 and *Staphylococcus aureus* ATCC 6538 in cheese slurries, 20 min of 400 MPa at 30 °C and of 600 MPa at 20 °C, respectively, were found to be sufficient [96]. Likewise, potential pathogenic food bacteria were inhibited due to HHP treatment. Studies on almonds, pressurised in water for 6 min at 414 MPa, followed by air drying at room temperature or 115 °C for 25 min, resulted in bacterial growth reduction of 4- and 6.7-log units, respectively [97]. The authors concluded that HHP treatments show great potential for microbial inactivation if the sample is suspended in the pressurizing medium.

With regards to fungal inhibition by HHP, Martínez-Rodríguez et al. [98] investigated the impact of HHP (300, 400, and 500 MPa, respectively) at 20 °C for 10 min on fungal mycelia development, spore viability, and enzymatic activity of *P. roqueforti*. Mycelia development was significantly reduced following all three treatments but in direct correlation with the applied pressure. Furthermore, the spore viability was notably reduced after exposure to 300 MPa and completely inhibited at higher pressures. Similarly, the total lipolytic activity of the samples decreased with increasing pressure. Researchers reported similar results for the inhibition of different food spoilage fungi, such as *Penicillium* spp., *Fusarium* spp., and *Aspergillus* spp., in a liquid medium and cheese [96,99]. This suggests that HHP treatments are a promising option for the decontamination of cereal grains in particular, as the grains are known to withstand pressures of 400 MPa without sensory or grain quality deterioration. Thus, potential spoilage fungi and their hydrolytic enzymes could be completely inhibited, without the need for classic heat treatments or chemicals. However, asco-spores of heat-resistant moulds were also reported to possess a high resistance to HHP. Hence, pressure treatments routinely applied to foods do not result in sufficient inhibition. However, HHP appears to sensitize asco-spores to subsequent heat treatments. Thus, a combination of heat and pressure treatment appears very promising [99].

Although the prevention of fungal growth is the best way to ensure mycotoxin-free crops, minor in-field contamination can result in mycotoxins present in otherwise good quality cereals. Thus, the in vitro and in situ degradation of mycotoxins is another relevant topic of research. However, few studies have investigated the sensitivity of mycotoxins to HHP treatments. The degradation of patulin in fruit juices was reported after treatment with 600 MPa for 300 s at 11 °C [100]. Unfortunately, there are no studies available regarding HHP treatment of cereals for microbial decontamination or degradation of mycotoxins. In addition, as observed previously by several researchers, the sensitivity of pathogenic and spoilage organisms and their metabolic products greatly depends on a number of factors, including the surrounding sample matrix, microbial strain, processing conditions, and moisture levels [92,95,96,99,101,102]. Therefore, without sufficient studies on cereal grains and investigations of typical cereal contaminants, it is impossible to predict the efficiency of HHP treatments on the microbial decontamination of cereal grains prior to storage.

In conclusion, the application of HHP appears to represent a promising approach for ensuring microbial safety without the need for chemical preservatives. However, HHP treatments require the sample to be suspended in a liquid medium. Otherwise, the pressure applied cannot be distributed evenly, leading to unsatisfactory results. This ultimately would require high moisture levels in the stored grains or would necessitate an additional drying step after the initial HHP treatment. HHP treatment has been shown to be effective in reducing the microbial load of foods for both pathogenic and spoilage microorganisms with minimal impact on the product quality. However, that the treatment is unsuitable for in-line procedures and must be performed in a batch process presents its biggest draw-back. Various parameters such as pressure, time, temperature, and pH have to be considered to optimise the process in terms of both microbial inactivation and in consideration of final product quality [103].

In particular, the combination of HHP with heating treatments requires further research to fully exploit its potential in the development of new products.

7. Conclusion and Future Trends

Scientific evidence for the potential of each treatment as a tool for microbial decontamination is available. In particular, novel technologies not currently used in industry were found to present several advantages over established ones. For example, the use of superheated steam combines a faster, more efficient microbial decontamination with less impact on the grain quality compared to conventional saturated steam or hot air treatments. In addition, the use of e-beam irradiation, high hydrostatic pressure, and microwaves, based on non-thermal inactivation mechanisms, presents several advantages over more established technologies, such as gamma rays or UV light. However, due to their novelty, particularly in terms of microbial decontamination of cereals, the side effects of these technologies have been sparsely investigated. Therefore, further research is required to better understand the impact on the treated grains and the effect on spoilage organisms after exposure to sub-lethal doses.

Another topic investigated in this review was the degradation of in-field produced and accumulated mycotoxins to prevent a potential consumer health hazard. All the evaluated treatments showed some potential for reducing the mycotoxin content in cereals. However, as a result of their structural diversity (Table 1) and higher intrinsic resistance against many treatments, when compared to the living organisms, the reduction of the myxotoxigenic load was found to be a major challenge. In many cases, the treatment time and intensity had to be much higher for mycotoxin degradation than for the inhibition of living organisms. Thus, successful degradation of these toxins is a major challenge without compromising the grain's quality and seed viability. In addition, major concern related to the decay of mycotoxins are the degradation products released. The vast majority of research has examined the reduction in the level of the original parent mycotoxin, paying little attention to the degradation products or mechanism of degradation. Therefore, the identity of the degradation products and their toxicity is unknown. As a result, the efficiency of mycotoxin degradation cannot be evaluated as the released compounds may potentially be equal or even more toxic compared to the parent toxin. Future research will need to understand the possible degradation mechanisms to identify the resulting compounds. Only then will it be possible to assess their toxicity and evaluate the success and efficiency of the treatments discussed in this review. Furthermore, concerns regarding a possible reformation of the toxins during subsequent processing steps and the formation of masked mycotoxins due to the treatments merits greater research interest.

For both purposes, microbial decontamination and detoxification, each treatment encompasses associated difficulties for the successful application to cereals. The even and homogeneous treatment of the whole sample appears to be the biggest challenge. In addition, the efficiency of a treatment depends on various influential factors. The sample matrix, target organism, moisture content, and water availability were the most frequently observed influencing factors within the available literature. Thus, the treatment conditions and setting must be optimised for each crop to make industrial application possible. However, even under ideal process conditions it appears unlikely that one physical treatment can result in sufficient microbial decontamination and detoxification without substantial grain quality deterioration. Consequently, the combination of several treatments appears to represent the most promising approach for optimal results. Future research should therefore focus on understanding and the optimisation of the synergies which are likely to be achievable through combinatory treatments. Only then will it be possible to produce products that meet the highest standards in terms of food quality and safety.

Acknowledgments: Financial support for this research was awarded by the Irish Government under the National Development Plan 2007–2013 through the research program FIRM/RSF/CoFoRD. This research was also partly funded by the Irish Department of Agriculture, Food and the Marine.

Author Contributions: M.S., E.Z. and E.K.A. conveived and designed the work; M.S. wrote the review; E.Z. and E.K.A. proof read and revised the article.

References

1. Freita-Silva, O.; de Oliveira, P.S.; Freire Júnior, M. Potential of Electron Beams to Control Mycotoxigenic Fungi in Food. *Food Eng. Rev.* **2014**, 160–170. [CrossRef]
2. Oerke, E.-C. Crop losses to pests. *J. Agric. Sci.* **2006**, *144*, 31. [CrossRef]
3. Siciliano, I.; Spadaro, D.; Prelle, A.; Vallauri, D.; Cavallero, M.C.; Garibaldi, A.; Gullino, M.L. Use of cold atmospheric plasma to detoxify hazelnuts from aflatoxins. *Toxins* **2016**, *8*, 125. [CrossRef] [PubMed]
4. Magan, N.; Hope, R.; Cairns, V.; Aldred, D. Post-harvest fungal ecology: Impact of fungal growth and mycotoxin accumulation in stored grain. *Eur. J. Plant Pathol.* **2003**, *109*, 723–730. [CrossRef]
5. Oliveira, P.M.; Zannini, E.; Arendt, E.K. Cereal fungal infection, mycotoxins, and lactic acid bacteria mediated bioprotection: From crop farming to cereal products. *Food Microbiol.* **2014**, *37*, 78–95. [CrossRef] [PubMed]

6. Magan, N.; Aldred, D. Post-Harvest Control Strategies: Minimizingmycotoxins in the Food Chain. *Int. J. Food Microbiol.* **2007**, *119*, 131–139. [CrossRef] [PubMed]
7. Schmidt, M.; Horstmann, S.; De Colli, L.; Danaher, M.; Speer, K.; Zannini, E.; Arendt, E.K. Impact of fungal contamination of wheat on grain quality criteria. *J. Cereal Sci.* **2016**, *69*, 95–103. [CrossRef]
8. Audenaert, K.; Monbaliu, S.; Deschuyffeleer, N.; Maene, P.; Vekeman, F.; Haesaert, G.; De Saeger, S.; Eeckhout, M. Neutralized electrolyzed water efficiently reduces *Fusarium* spp. in vitro and on wheat kernels but can trigger deoxynivalenol (DON) biosynthesis. *Food Control* **2012**, *23*, 515–521. [CrossRef]
9. Cheli, F.; Pinotti, L.; Rossi, L.; Dell'Orto, V. Effect of milling procedures on mycotoxin distribution in wheat fractions: A review. *LWT—Food Sci. Technol.* **2013**, *54*, 307–314. [CrossRef]
10. Vidal, A.; Marín, S.; Ramos, A.J.; Cano-Sancho, G.; Sanchis, V. Determination of aflatoxins, deoxynivalenol, ochratoxin A and zearalenone in wheat and oat based bran supplements sold in the Spanish market. *Food Chem. Toxicol.* **2013**, *53*, 133–138. [CrossRef] [PubMed]
11. Magan, N.; Aldred, D. *Food Spoilage Microorganisms*; Woodhead Publishing: Sawston, UK, 2006.
12. Balasubramaniam (Bala), V.M.; Martínez-Monteagudo, S.I.; Gupta, R. Principles and Application of High Pressure–Based Technologies in the Food Industry. *Annu. Rev. Food Sci. Technol.* **2015**, *6*, 435–462. [CrossRef] [PubMed]
13. Crowley, S.; Mahony, J.; Van Sinderen, D. Current perspectives on antifungal lactic acid bacteria as natural bio-preservatives. *Trends Food Sci. Technol.* **2013**, *33*, 93–109. [CrossRef]
14. Pawlowska, A.M.; Zannini, E.; Coffey, A.; Arendt, E.K. "Green Preservatives": Combating Fungi in the Food and Feed Industry by Applying Antifungal Lactic Acid Bacteria. *Adv. Food Nutr. Res.* **2012**, *66*, 217–238. [CrossRef] [PubMed]
15. Magan, N.; Lacey, J. Effects of gas composition and water activity on growth of field and storage fungi and their interactions. *Trans. Br. Mycol. Soc.* **1984**, *82*, 305–314. [CrossRef]
16. Taniwaki, M.H.; Hocking, A.D.; Pitt, J.I.; Fleet, G.H. Growth of fungi and mycotoxin production on cheese under modified atmospheres. *Int. J. Food Microbiol.* **2001**, *68*, 125–133. [CrossRef]
17. Gupta, A.; Sinha, S.N.; Atwal, S.S. Modified Atmosphere Technology in Seed Health Management: Laboratory and Field Assay of Carbon Dioxide against Storage Fungi in Paddy. *Plant Pathol. J.* **2014**, *13*, 193–199. [CrossRef]
18. Savi, G.D.; Scussel, V.M. Effects of Ozone Gas Exposure on Toxigenic Fungi Species from *Fusarium*, *Aspergillus*, and *Penicillium* Genera. *Ozone Sci. Eng. J. Int. Ozone Assoc.* **2014**, *36*, 144–152. [CrossRef]
19. O'Donnell, C.P.; Tiwari, B.K.; Bourke, P.; Cullen, P.J. Effect of ultrasonic processing on food enzymes of industrial importance. *Trends Food Sci. Technol.* **2010**, *21*, 358–367. [CrossRef]
20. Klein, J.D.; Lurie, S. Postharvest heat treatment and fruit quality. *Postharvest News Inf.* **1991**, *2*, 15–19.
21. Lan, S. Effects of Post-Harvest Treatment and Heat Stress on the Antioxidant Properties of Wheat. Master's Thesis, University of Maryland, College Park, MD, USA, 3 August 2006.
22. Lehtinen, P.; Kiiliäinen, K.; Lehtomäki, I.; Laakso, S. Effect of Heat Treatment on Lipid Stability in Processed Oats. *J. Cereal Sci.* **2003**, *37*, 215–221. [CrossRef]
23. Rose, D.J.; Bianchini, A.; Martinez, B.; Flores, R.A. Methods for reducing microbial contamination of wheat flour and effects on functionality. *Cereal Foods World* **2012**, *57*, 104–109. [CrossRef]
24. Bari, L.; Ohki, H.; Nagakura, K.; Ukai, M. Application of Ultra Superheated Steam Technology (USST) to Food Grain Preservation at Ambient Temperature for Extended Periods of Time. *Adv. Food Technol. Nutr. Sci.* **2015**, *SE1*, S14–S21. [CrossRef]
25. Gilbert, J.; Woods, S.M.; Turkington, T.K.; Tekauz, A. Effect of heat treatment to control *Fusarium graminearum* in wheat seed. *Can. J. Plant Pathol.* **2005**, *27*, 448–452. [CrossRef]
26. Chang, Y.; Li, X.-P.; Liu, L.; Ma, Z.; Hu, X.; Zhao, W.; Gao, G. Effect of Processing in Superheated Steam on Surface Microbes and Enzyme Activity of Naked Oats. *J. Food Process. Preserv.* **2015**, *39*, 2753–2761. [CrossRef]
27. Hu, Y.; Nie, W.; Hu, X.; Li, Z. Microbial decontamination of wheat grain with superheated steam. *Food Control* **2016**, *62*, 264–269. [CrossRef]
28. Ban, G.-H.; Kang, D.-H. Effectiveness of superheated steam for inactivation of *Escherichia coli* O157:H7, *Salmonella* Typhimurium, *Salmonella* Enteritidis phage type 30, and *Listeria monocytogenes* on almonds and pistachios. *Int. J. Food Microbiol.* **2016**, *220*, 19–25. [CrossRef] [PubMed]

29. Cenkowski, S.; Pronyk, C.; Zmidzinska, D.; Muir, W.E. Decontamination of food products with superheated steam. *J. Food Eng.* **2007**, *83*, 68–75. [CrossRef]
30. Clear, R.M.; Patrick, S.K.; Wallis, R.; Turkington, T.K. Effect of dry heat treatment on seed-borne *Fusarium graminearum* and other cereal pathogens. *Can. J. Plant Pathol.* **2002**, *24*, 489–498. [CrossRef]
31. Bond, W.W.; Favero, M.S.; Petersen, N.J.; Marshall, J.H. Dry-heat inactivation kinetics of naturally occurring spore populations. *Appl. Microbiol.* **1970**, *20*, 573–578. [PubMed]
32. Nielsen, K.F.; Holm, G.; Uttrup, L.P.; Nielsen, P.A. Mould growth on building materials under low water activities. Influence of humidity and temperature on fungal growth and secondary metabolism. *Int. Biodeterior. Biodegrad.* **2004**, *54*, 325–336. [CrossRef]
33. Miller, J.D.; Trenholm, H.L. *Mycotoxins in Grain Compounds Other than Aflatoxin*; Eagan Press: Saint Paul, MN, USA, 1997.
34. Bretz, M.; Knecht, A.; Göckler, S.; Humpf, H.U. Structural elucidation and analysis of thermal degradation products of the *Fusarium* mycotoxin nivalenol. *Mol. Nutr. Food Res.* **2005**, *49*, 309–316. [CrossRef] [PubMed]
35. Vidal, A.; Sanchis, V.; Ramos, A.J.; Marín, S. Thermal stability and kinetics of degradation of deoxynivalenol, deoxynivalenol conjugates and ochratoxin A during baking of wheat bakery products. *Food Chem.* **2015**, *178*, 276–286. [CrossRef] [PubMed]
36. Boudra, H.; Lebars, P.; Lebars, J. Thermostability of Ochratoxin A in Wheat under 2 Moisture Conditions. *Appl. Environ. Microbiol.* **1995**, *61*, 1156–1158. [PubMed]
37. Syamaladevi, R.M.; Tang, J.; Villa-Rojas, R.; Sablani, S.; Carter, B.; Campbell, G. Influence of Water Activity on Thermal Resistance of Microorganisms in Low-Moisture Foods: A Review. *Compr. Rev. Food Sci. Food Saf.* **2016**, *15*, 353–370. [CrossRef]
38. Ban, G.H.; Yoon, H.; Kang, D.H. A comparison of saturated steam and superheated steam for inactivation of *Escherichia coli* O157: H7, *Salmonella* Typhimurium, and *Listeria monocytogenes* biofilms on polyvinyl chloride and stainless steel. *Food Control* **2014**, *40*, 344–350. [CrossRef]
39. Alfy, A.; Kiran, B.V.; Jeevitha, G.C.; Hebbar, H.U. Recent Developments in Superheated Steam Processing of Foods—A Review. *Crit. Rev. Food Sci. Nutr.* **2016**, *56*, 2191–2208. [CrossRef] [PubMed]
40. Jalili, M. A Review on Aflatoxins Reduction in Food. *Iran. J. Health Saf. Environ.* **2015**, *3*, 445–459.
41. Nemţanu, M.R.; Braşoveanu, M.; Karaca, G.; Erper, I. Inactivation effect of electron beam irradiation on fungal load of naturally contaminated maize seeds. *J. Sci. Food Agric.* **2014**, *94*, 2668–2673. [CrossRef] [PubMed]
42. Dev, S.R.S.; Birla, S.L.; Raghavan, G.S.V.; Subbiah, J. Microbial decontamination of food by microwave (MW) and radiao frequency (RF). In *Microbial Decontamination in the Food Industry*; Novel Methods and Applications; Woodhead Publishing: Sawston, UK, 2012; pp. 274–299.
43. FAO/IAEA Training Manual on Food Irradiation Technology and Techniques. In *Technical Reports Series, Proceedings of the International Atomic Energy Commission*; IAEA Publications: Vienna, Austria, 1982; p. 224.
44. Mahmoud, N.S.; Awad, S.H.; Madani, R.M.A.; Osman, F.A.; Elmamoun, K.; Hassan, A.B. Effect of γ radiation processing on fungal growth and quality characteristcs of millet grains. *Food Sci. Nutr.* **2016**, *4*, 342–347. [CrossRef] [PubMed]
45. D'Ovidio, K.L.; Trucksess, M.W.; Devries, J.W.; Bean, G. Effects of irradiation on fungi and fumonisin B1 in corn, and of microwave-popping on fumonisins in popcorn. *Food Addit. Contam.* **2007**, *24*, 735–743. [CrossRef] [PubMed]
46. Lung, H.-M.; Cheng, Y.-C.; Chang, Y.-H.; Huang, H.-W.; Yang, B.B.; Wang, C.-Y. Microbial decontamination of food by electron beam irradiation. *Trends Food Sci. Technol.* **2015**, *44*, 66–78. [CrossRef]
47. Supriya, P.; Sridhar, K.R.; Ganesh, S. Fungal decontamination and enhancement of shelf life of edible split beans of wild legume Canavalia maritima by the electron beam irradiation. *Radiat. Phys. Chem.* **2014**, *96*, 5–11. [CrossRef]
48. Salem, E.A.; Soliman, S.A.; El-Karamany, A.M.; El-shafea, Y.M.A. Effect of Utilization of Gamma Radiation Treatment and Storage on Total Fungal Count, Chemical Composition and Technological Properties Wheat Grain. *Egypt. J. Biol. Pest Control* **2016**, *26*, 163–171.
49. Aziz, N.H.; El-Far, F.M.; Shahin, A.A.M.; Roushy, S.M. Control of *Fusarium* moulds and fumonisin B1 in seeds by gamma-irradiation. *Food Control* **2007**, *18*, 1337–1342. [CrossRef]

50. Carocho, M.; Antonio, A.L.; Barreira, J.C.M.; Rafalski, A.; Bento, A.; Ferreira, I.C.F.R. Validation of Gamma and Electron Beam Irradiation as Alternative Conservation Technology for European Chestnuts. *Food Bioprocess Technol.* **2014**, *7*, 1917–1927. [CrossRef]
51. Carocho, M.; Barros, L.; Antonio, A.L.; Barreira, J.C.M.; Bento, A.; Kaluska, I.; Ferreira, I.C.F.R. Analysis of organic acids in electron beam irradiated chestnuts (*Castanea sativa* Mill.): Effects of radiation dose and storage time. *Food Chem. Toxicol.* **2013**, *55*, 348–352. [CrossRef] [PubMed]
52. Akueche, E.C.; Anjorin, S.T.; Harcourt, B.I.; Kana, D. Studies on fungal load, total aflatoxins and ochratoxin a contents of gamma-irradiated and non-irradiated Sesamum indicum grains from Abuja markets, Nigeria. *Kasetsart J. Nat. Sci.* **2012**, *46*, 371–382.
53. Herzallah, S.; Alshawabkeh, K.; Al Fataftah, A. Aflatoxin decontamination of artificially contaminated feeds by sunlight, γ-radiation, and microwave heating. *J. Appl. Poult. Res.* **2008**, *17*, 515–521. [CrossRef]
54. Jalili, M.; Jinap, S.; Noranizan, M.A. Aflatoxins and ochratoxin a reduction in black and white pepper by gamma radiation. *Radiat. Phys. Chem.* **2012**, *81*, 1786–1788. [CrossRef]
55. Mehrez, A.; Maatouk, I.; Romero-González, R.; Ben Amara, A.; Kraiem, M.; Garrido Frenich, A.; Landoulsi, A. Assessment of ochratoxin A stability following gamma irradiation: Experimental approaches for feed detoxification perspectives. *World Mycotoxin J.* **2016**, *9*, 289–298. [CrossRef]
56. Hooshmand, H.; Klopfenstein, C.F. Effects of gamma irradiation on mycotoxin disappearance and amino acid contents of corn, wheat, and soybeans with different moisture contents. *Plant Foods Hum. Nutr.* **1995**, *47*, 227–238. [CrossRef] [PubMed]
57. Carocho, M.; Barreira, J.C.; Antonio, A.L.; Bento, A.; Kaluska, I.; Ferreira, I.C. Effects of electron beam radiation on nutritional parameters of Portuguese chestnuts (*Castanea sativa* mill.). *J. Agric. Food Chem.* **2012**, *60*, 7754–7760. [CrossRef] [PubMed]
58. El-Naggar, S.M.; Mikhaiel, A.A. Disinfestation of stored wheat grain and flour using gamma rays and microwave heating. *J. Stored Prod. Res.* **2011**, *47*, 191–196. [CrossRef]
59. Melki, M.; Marouani, A. Effects of gamma rays irradiation on seed germination and growth of hard wheat. *Environ. Chem. Lett.* **2010**, *8*, 307–310. [CrossRef]
60. Deberghes, P.; Betbeder, A.M.; Boisard, F.; Blanc, R.; Delaby, J.F.; Krivobok, S.; Steiman, R.; Seigle-Murandi, F.; Creppy, E.E. Detoxification of ochratoxin A, a food contaminant: Prevention of growth of *Aspergillus ochraceus* and its production of ochratoxin A. *Mycotoxin Res.* **1995**, *11*, 37–47. [CrossRef] [PubMed]
61. Di Stefano, V.; Pitonzo, R.; Cicero, N.; D'Oca, M.C. Mycotoxin contamination of animal feedingstuff: Detoxification by gamma-irradiation and reduction of aflatoxins and ochratoxin A concentrations. *Food Addit. Contam. Part A* **2014**, *31*, 2034–2039. [CrossRef] [PubMed]
62. Aquino, S.; Ferreira, F.; Ribeiro, D.H.B.; Corrêa, B.; Greiner, R.; Villavicencio, A.L.C.H. Evaluation of viability of *Aspergillus flavus* and aflatoxins degradation in irradiated samples of maize. *Braz. J. Microbiol.* **2005**, *36*, 352–356. [CrossRef]
63. Farag, R.S.; El-Baroty, G.S.; Abo-Hagger, A.A. Aflatoxin destruction and residual toxicity of contaminated-irradiated yellow corn and peanuts on rats. *Adv. Food Sci.* **2004**, *26*, 122–129.
64. Prado, G.; de Carvalho, E.P.; Oliveira, M.S.; Madeira, J.G.C.; Morais, V.D.; Correa, R.F.; Cardoso, V.N.; Soares, T.V.; da Silva, J.F.M.; Gonçalves, R.C.P. Effect of gamma irradiation on the inactivation of aflatoxin B1 and fungal flora in peanut. *Braz. J. Microbiol.* **2003**, *34*, 138–140. [CrossRef]
65. Wang, F.; Xie, F.; Xue, X.; Wang, Z.; Fan, B.; Ha, Y. Structure elucidation and toxicity analyses of the radiolytic products of aflatoxin B_1 in methanol-water solution. *J. Hazard. Mater.* **2011**, *192*, 1192–1202. [CrossRef] [PubMed]
66. Kume, T.; Furuta, M.; Todoriki, S.; Uenoyama, N.; Kobayashi, Y. Status of food irradiation in the world. *Radiat. Phys. Chem.* **2009**, *78*, 222–226. [CrossRef]
67. Kottapalli, B.; Wolf-Hall, C.E.; Schwarz, P. Effect of electron-beam irradiation on the safety and quality of *Fusarium*-infected malting barley. *Int. J. Food Microbiol.* **2006**, *110*, 224–231. [CrossRef] [PubMed]
68. Stepanik, T.; Kost, D.; Nowicki, T.; Gaba, D. Effects of electron beam irradiation on deoxynivalenol levels in distillers dried grain and solubles and in production intermediates. *Food Addit. Contam.* **2007**, *24*, 1001–1006. [CrossRef] [PubMed]
69. Lanza, C.M.; Mazzaglia, A.; Paladino, R.; Auditore, L.; Barnà, D.; Loria, D.; Trifirò, A.; Trimarchi, M.; Bellia, G. Characterization of peeled and unpeeled almond (*Prunus amygdalus*) flour after electron beam processing. *Radiat. Phys. Chem.* **2013**, *86*, 140–144. [CrossRef]

70. Schoeller, N.P.; Ingham, S.C.; Ingham, B.H. Assessment of the Potential for *Listeria monocytogenes* Survival and Growth during Alfalfa Sprout Production and Use of Ionizing Radiation as a Potential Intervention Treatment. *J. Food Prot.* **2002**, *8*, 1259–1266. [CrossRef]
71. Kikuchi, O.K.; Todoriki, S.; Saito, M.; Hayashi, T. Efficacy of soft-electron (low-energy electron beam) for soybean decontamination in comparison with gamma-rays. *J. Food Sci.* **2003**, *68*, 649–652. [CrossRef]
72. Farkas, J.; Mohacsi-Farkas, C. History and future of food irradiation. *Trends Food Sci. Technol.* **2011**, *22*, 121–126. [CrossRef]
73. Oms-Oliu, G.; Martín-Belloso, O.; Soliva-Fortuny, R. Pulsed light treatments for food preservation. A review. *Food Bioprocess Technol.* **2010**, *3*, 13–23. [CrossRef]
74. Aron Maftei, N.; Ramos-Villarroel, A.Y.; Nicolau, A.I.; Martín-Belloso, O.; Soliva-Fortuny, R. Pulsed light inactivation of naturally occurring moulds on wheat grain. *J. Sci. Food Agric.* **2014**, *94*, 721–726. [CrossRef] [PubMed]
75. Nicorescu, I.; Nguyen, B.; Moreau-Ferret, M.; Agoulon, A.; Chevalier, S.; Orange, N. Pulsed light inactivation of Bacillus subtilis vegetative cells in suspensions and spices. *Food Control* **2013**, *31*, 151–157. [CrossRef]
76. Schmidt-Heydt, M.; Cramer, B.; Graf, I.; Lerch, S.; Hunpf, H.-U.; Geisen, R. Wavelength-dependent degradation of ochratoxin and citrinin by light in vitro and in vivo and its implications on *Penicillium*. *Toxins* **2012**, *4*, 1535–1551. [CrossRef] [PubMed]
77. Jubeen, F.; Bhatti, I.A.; Khan, M.Z.; Shahid, M. Effect of UVC Irradiation on Aflatoxins in Ground Nut (*Arachis hypogea*) and Tree Nuts (*Juglans regia*, *Prunus duclus* and *Pistachio vera*). *Chem. Soc. Pak.* **2012**, *34*, 1–10.
78. Liu, R.; Jin, Q.; Tao, G.; Shan, L.; Huang, J.; Liu, Y.; Wang, X.; Mao, W.; Wang, S. Photodegradation kinetics and byproducts identification of the Aflatoxin B1 in aqueous medium by ultra-performance liquid chromatography-quadrupole time-of-flight mass spectrometry. *J. Mass Spectrom.* **2010**, *45*, 553–559. [CrossRef] [PubMed]
79. Liu, R.; Chang, M.; Jin, Q.; Huang, J.; Liu, Y.; Wang, X. Degradation of aflatoxin B1 in aqueous medium through UV irradiation. *Eur. Food Res. Technol.* **2011**, *233*, 1007–1012. [CrossRef]
80. Fang, Y.; Hu, J.; Xiong, S.; Zhao, S. Effect of low-dose microwave radiation on *Aspergillus parasiticus*. *Food Control* **2011**, 22, 1078–1084. [CrossRef]
81. Ursu, M.-P. Usage of Microwaves for Decontamination of Sensible Materials and Cereal Seeds. *Rev. Tehnol. Neconv.* **2015**, *19*, 60–64.
82. Kabak, B.; Dobson, A.D.; Var, I. Strategies to Prevent Mycotoxin Contamination of Food and Animal Feed: A Review. *Crit. Rev. Food Sci. Nutr.* **2006**, *46*, 593–619. [CrossRef] [PubMed]
83. Basaran, P.; Akhan, Ü. Microwave irradiation of hazelnuts for the control of aflatoxin producing *Aspergillus parasiticus*. *Innov. Food Sci. Emerg. Technol.* **2010**, *11*, 113–117. [CrossRef]
84. Feng, H.; Yang, W.; Hielscher, T. Power Ultrasound. *Food Sci. Technol. Int.* **2008**, *14*, 433–436. [CrossRef]
85. Butz, P.; Tauscher, B. Emerging technologies: Chemical aspects. *Food Res. Int.* **2002**, *35*, 279–284. [CrossRef]
86. Chemat, F.; Zill-E-Huma; Khan, M.K. Applications of ultrasound in food technology: Processing, preservation and extraction. *Ultrason. Sonochem.* **2011**, *18*, 813–835. [CrossRef] [PubMed]
87. Bilek, S.E.; Turantaş, F. Decontamination efficiency of high power ultrasound in the fruit and vegetable industry, a review. *Int. J. Food Microbiol.* **2013**, *166*, 155–162. [CrossRef] [PubMed]
88. Scouten, A.J.; Beuchat, L.R. Combined effects of chemical, heat and ultrasound treatments to kill *Salmonella* and *Escherichia coli* O157:H7 on alfalfa seeds. *J. Appl. Microbiol.* **2002**, *92*, 668–674. [CrossRef] [PubMed]
89. Seymour, I.J.; Burfoot, D.; Smith, R.L.; Cox, L.A.; Lockwood, A. Ultrasound decontamination of minimally processed fruits and vegetables. *Int. J. Food Sci. Technol.* **2002**, *37*, 547–557. [CrossRef]
90. Herceg, Z.; Jambrak, R.R.; Vukušić, T.; Stulić, V.; Stanzer, D.; Milošević, S. The effect of high-power ultrasound and gas phase plasma treatment on *Aspergillus* spp. and *Penicillium* spp. count in pure culture. *J. Appl. Microbiol.* **2015**, *118*, 132–141. [CrossRef] [PubMed]
91. Lindner, W.; Hasenhuti, K. Decontamination and Detoxification of Corn Which Was Contaminated with Trichothecenes Applying Ultrasonication (Abstr.). In Proceedings of the IX Internat IUPAC Symposium on Mycotoxins and Phytotoxins, Rome, Italy, 7–31 May 1996; p. 182.
92. Heinz, V.; Buckow, R. Food preservation by high pressure. *J. Verbrauch. Lebensmittelsich.* **2009**, *5*, 73–81. [CrossRef]
93. Polydera, A.C.; Stoforos, N.G.; Taoukis, P.S. Comparative shelf life study and vitamin C loss kinetics in pasteurised and high pressure processed reconstituted orange juice. *J. Food Eng.* **2003**, *60*, 21–29. [CrossRef]

94. Wannasawat Ratphitagsanti, M. *Approaches for Enhancing Lethality of Bacterial Spores Treated by Pressure-Assisted Thermal Processing*; ProQuest Dissertations Publishing: Ann Arbor, MI, USA, 2009.
95. Patterson, M.F. Microbiology of pressure-treated foods. *J. Appl. Microbiol.* **2005**, *98*, 1400–1409. [CrossRef] [PubMed]
96. O'Reilly, C.E.; O'Connor, P.M.; Kelly, A.L.; Beresford, T.P.; Murphy, P.M. Use of hydrostatic pressure for inactivation of microbial contaminants in cheese. *Appl. Environ. Microbiol.* **2000**, *66*, 4890–4896. [CrossRef] [PubMed]
97. Willford, J.; Mendonca, A.; Goodridge, L. Water Pressure Effectively Reduces Salmonella enterica Serovar Enteritidis on the Surface of Raw Almonds. *J. Food Prot.* **2008**, *4*, 825–829. [CrossRef]
98. Bello, E.F.T.; Martínez, G.G.; Klotz Ceberio, B.F.; Rodrigo, D.; López, A.M. High Pressure Treatment in Foods. *Foods* **2014**, *3*, 476–490. [CrossRef] [PubMed]
99. Black, E.P.; Setlow, P.; Hocking, A.D.; Stewart, C.M.; Kelly, A.L.; Hoover, D.G. Response of spores to high-pressure processing. *Compr. Rev. Food Sci. Food Saf.* **2007**, *6*, 103–119. [CrossRef]
100. Hao, H.; Zhou, T.; Koutchma, T.; Wu, F.; Warriner, K. High hydrostatic pressure assisted degradation of patulin in fruit and vegetable juice blends. *Food Control* **2016**, *62*, 237–242. [CrossRef]
101. Martínez-Rodríguez, Y.; Acosta-Muñiz, C.; Olivas, G.I.; Guerrero-Beltrán, J.; Rodrigo-Aliaga, D.; Mujica-Paz, H.; Welti-Chanes, J.; Sepulveda, D.R. Effect of high hydrostatic pressure on mycelial development, spore viability and enzyme activity of *Penicillium Roqueforti. Int. J. Food Microbiol.* **2014**, *168–169*, 42–46. [CrossRef] [PubMed]
102. Smith, K.; Mendonca, A.; Jung, S. Impact of high-pressure processing on microbial shelf-life and protein stability of refrigerated soymilk. *Food Microbiol.* **2009**, *26*, 794–800. [CrossRef] [PubMed]
103. Torres, J.A.; Saraiva, J.A.; Guerra-Rodríguez, E.; Aubourg, S.P.; Vázquez, M. Effect of combining high-pressure processing and frozen storage on the functional and sensory properties of horse mackerel (*Trachurus trachurus*). *Innov. Food Sci. Emerg. Technol.* **2014**, *21*, 2–11. [CrossRef]

9

Fat Replacers in Baked Food Products

Kathryn Colla, Andrew Costanzo and Shirani Gamlath *

Centre for Advanced Sensory Sciences, School of Exercise and Nutrition Sciences, Deakin University, 1 Gheringhap Street, Geelong 3220, Australia; k.colla@deakin.edu.au (K.C.); andrew.costanzo@deakin.edu.au (A.C.)

* Correspondence: shirani.gamlath@deakin.edu.au

Abstract: Fat provides important sensory properties to baked food products, such as colour, taste, texture and odour, all of which contribute to overall consumer acceptance. Baked food products, such as crackers, cakes and biscuits, typically contain high amounts of fat. However, there is increasing demand for healthy snack foods with reduced fat content. In order to maintain consumer acceptance whilst simultaneously reducing the total fat content, fat replacers have been employed. There are a number of fat replacers that have been investigated in baked food products, ranging from complex carbohydrates, gums and gels, whole food matrices, and combinations thereof. Fat replacers each have different properties that affect the quality of a food product. In this review, we summarise the literature on the effect of fat replacers on the quality of baked food products. The ideal fat replacers for different types of low-fat baked products were a combination of polydextrose and guar gum in biscuits at 70% fat replacement (FR), oleogels in cake at 100% FR, and inulin in crackers at 75% FR. The use of oatrim (100% FR), bean puree (75% FR) or green pea puree (75% FR) as fat replacers in biscuits were equally successful.

Keywords: fat replacers; baked products; carbohydrates; gums; gels; whole foods

---

1. Introduction

Dietary fat has an important role within food matrices beyond basic nutrition. It contributes to many sensory and quality properties of a food including physical, textural and olfactory factors which all influence overall palatability. Many snack foods, in particular, rely on dietary fat to fulfil these palatable qualities in order to maintain consumer acceptance and consumption. The World Health Organisation [1], along with many national health authorities [2–5], recommends decreasing consumption of discretionary snack foods due to their poor nutritional content. Excess dietary fat intake, notably from discretionary snack foods, is one of the key contributors to excess energy intake and therefore weight gain [6]. Prevalence of overweight and obesity is rising worldwide [7,8] which is cause for concern as obesity is associated with increased risk of cardiovascular disease [9], type 2 diabetes mellitus [10], and some cancers [11].

Despite consumer awareness and product labelling [12,13], consumption of snack foods is relatively high with little compensation for the increased energy intake [14–16]. Many promoters have been attributed to increased snack food intake, such as convenience, taste, marketing and pricing [16,17]. In order to respond to these recommendations and consumer demands, manufacturing companies are increasingly developing snacks which are more nutrient dense than traditional snacks such as chips and cakes, which are typically high in added fat, sugar and sodium. Some examples of these types of innovative snacks include yoghurts, bars, puddings, crackers and chips which contain popular health foods (or superfoods) such as seeds, nuts, ancient grains, other wholegrains, dietary fibres, legumes, fruits and vegetables. While many of these snacks may be high in protein and dietary fibre, many also typically contribute large amounts of fat, sugar and sodium to the consumers' diet [18].

Efforts must be made to develop appealing snacks which are both high in protein and dietary fibre while not contributing large amounts of sodium, sugar and fat. Snack food categories such as cakes and muffins are yet to see significant innovation in creating high protein or high fibre alternatives [16]. In addition, there are still limited reduced fat options of these baked products on the market, likely attributed to the technological difficulty in producing such products. Ultimately, there is a need to increase the number of nutritious snack options available that satisfy the above drivers, while reducing fat composition and therefore total energy intake. Baked snack foods that omit dietary fat as a "low-fat" alternative often have poor sensory properties, such as crumbliness, dryness, poor mouthfeel and overall reduced consumer acceptance [19–23]. A number of potential "fat replacers" have been purported in order to reduce the fat content in food matrices whilst maintaining the sensory properties that are usually attributed to dietary fat. Fat replacers are subcategorised as either fat substitutes or fat mimetics. Fat substitutes replicate the functional and sensory properties of fat in a food, usually contain no energy or less energy than fat, and may be used to replace some or all of the fat normally present in a product [24,25]. Fat mimetics are protein- or carbohydrate-based ingredients that are not used to fully substitute the use of fat, but rather replicate some of the properties that fat provides within a food [24,25]. Many baked products on the market currently utilise fat replacers in order to reduce the total energy or fat content whilst maintaining consumer acceptance. This review aims to summarise the current evidence for application of fat replacers in biscuits, crackers, muffins, cakes and bread, and their effect on quality and sensory properties.

2. Application of Fat Replacers in Baked Products

Fat replacers are defined by the American Dietetic Association as "an ingredient that can be used to provide some or all of the functions of fat, yielding fewer calories than fat" [24]. A wide range of products in the food industry uses fat replacers, some of which include meat, dairy and baked products [24]. It is important for product developers and food technologists to understand how different fat replacers influence the sensory and physical quality of snacks in order to guide the development of healthier alternative products. For example, in cakes, fat can contribute to increased leavening, tenderness and a finer crumb through a combined effect of trapping air cells during the creaming process [26]. This structure is then set during baking due to starch gelatinisation and coagulation of egg proteins [26]. Fat is typically used in biscuits to lubricate and coat the flour granules to prevent water absorption, and the development of starch and gluten in order to achieve a fine crumb (crumbly texture) and soft, tender mouthfeel [27]. Fat also contributes other important functions to cakes, biscuits and crackers such as flavour delivery and shelf life which is achieved through delaying water absorption by starch granules [28–31].

Fat replacers can be ingredients which are of carbohydrate, protein or fat origin, with many different types of fat replacers with different structures and functions within each group. We have not differentiated fat substitutes and fat mimetics in this review as the majority of fat replacers used in baked food products are fat mimetics. Instead, we have categorised fat replacers in this review as complex carbohydrate powders, gums and gels, whole food purees and products, or a combination thereof. This categorisation is based on their functional and industrial applications rather than their chemical properties.

(a) Complex carbohydrates are typically successful fat replacers due to their ability to bind water to form a paste which can mimic the texture and viscosity of fats in food products through providing lubricant or flow properties similar to fat in some food systems [28,32]. Examples of carbohydrate based fat replacers include inulin, maltodextrin and plant fibres.

(b) Gums and gels work similarly in function to complex carbohydrates, in that they bind with water to form gels which mimic the texture and viscosity of fats [28]. While some gums and gels are made up of complex carbohydrates, this is not specific as there are some protein- and fat-based gums and gels. Examples of gums and gels used as fat replacers include pectins, oleogels and whey protein.

(c) Whole foods are complete or partial food matrices that are included in a food product as fat replacers. Recently, many products have utilised whole foods such as fruits and vegetables, legumes or cereal based ingredients as fat replacers. These foods are typically successful due to their highly creamy texture when mashed or processed. Foods such as avocado can achieve this due to its oil composition, banana for its high starch content, and legumes for their high starch and protein contents.

(d) Combinations of the above fat replacers are useful as they can potentially replicate multiple sensory qualities of dietary fat. In addition, complexes formed from these combinations, such as emulsions and esters, may have a greater fat replacing effect than the sum of their parts.

3. Summary of the Current Fat Replacers Used in Baked Products

Complex carbohydrate fat replacers range from digestible starches to non-digestible plant fibres (Table 1). It should be noted that the replacement of dietary fat with complex carbohydrates reduced energy density of all the food products in Table 1, regardless of fibre status, due to complex carbohydrate being less energy dense than fat. The use of fibres instead of starches could have an advantage on the market, as foods may meet criteria for fibre content claims. Inulin, a non-digestible dietary fibre typically derived from chicory root, was observed to have the greatest success in replacing dietary fat in baked products, where a fat replacement (FR) level of up to 75% in legume crackers and cake (1:1, inulin: water; and 1:2 inulin: water, respectively) was able to reduce total energy without any changes in consumer acceptance [33,34]. It should be noted that the addition of inulin did change the textural and physical properties of the cracker and cake products. While acceptance was not measured for the use of inulin in muffins, 50% FR had the least sensory and physical changes compared to 75% and 100% FR [35]. In addition, Zahn et al. tested the use of four commercial inulin formulations in muffins which varied in inulin to water ratio and solubility, but the outcomes for each were similar [35]. Maltodextrin was also successful at 75% fat replacer level in legume crackers and at 66% FR in muffins, although there were changes noted in aroma, appearance, taste and texture [33,36]. Total FR of inulin or maltodextrin (100%) had a significant decrease in consumer acceptance, so it is not recommended to fully replace fat in a baked food product. Results were also promising for inulin used as a fat replacer in biscuits, although there was some notable changes to textural and physical properties [33–35,37–39]. Other complex carbohydrates used as fat replacers in biscuits included lupine extract, maltodextrin, corn fibre, and rice starch, although all of these had significant effects on sensory properties of the biscuits except rice starch [33,36,40–43]. Rice starch has no significant effects on sensory properties, but was only tested at 20% FR. All complex carbohydrate fat replacers had a significant effect on the physical properties of doughs and their baked products, with significant increases in density, toughness, breaking strength, moisture, and decreases in volume for nearly all tested products [33–46].

Of all the complex carbohydrate fat replacers, inulin had the greatest success at reducing total fat and energy of the food product, with the least impact on sensory qualities and consumer acceptance, particularly in the legume crackers. Long chain inulin has the ability to form microcrystals which in turn aggregate together, interact with water, and eventually agglomerate creating a gel network [47]. To some extent, this gel network seems to have the ability to mimic the functions of fat in baked products such as being able to lubricate dry ingredients (through surrounding starch and protein), assisting in maintaining a shortening effect. Maltodextrin was also a successful fat replacer in legume crackers, although it was not as successful at replacing fat in biscuits compared to inulin. Inulin is also a good source of fibre, has promising gut health properties due to its prebiotic nature, and may increase absorption of nutrients such as calcium [48]. Moreover, inulin may benefit from marketing with fibre content claims, which may be appealing to consumers. Therefore, we recommend inulin as a reasonably high level fat replacer in crackers, cakes, biscuits and muffins [48].

Table 1. Summary of quality changes of complex carbohydrate fat replacers in baked food products.

Fat Replacer	Food(s)	FR Tested	Quality Changes
Inulin	Legume Cracker [33] Cake [34] Biscuit [37–39] Muffin [35]	25–100% 9.3–50% 35–100% 50–100%	Physical: ↓ cell density, aW, volume; ↑ breaking strength, dough consistency, moisture, crumb density, firmness, springiness; NSC cohesiveness Sensory: ↓ buttery flavour, crumbliness, acceptance (100% FR), embrowning (muffin: 50%), open surface, arched shape, typical smell, sweetness, typical taste; ↑ toasted flavour, chewiness, adhesiveness, springiness (100% FR), crispiness, crunchiness, dryness, toughness hardness, glossiness; NSC acceptance (50–75% FR)
Lupine Extract	Biscuit [40]	30–40%	Physical: ↓ volume, lightness; ↑ breaking strength, dough consistency, aW, moisture Sensory: ↓ sweetness; ↑ firmness, dryness, chewing time, roasted flavour
Maltodextrin	Biscuit [40,41] Legume Cracker [33] Muffin [36] Croissant [42]	30–40% 25–100% 66% 25–100%	Physical: ↓ volume, spread ratio; ↑ breaking strength, dough consistency, aW, moisture, cohesiveness, chewiness; NSC hardness, springiness Sensory: ↓ sweetness, overall flavour, aroma, colour, appearance, texture, taste, flavor, overall acceptance (muffin); ↑ firmness, dryness, chewing time; NSC acceptance (legumes cracker: 50–75% FR), mouthfeel
Corn Fibre	Biscuit [40]	30–40%	Physical: ↓ volume; ↑ breaking strength, dough consistency, aW, moisture Sensory: ↓ sweetness; ↑ firmness, dryness, chewing time
Rice Starch	Biscuit [43] Muffin [43]	20% 20%	Physical: ↓ volume, height (muffins); ↑ thickness (biscuit) Sensory: NSC all sensory qualities
Resistant Starch	Biscuit [34]	40%	Physical: ↓ hardness; ↑ spread ratio
Polydextrose	Biscuit [41,45,46]	11.5–50%	Physical: ↑ hardness, brittleness, aW, breaking strength; ↓ penetration distance, spread ratio [41] Sensory: ↑ hardness, ↓ overall flavour, appearance, texture, taste, acceptance, NSC colour

aW: Water activity; FR: Fat replacement; NSC: No significant change; ↓: decrease; ↑: increase.

Gum and gel fat replacers, while mostly being carbohydrates, also include lipid-based and protein-based gums and gels (Table 2). Some of these fat replacers may also increase suitability for nutrition content claims, such as sources of fibre or protein. Guar gum and xanthan gum had relatively little effect on the physical properties of the cake product when used as fat replacers [49]. While sensory measures were not compared to a control, both types of cakes were rated as acceptable with a greater acceptance in the cake containing xanthan gum, and 50% FR was considered ideal [49]. Oatrim (a tasteless white powder derived from oats, comprised of amylodextrins and 5–10% β-glucan soluble fiber; incorporated as a powder or gel), caused significant changes to the physical properties of cake, croissants and biscuits [50–52]. However, this did not appear to have any impact on the sensory properties of these foods, even at 100% FR. Pectin also caused significant changes to the physical properties of cake, croissants and biscuits, specifically increasing the hardness and reducing the volume of these foods, which was paralleled by increased perception of hardness and reduced flavour from sensory evaluations [42,46,53,54]. This is notable as pectin was tested at a relatively low FR level in cake and biscuits (10–30%), suggesting it is not an ideal fat replacer in baked products. Hydroxypropyl methylcellulose (HPMC) had significant effects on physical and sensory properties of crackers and biscuits, even at relatively low FR levels [33,55]. While consumer acceptance was not tested on crackers due to being considered unacceptable by a focus group [33], HPMC in biscuits was considered significantly less acceptable compared to control biscuits containing 18% canola oil suggesting it is also not an ideal fat replacer in these foods.

Oleogels are products of solidifying vegetable oils using natural wax esters [56–59]. The oleogelation process forms waxy crystal structure which hold liquid oil within a solid matrix, which allows the use of liquid vegetable oils in place of shortening. While this does not necessarily reduce the total fat content of a food product, it is useful in reducing saturated fat content. It should be noted that all oleogels studies reviewed in this paper did reduce overall fat content of their tested foods [56–59]. However, oleogels were not successful as fat replacers in these studies as they made biscuit and cake denser and harder. Sensory properties seemed to be promising with an increase in taste and no difference in acceptance compared to the control foods. Lastly, whey protein was also not an ideal fat replacer for biscuits as it resulted in a decrease in overall flavour and acceptance [45,46].

Overall, gums and gels were not very successful as fat replacers in baked goods. Oatrim appeared to be the most successful as there were no significant changes to the sensory properties of cake and biscuits, although there were a large range of physical changes to these foods which might have an impact on industrial applications. Xanthan gum and guar gum might potential be useful fat replacers in cake as they had little impact on physical properties, although more robust sensory evaluations are needed in future studies.

Table 2. Summary of quality changes of gum and gel fat replacers in baked food products.

Fat Replacer	Food(s)	FR Tested	Quality Changes
Xanthan Gum	Cake [49]	25–100%	Physical: ↓ volume (100% FR), elasticity; ↑ dough density; NSC aW, firmness
Guar Gum	Cake [49]	25–100%	Physical: ↓ volume (100% FR), elasticity; ↑ dough density; NSC aW, firmness
Oatrim	Cake [50] Biscuit [51,52]	20–60% 50–100%	Physical: ↓ air bubbles, viscosity, spread ratio, moisture, hardness (biscuits), brittleness; ↑ specific gravity, dough pH, height, hardness (cake), cohesiveness, springiness, aW Sensory: NSC colour, appearance, tenderness, sweetness, flavour, aftertaste, overall
Pectin	Cake [53] Biscuit [46,54] Croissant [42]	10–30% 10–100% 25–100%	Physical: ↓ spread ratio, penetration distance, volume; ↑ weight, aW, breaking strength, specific gravity, moisture, hardness Sensory: ↑ hardness, lightness, bitterness (biscuit: 100%); ↓ overall flavour, acceptance, colour, texture, cell size, taste, mouthfeel
Hydroxypropyl Methylcellulose (HPMC)	Legume Cracker [33] Biscuit [55]	25–100% 15–30%	Physical: ↓ lightness, yellowness; ↑ moisture, hardness, breaking strength; NSC aW Sensory: ↑ hardness, crispness; ↓ overall acceptance, yellowness, buttery flavour
Oleogels	Biscuit [56] Cake [57–59]	40–70% 25–100%	Physical: ↓ spread ratio, breaking strength, specific volume, fragmentation, porosity; ↑ hardness, specific gravity; NSC cell structure Sensory: ↑ hardness, chewiness, springiness, lightness (crust), colour (crust), overall taste; ↓ cohesiveness; NSC overall smell, overall acceptability
Whey Protein	Biscuit [45,46]	11.5–50%	Physical: ↓ hardness, weight; ↑ aW; NSC spread ratio Sensory: ↑ hardness; ↓ overall flavour, acceptance

aW: Water activity; FR: Fat reduction; NSC: No significant change; ↓: decrease; ↑: increase.

The interest in using whole food fat replacers has increased in recent years. These fat replacers are beneficial as they have a range of carbohydrates, lipids and proteins that may aid in the rheological properties of baked products, making them potentially more suitable than simple extracts and isolates. Overall, whole food fat replacers had the least effect on the physical and sensory properties of baked products, and in some cases increased the consumer acceptance (Table 3). Apricot kernel flour was a successful fat replacer with little impact on the physical and sensory properties of biscuits at a maximum of 50% FR [60,61]. Chia seed mucilage also had little impact on physical properties of cake and bread up to 100% FR [62,63], although sensory properties were not tested in these studies.

High oleic sunflower oil (HOSO) did not significantly decrease the amount of total fat in biscuits, but did reduce the saturated fat content [64]. However, the use of HOSO as a fat replacer was not considered successful as it has significant impact on the volume, colour and texture of the biscuits. The use of avocado puree as a fat replacer in cake and biscuits was successful at 50% FR, as it did not impact consumer acceptance [51,65]. However, at 75–100% FR, acceptance of the low-fat cake decreased compared to the control cake containing shortening [65]. Apple puree or pomace was the only whole food fat replacer to result in a reduction in sensory quality and consumer acceptance, even at low FR levels (10%) [66,67]. Therefore, apple puree is not recommended as a fat replacer in biscuits. Bean puree and green pea puree had very similar effects on the sensory properties of biscuits with increases in sensory qualities at 25–75% FR [68,69]. The use of green pea puree at FR of 25% in biscuits was considered ideal, whereas a FR of 100% resulted in reduced consumer acceptance [69]. Lastly, a high β-glucan product derived from oats or oat bran had significant impact on texture, colour and moisture of biscuits [45,54,70]. Although sensory properties were not tested in these studies, this suggests that the high β-glucan product was not a successful replacer for shortening in biscuits.

Whole foods may be the most suitable candidates for fat replacers in baked foods as they appeared to have the least impact on physical and sensory properties. In addition, they may also be beneficial as they may contain phytochemicals and micronutrients which could increase the health benefits and marketing potential of baked foods products, leading to novel functional foods. Lastly, consumer are more likely to accept foods with ingredients or additives that are made from natural, whole food products [71]. Bean and pea purees were the most successful fat replacers for biscuits at 25–75% FR, and avocado puree was successful at reducing fat in cake at 50% FR. However, more studies on whole food fat replacers in biscuits and bread is needed before they can be recommended as reliable fat replacers.

Table 3. Summary of quality changes of whole food fat replacers in baked food products.

Fat Replacer	Food(s)	FR Tested	Quality Changes
Apricot Kernel Flour	Biscuit [60,61]	10–50%	Physical: ↓ spread ratio, yellowness; ↑ hardness, lightnessSensory: NSC overall sensory score
Chia Seed Mucilage	Cake [62,63] Bread [63]	25–100% 25–100%	Physical: ↓ lightness, yellowness; ↑ firmness; NSC volume, symmetry, uniformity, redness, moisture, aW, breaking strength
High Oleic Sunflower Oil (HOSO)	Biscuit [64]	100%	Physical: ↓ volume, moisture, lightness, yellowness; ↑ biscuit density, breaking strength, redness; NSC dough density
Avocado Puree	Biscuit [51] Cake [65]	50% 50–100%	Physical: ↓ spread ratio, moisture, stiffness, hardness; ↑ aW, brittleness Sensory: ↓ appearance, acceptance (75–100%); NSC colour, tenderness, sweetness, flavour, aftertaste, acceptance (50%), overall sensory score
Apple Puree/Pomace	Biscuit [66,67]	10–100%	Physical: ↓ spread ratio, brittleness, hardness, yellowness; ↑ moisture Sensory: ↓ appearance, texture, chewiness, sweetness, moistness (100%), flavour, aftertaste, overall sensory score; ↑ moistness (50%); NSC colour
Bean Puree	Biscuit [68]	25–75%	Sensory: ↑ appearance, colour, flavour, texture, acceptance
Green Pea Puree	Biscuit [69]	25–100%	Physical: ↑ moisture Sensory: ↓ flavour, aftertaste, acceptance (100%); ↑ colour, moistness, flavour (25–75%), acceptance (25%); NSC smell
Oat Bran/High β-Glucan Oat Product	Biscuit [45,54,70]	10–100%	Physical: ↓ spread ratio, hardness [59], redness, yellowness; ↑ hardness [37], brittleness, moisture, aW, lightness, volume

aW: Water activity; FR: Fat reduction; NSC: No significant change; ↓: decrease; ↑: increase.

Fat replacers in combination with additional ingredients may provide better fat-like qualities as the additional ingredients are usually designed to supplement the unwanted effects of individual fat replacers, as seen above (Tables 1–3). These additional ingredients are usually other types of fat replacers, but can also be enzymes or emulsifiers. Few studies have assessed combined fat replacers in baked products, although the results appear promising (Table 4). Polydextrose and guar gum were successful fat replacers in biscuits at a relatively high level of FR (70%), with an increase in perceived taste, flavour and consumer acceptance [72]. Maltodextrin and xanthan gum yielded increased moisture, hardness and chewiness in 66% FR muffins, but sensory analysis was not conducted in these samples [36]. Kel-Lite BK, a commercial fat replacer containing xanthan gum, guar gum, cellulose gel, sodium stearoyl lactylate, gum Arabic, dextrin, lecithin, and mono- and diglyceride, resulted in increased bitterness and, oddly increased both crumb firmness and softness in biscuits at 33%, 66% and 100% FR [54]. HOSO and inulin were also successful fat replacers in biscuits at 100% FR [64,73], although HOSO does contain lipids so the biscuits only had reduced saturated fat rather than total fat. However, HOSO and inulin resulted in decreased appearance, flavour, odour, texture, and consumer acceptance in cakes, croissants and muffins [73]. Therefore, HOSO and inulin may only be suitable for use as fat replacers in biscuits. HOSO and β-Glucan may also be a useful fat replacer at 100% FR as this had little impact on physical properties in biscuits, although sensory evaluations were not conducted [64]. A combination of emulsion filled gel based on inulin and extra virgin olive oil (EVOO) has also been trialed as a fat mimetic in biscuits [74]. At 50% FR, there were no changes to the physical properties and the overall consumer acceptance of the biscuit compared to the control biscuit containing 20% butter, although there was a decrease in overall flavour. However, consumer acceptance was not maintained at 100% FR. Inulin, lipase and a commercial emulsifier ("Colco"; a type of alpha-gel emulsifier containing glycerol monostearate and polyglycerol esters of fatty acids) had little impact on physical properties of cake at 50–70% FR, although no sensory evaluation was conducted for this combined fat replacer either [75]. One study assessed the double, but not triple, combinations of corn fibre, maltodextrin and lupine extract in biscuits, each at 30–40% FR [40]. All combinations had little impact on the physical properties of the biscuits compared to the control biscuit containing 33% margarine. However, consumer preference for corn fibre and lupine extract was significant lower than the control, whereas corn fibre and maltodextrin was significant higher than the control [40]. This suggests that the combination of corn fibre and maltodextrin may be an ideal fat replacement in biscuits at a moderate FR level. Tapioca dextrin, tapioca starch and resistant starch as a combination fat replacer had an impact on a wide range of sensory properties in biscuits [76]. However, overall consumer acceptance decreased, even at relatively low FR levels (10–20%), so we do not recommend the use of this combination fat replacer in biscuits.

Overall, combination fat replacers may be potential candidates for ingredients in low-fat baked products. The use of polydextrose and guar gum appears to be a reasonably effective fat replacer in biscuits. However, with the limited evidence currently available, recommendations cannot be made for the use of combination fat replacers in other baked products.

Table 4. Summary of quality changes of combined fat replacers in baked food products.

Fat Replacer	Food(s)	FR Tested	Quality Changes
Polydextrose and Guar Gum	Biscuit [72]	70%	Physical: ↑ spread ratio, hardness, stress-strain ratio, moisture Sensory: ↑ overall taste, overall flavour, acceptance
Maltodextrin and Xanthan Gum	Muffin [36]	66%	Physical: ↑ aW, moisture, hardness, chewiness; ↓ volume; NSC springiness, cohesiveness
Kel-Lite BK	Biscuit [54]	33–100%	Physical: ↑ crumb firmness, crumb softness; NSC volume Sensory: ↑ bitterness

Table 4. *Cont.*

Fat Replacer	Food(s)	FR Tested	Quality Changes
HOSO and Inulin	Biscuit [64,73] Cake [73] Croissant [73] Muffin [73]	100%	Physical: NSC dough density, biscuit density, volume, moisture, breaking strength, lightness, colour Sensory: ↓ appearance (croissant and muffin), odour (croissant and muffin), texture (cake and croissant), flavour (cake and muffin), acceptance (cake, croissant and muffin), purchase intent (cake), preference (cake and muffin)
HOSO and β-Glucan	Biscuit [64]	100%	Physical: ↓ volume, lightness; ↑ biscuit density; NSC dough density, moisture, breaking strength, colour
EVOO and EFG based on Inulin	Biscuit [74]	50–100%	Physical: ↓ breaking strength (100%), porosity (100%); Sensory: ↓ caramel odour, buttery odour and flavour, sweetness, crunchiness, crush, dryness, acceptance (100%); ↑ consistency; NSC grain odour and flavour, saltiness
Inulin, Lipase and Emulsifier	Cake [75]	50–70%	Physical: ↓ batter density; ↑ cohesiveness; NSC volume, cell structure, hardness, chewiness, springiness
Corn Fibre, Maltodextrin and/or Lupine Extract	Biscuit [40]	30–40%	Physical: ↓ lightness, volume; ↑ breaking strength Sensory: ↓ preference (corn fibre and lupine extract); ↑ preference (corn fibre and maltodextrin)
Tapioca Dextrin, Tapioca Starch and Resistant Starch	Biscuit [76]	10–20%	Physical: ↓ spread ratio; ↑ breaking strength Sensory: ↓ buttery taste, crunchiness, hardness, colour, buttery odour, appearance, texture, taste, sweetness, acceptance; ↑ shape homogeneity, floury taste, pastiness, floury odour

aW: Water activity; FR: Fat reduction; NSC: No significant change; ↓: decrease; ↑: increase, HOSO: High Oleic Sunflower Oil; EVOO: Extra Virgin Olive Oil; EFG: Emulsion Filled Gel.

4. Industry Recommendations and Conclusions

It should be noted that there is limited literature on the use of fat replacers in low-fat baked products. Many of the reviewed fat replacers have only been assessed once, and also only in one type of food. There is a need for additional replicate studies using a variety of recipes. Also, while we have reviewed the current literature here, we cannot compare physical and sensory properties between studies. Therefore, while we can summarise which fat replacers were successful within a certain baked product, it is difficult to determine which fat replacer is best. In addition, the use of fat replacers in bread, muffins and croissants were only assessed in few studies each. Therefore, there is not enough information to make a recommendation of the best type of fat replacer for these products. Below is our recommendations for the best currently assessed fat replacers in a range of baked food products:

Biscuit—Oatrim was the most successful fat replacer in biscuits as it was able to retain most sensory properties of a traditional biscuit even at 100% FR, although there was a decrease in hardness and brittleness [51,52]. However, it should also be noted that both bean puree and green pea puree were able to increase the sensory qualities and consumer acceptance of biscuits at 75% FR with less of an impact on the physical properties compared to oatrim [68,69]. Legume purees might also have an advantage over oatrim as they may aid the marketability of food products due to potential nutrition claims such as vegetable and protein content. However, legume purees should not be used at 100% FR. Overall, we recommend the use of either oatrim or legume purees as fat replacers in biscuits.

Cake—Oleogels appeared to be the most successful fat replacer in cake, with no changes to the sensory qualities at 100% FR [57–59]. However, there were significant changes to the physical properties of cake when using oleogels at FR levels ≥50% [58] which might lead to difficulty during cake production. An alternative could be avocado puree which was only successful at 50% FR but had less of an impact on the physical properties of cake [65], or inulin which was successful up to 75% FR but had an impact on the physical and textural properties of cake [34].

Cracker—While there was only one study on the use of fat replacers in crackers [33], it assessed and compared a range of fat replacers in the one study. Inulin appeared to be the most successful fat replacer in these crackers, reaching an acceptable level of FR at 75%. The additional benefits of using inulin is that it may aid the marketability of food products due to potential high fibre claims.

Author Contributions: K.C. and A.C. collated the literature and wrote the manuscript. S.G. conceived the original idea, designed the format, reviewed the manuscript and provided critical feedback.

References

1. World Health Organisation. *Prevention of Cardiovascular Disease*; World Health Organisation: Geneva, Switzerland, 2007.
2. Department of Health and Human Services, Department of Agriculture. *2015–2020 Dietary Guidelines for Americans*, 8th ed.; Department of Health and Human Services: Washington, DC, USA, 2015.
3. Health Canada. *Eating Well with Canada's Food Guide*; Health Canada: Ottawa, ON, Canada, 2011.
4. National Health and Medical Research Council. *Nutrient Reference Values for Australia and New Zealand Including Recommended Dietary Intakes*; National Health and Medical Research Council: Canberra, Australia, 2006.
5. Public Health England. *The Eatwell Guide*; Public Health England: London, UK, 2016.
6. Hooper, L.; Abdelhamid, A.; Bunn, D.; Brown, T.; Summerbell, C.D.; Skeaff, C.M. Effects of total fat intake on body weight. *Cochrane Database Syst. Rev.* **2015**, *8*, CD011834. [CrossRef] [PubMed]
7. Aune, D.; Sen, A.; Prasad, M.; Norat, T.; Janszky, I.; Tonstad, S.; Romundstad, P.; Vatten, L.J. BMI and all cause mortality: Systematic review and non-linear dose-response meta-analysis of 230 cohort studies with 3.74 million deaths among 30.3 million participants. *BMJ* **2016**, *353*, i2156. [CrossRef] [PubMed]
8. Ng, M.; Fleming, T.; Robinson, M.; Thomson, B.; Graetz, N.; Margono, C.; Mullany, E.C.; Biryukov, S.; Abbafati, C.; Abera, S.F.; et al. Global, regional, and national prevalence of overweight and obesity in children and adults during 1980–2013: A systematic analysis for the Global Burden of Disease Study 2013. *Lancet* **2014**, *384*, 766–781. [CrossRef]
9. Whitlock, G.; Lewington, S.; Sherliker, P.; Clarke, R.; Emberson, J.; Halsey, J.; Qizilbash, N.; Collins, R.; Peto, R. Body-mass index and cause-specific mortality in 900,000 adults: Collaborative analyses of 57 prospective studies. *Lancet* **2009**, *373*, 1083–1096. [PubMed]
10. Abdullah, A.; Peeters, A.; de Courten, M.; Stoelwinder, J. The magnitude of association between overweight and obesity and the risk of diabetes: A meta-analysis of prospective cohort studies. *Diabetes Res. Clin. Pract.* **2010**, *89*, 309–319. [CrossRef] [PubMed]
11. Renehan, A.G.; Tyson, M.; Egger, M.; Heller, R.F.; Zwahlen, M. Body-mass index and incidence of cancer: A systematic review and meta-analysis of prospective observational studies. *Lancet* **2008**, *371*, 569–578. [CrossRef]
12. Bucher, T.; Collins, C.; Rollo, M.E.; McCaffrey, T.A.; De Vlieger, N.; Van der Bend, D.; Truby, H.; Perez-Cueto, F.J. Nudging consumers towards healthier choices: A systematic review of positional influences on food choice. *Br. J. Nutr.* **2016**, *115*, 2252–2263. [CrossRef] [PubMed]
13. Krystallis, A.; Chrysochou, P. Do health claims and prior awareness influence Consumers' preferences for unhealthy foods? The case of functional Children's snacks. *Agribusiness* **2012**, *28*, 86–102. [CrossRef]
14. Pearson, N.; Biddle, S.J. Sedentary behavior and dietary intake in children, adolescents, and adults. *Am. J. Prevent. Med.* **2011**, *41*, 178–188. [CrossRef] [PubMed]
15. Piernas, C.; Popkin, B.M. Trends in snacking among US children. *Health Aff.* **2010**, *29*, 398–404. [CrossRef] [PubMed]
16. Forbes, S.L.; Kahiya, E.; Balderstone, C. Analysis of snack food purchasing and consumption behavior. *J. Food Prod. Market.* **2016**, *22*, 65–88. [CrossRef]
17. Chandon, P.; Wansink, B. Does food marketing need to make us fat? A review and solutions. *Nutr. Rev.* **2012**, *70*, 571–593. [CrossRef] [PubMed]
18. Block, G. Foods contributing to energy intake in the US: Data from NHANES III and NHANES 1999–2000. *J. Food Composit. Anal.* **2004**, *17*, 439–447. [CrossRef]
19. Frye, A.M.; Setser, C.S. Optimizing texture of reduced-calorie yellow layer cakes. *Cereal Chem.* **1992**, *69*, 338–343.
20. Drewnowski, A.; Nordensten, K.; Dwyer, J. Replacing sugar and fat in biscuits: Impact on product quality and preference. *Food Qual. Prefer.* **1998**, *9*, 13–20. [CrossRef]

21. Siro, I.; Kapolna, E.; Kapolna, B.; Lugasi, A. Functional food. Product development, marketing and consumer acceptance—A review. *Appetite* **2008**, *51*, 456–467. [CrossRef] [PubMed]
22. Tepper, B.J.; Trail, A.C. Taste or health: A study on consumer acceptance of corn chips. *Food Qual. Pref.* **1998**, *9*, 267–272. [CrossRef]
23. Hamilton, J.; Knox, B.; Hill, D.; Parr, H. Reduced fat products–consumer perceptions and preferences. *Br. Food J.* **2000**, *102*, 494–506. [CrossRef]
24. Richard, D.M. Position of the American Dietetic Association fat replacer. *J. Am. Diet. Assoc.* **1998**, *98*, 463–468.
25. Akoh, C.C. Fat replacers. *Food Technol.* **1998**, *52*, 47–53.
26. Wilderjans, E.; Luyts, A.; Brijs, K.; Delcour, J.A. Ingredient functionality in batter type cake making. *Trends Food Sci. Technol.* **2013**, *30*, 6–15. [CrossRef]
27. Maache-Rezzoug, Z.; Bouvier, J.M.; Allaf, K.; Patras, C. Effect of principal ingredients on rheological behaviour of biscuit dough and on quality of biscuits. *J. Food Eng.* **1998**, *35*, 23–42. [CrossRef]
28. Lucca, P.A.; Tepper, B.J. Fat replacers and the functionality of fat in foods. *Trends Food Sci. Technol.* **1994**, *5*, 12–19. [CrossRef]
29. Berenzon, S.; Saguy, I.S. Oxygen absorbers for extension of crackers shelf-life. *LWT-Food Sci. Technol.* **1998**, *31*, 1–5. [CrossRef]
30. Manley, D. *Manley's Technology of Biscuits, Crackers and Biscuits*; Woodhead Publishing: Cambridge, UK, 2011.
31. Nasir, M.; Butt, M.S.; Anjum, F.M.; Sharif, K.A.; Minhas, R. Effect of moisture on the shelf life of wheat flour. *Int. J. Agric. Biol.* **2003**, *5*, 458–459.
32. Voragen, A.G. Technological aspects of functional food-related carbohydrates. *Trends in Food Sci. Technol.* **1998**, *9*, 328–335. [CrossRef]
33. Colla, K.; Gamlath, S. Inulin and maltodextrin can replace fat in baked savoury legume snacks. *Int. J. Food Sci. Technol.* **2015**, *50*, 2297–2305. [CrossRef]
34. Rodríguez-García, J.; Puig, A.; Salvador, A.; Hernando, I. Optimization of a sponge cake formulation with inulin as fat replacer: Structure, physicochemical, and sensory properties. *J. Food Sci.* **2012**, *77*, C189–C197. [CrossRef] [PubMed]
35. Zahn, S.; Pepke, F.; Rohm, H. Effect of inulin as a fat replacer on texture and sensory properties of muffins. *Int. J. Food Sci. Technol.* **2010**, *45*, 2531–2537. [CrossRef]
36. Khouryieh, H.A.; Aramouni, F.M.; Herald, T.J. Physical and sensory characteristics of no-sugar-added/low-fat muffin. *J. Food Qual.* **2005**, *28*, 439–451. [CrossRef]
37. Błońska, A.; Marzec, A.; Błaszczyk, A. Instrumental Evaluation of Acoustic and Mechanical Texture Properties of Short-Dough Biscuits with Different Content of Fat and Inulin. *J. Texture Stud.* **2014**, *45*, 226–234. [CrossRef]
38. Rodríguez-García, J.; Laguna, L.; Puig, A.; Salvador, A.; Hernando, I. Effect of fat replacement by inulin on textural and structural properties of short dough biscuits. *Food Bioprocess Technol.* **2013**, *6*, 2739–2750. [CrossRef]
39. Krystyjan, M.; Gumul, D.; Ziobro, R.; Sikora, M. The effect of inulin as a fat replacement on dough and biscuit properties. *J. Food Qual.* **2015**, *38*, 305–315. [CrossRef]
40. Forker, A.; Zahn, S.; Rohm, H. A combination of fat replacers enables the production of fat-reduced shortdough biscuits with high-sensory quality. *Food Bioprocess Technol.* **2012**, *5*, 2497–2505. [CrossRef]
41. Sudha, M.L.; Srivastava, A.K.; Vetrimani, R.; Leelavathi, K. Fat replacement in soft dough biscuits: Its implications on dough rheology and biscuit quality. *J. Food Eng.* **2007**, *80*, 922–930. [CrossRef]
42. Shouk, A.A.; El-Faham, S.Y. Effect of fat replacers and hull-less barley flour on low-fat croissant quality. *Pol. J. Food Nutr. Sci.* **2005**, *14*, 287–292.
43. Lee, Y.T.; Puligundla, P. Characteristics of reduced-fat muffins and biscuits with native and modified rice starches. *Emir. J. Food Agric.* **2016**, *28*, 311–316. [CrossRef]
44. Basman, A.; Ozturk, S.; Kahraman, K.; Koksel, H. Emulsion and pasting properties of resistant starch with locust bean gum and their utilization in low fat biscuit formulations. *Int. J. Food Prop.* **2008**, *11*, 762–772. [CrossRef]
45. Zoulias, E.I.; Oreopoulou, V.; Tzia, C. Textural properties of low-fat biscuits containing carbohydrate-or protein-based fat replacers. *J. Food Eng.* **2002**, *55*, 337–342. [CrossRef]
46. Zoulias, E.I.; Oreopoulou, V.; Tzia, C. Effect of fat mimetics on physical, textural and sensory properties of biscuits. *Int. J. Food Prop.* **2000**, *3*, 385–397. [CrossRef]

47. Bayarri, S.; González-Tomás, L.U.; Hernando, I.; Lluch, M.A.; Costell, E. Texture perceived on inulin-enriched low-fat semisolid dairy desserts. Rheological and structural basis. *J. Texture Stud.* **2011**, *42*, 174–184. [CrossRef]
48. Shoaib, M.; Shehzad, A.; Omar, M.; Rakha, A.; Raza, H.; Sharif, H.R.; Shakeel, A.; Ansari, A.; Niazi, S. Inulin: Properties, health benefits and food applications. *Carbohydr. Polym.* **2016**, *147*, 444–454. [CrossRef] [PubMed]
49. Zambrano, F.; Despinoy, P.; Ormenese, R.C.; Faria, E.V. The use of guar and xanthan gums in the production of 'light'low fat cakes. *Int. J. Food Sci. Technol.* **2004**, *39*, 959–966. [CrossRef]
50. Lee, S.; Kim, S.; Inglett, G.E. Effect of shortening replacement with oatrim on the physical and rheological properties of cakes. *Cereal Chem.* **2005**, *82*, 120–124. [CrossRef]
51. Wekwete, B.; Navder, K.P. Effects of avocado fruit puree and oatrim as fat replacers on the physical, textural and sensory properties of oatmeal biscuits. *J. Food Qual.* **2008**, *31*, 131–141. [CrossRef]
52. Swanson, R.B.; Garen, L.A.; Parks, S.S. Effect of a carbohydrate-based fat substitute and emulsifying agents on reduced-fat peanut butter biscuits. *J. Food Qual.* **1999**, *22*, 19–29. [CrossRef]
53. Lim, J.; Ko, S.; Lee, S. Use of Yuja (Citrus junos) pectin as a fat replacer in baked foods. *Food Sci. Biotechnol.* **2014**, *23*, 1837–1841. [CrossRef]
54. Conforti, F.D.; Charles, S.A.; Duncan, S.E. Evaluation of a carbohydrate-based fat replacer in a fat-reduced baking powder biscuit. *J. Food Qual.* **1997**, *20*, 247–256. [CrossRef]
55. Laguna, L.; Primo-Martín, C.; Varela, P.; Salvador, A.; Sanz, T. HPMC and inulin as fat replacers in biscuits: Sensory and instrumental evaluation. *LWT-Food Sci. Technol.* **2014**, *56*, 494–501. [CrossRef]
56. Mert, B.; Demirkesen, I. Reducing saturated fat with oleogel/shortening blends in a baked product. *Food Chem.* **2016**, *199*, 809–816. [CrossRef] [PubMed]
57. Kim, J.Y.; Lim, J.; Lee, J.; Hwang, H.S.; Lee, S. Utilization of oleogels as a replacement for solid fat in aerated baked goods: Physicochemical, rheological, and tomographic characterization. *J. Food Sci.* **2017**, *82*, 445–452. [CrossRef] [PubMed]
58. Amoah, C.; Lim, J.; Jeong, S.; Lee, S. Assessing the effectiveness of wax-based sunflower oil oleogels in cakes as a shortening replacer. *LWT-Food Sci. Technol.* **2017**, *86*, 430–437.
59. Pehlivanoglu, H.; Ozulku, G.; Yildirim, R.M.; Demirci, M.; Toker, O.S.; Sagdic, O. Investigating the usage of unsaturated fatty acid-rich and low-calorie oleogels as a shortening mimetics in cake. *J. Food Process. Preserv.* **2018**, *42*, e13621. [CrossRef]
60. Seker, I.T.; Ozboy-Ozbas, O.; Gokbulut, I.; Ozturk, S.; Koksel, H. Utilization of apricot kernel flour as fat replacer in biscuits. *J. Food Process. Preserv.* **2010**, *34*, 15–26. [CrossRef]
61. Özboy-Özbaş, Ö.; Seker, I.T.; Gökbulut, I. Effects of resistant starch, apricot kernel flour, and fiber-rich fruit powders on low-fat biscuit quality. *Food Sci. Biotechnol.* **2010**, *19*, 979–986. [CrossRef]
62. Felisberto, M.H.; Wahanik, A.L.; Gomes-Ruffi, C.R.; Clerici, M.T.; Chang, Y.K.; Steel, C.J. Use of chia (*Salvia hispanica* L.) mucilage gel to reduce fat in pound cakes. *LWT-Food Sci. Technol.* **2015**, *63*, 1049–1055. [CrossRef]
63. Fernandes, S.S.; de las Mercedes Salas-Mellado, M. Addition of chia seed mucilage for reduction of fat content in bread and cakes. *Food Chem.* **2017**, *227*, 237–244. [CrossRef] [PubMed]
64. Onacik-Gür, S.; Żbikowska, A.; Jaroszewska, A. Effect of high-oleic sunflower oil and other pro-health ingredients on physical and sensory properties of biscuits. *CyTA-J. Food* **2015**, *13*, 621–628. [CrossRef]
65. Nguyen, D.; Carotenuto, M.; Khan, S.; Bhaduri, S.; Ghatak, R.; Navder, K.P. Effect of Avocado Fruit Puree as Fat Replacer on the Physical, Textural and Sensory Properties of Shortened Cakes. *J. Acad. Nutr. Diet.* **2013**, *113*, A59. [CrossRef]
66. Min, B.; Bae, I.Y.; Lee, H.G.; Yoo, S.H.; Lee, S. Utilization of pectin-enriched materials from apple pomace as a fat replacer in a model food system. *Bioresour. Technol.* **2010**, *101*, 5414–5418. [CrossRef] [PubMed]
67. Hayek, S.A.; Ibrahim, S.A. Consumer acceptability of chocolate chip biscuits using applesauce as a fat (butter) substitute. *Emir. J. Food Agric.* **2013**, 159–168.
68. Rankin, L.L.; Bingham, M. Acceptability of oatmeal chocolate chip biscuits prepared using pureed white beans as a fat ingredient substitute. *J. Acad. Nutr. Diet.* **2000**, *100*, 831–833.
69. Romanchik-Cerpovicz, J.E.; Jeffords, M.J.; Onyenwoke, A.C. College student acceptance of chocolate bar biscuits containing puree of canned green peas as a fat-ingredient substitute. *J. Culin. Sci. Technol.* **2018**. [CrossRef]

70. Lee, S.; Inglett, G.E. Rheological and physical evaluation of jet-cooked oat bran in low calorie biscuits. *Int. J. Food Sci. Technol.* **2006**, *41*, 553–559. [CrossRef]
71. Aschemann-Witzel, J.; Varela, P.; Peschel, A.O. Consumers' categorization of food ingredients: Do consumers perceive them as 'clean label' producers expect? An exploration with projective mapping. *Food Qual. Prefer.* **2019**, *71*, 117–128. [CrossRef]
72. Chugh, B.; Singh, G.; Kumbhar, B.K. Development of low-fat soft dough biscuits using carbohydrate-based fat replacers. *Int. J. Food Sci.* **2013**, *2013*, 576153. [CrossRef] [PubMed]
73. Doménech-Asensi, G.; Merola, N.; López-Fernández, A.; Ros-Berruezo, G.; Frontela-Saseta, C. Influence of the reformulation of ingredients in bakery products on healthy characteristics and acceptability of consumers. *Int. J. Food Sci. Nutr.* **2016**, *67*, 74–82. [CrossRef] [PubMed]
74. Giarnetti, M.; Paradiso, V.M.; Caponio, F.; Summo, C.; Pasqualone, A. Fat replacement in shortbread cookies using an emulsion filled gel based on inulin and extra virgin olive oil. *LWT-Food Sci. Technol.* **2015**, *63*, 339–345. [CrossRef]
75. Rodríguez-García, J.; Sahi, S.S.; Hernando, I. Functionality of lipase and emulsifiers in low-fat cakes with inulin. *LWT-Food Sci. Technol.* **2014**, *58*, 173–182. [CrossRef]
76. Laguna, L.; Varela, P.; Salvador, A.N.; Sanz, T.; Fiszman, S.M. Balancing texture and other sensory features in reduced fat short-dough biscuits. *J. Texture Stud.* **2012**, *43*, 235–245. [CrossRef]

10

Production of Barbari Bread (Traditional Iranian Bread) using Different Levels of Distillers Dried Grains with Solubles (DDGS) and Sodium Stearoyl Lactate (SSL)

Shirin Pourafshar [1], Kurt A. Rosentrater [2,3,*] and Padmanaban G. Krishnan [1]

1 Dairy and Food Science Department, South Dakota State University, Brookings, SD 57007, USA; SP8DS@hscmail.mcc.virginia.edu (S.P.); Padmanaban.Krishnan@sdstate.edu (P.G.K.)
2 Department of Agriculture and Biosystems Engineering, Iowa State University, Ames, IA 50011, USA
3 Department of Food Science and Human Nutrition, Iowa State University, Ames, IA 50011, USA
* Correspondence: karosent@iastate.edu

Abstract: Bread is one of the oldest foods known throughout history and even though it is one of the principal types of staple around the world, it usually lacks enough nutrients, including protein and fiber. As such, fortification is one of the best solutions to overcome this problem. Thus, the objective this study was to examine the effect of three levels of distillers dried grains with solubles (DDGS) (0%, 10% and 20%) in conjunction with three levels of SSL (sodium stearoyl lactate) (0%, 2% and 5%) on physical and chemical properties of Barbari bread (traditional Iranian bread). To the best of our knowledge, this is the first study to evaluate DDGS and Sodium Stearoyl-2-Lactilate (SSL), as sources of fortification in Barbari bread. The results showed that incorporation of 20% of DDGS and 0% SSL caused a significant increase in the amount of fiber and protein. As for the physical attributes, using higher amount of DDGS caused a darker color, and as for the texture parameters, the highest firmness was measured when 10% DDGS and 5% of SSL were used. Different Mixolab and Rapid Visco Analyzer (RVA) parameters also were measured with varying results. The findings of this study show that DDGS can be a valuable source of fiber and protein, which can be used as a cost effective source to fortify cereal-based products.

Keywords: distillers dried grains with solubles; fortification; sodium stearoyl sactate

---

1. Introduction

Cereals are the edible seeds or grains of the grass family, *Gramineae*. Because cereals are inexpensive and readily available, humans in almost every country have used them as major food staples for centuries. Cereals and cereal products are an important source of energy, protein and fiber [1]. Wheat is the most important cereal, and is commonly consumed worldwide. Historians do not know exactly where wheat was first cultivated, but sources point to either Syria-Palestine or southern parts of Anatolia. Wheat cultivation spread from Palestine to Egypt and then from northern Mesopotamia to Persia, where bread was first developed. From there, the growth of wheat and bread spread in all directions [2]. Although whole wheat as a food component has high nutritional value, a considerable proportion of the grain's nutrients are lost during the milling processes. Thus, the importance of adding value to those products made with all-purpose flour or other wheat flours increases. Since bread is the most consumed cereal product, fortification can help combat problems such as malnutrition.

One way of fortifying cereal products, especially breads, may be through the use of distillers dried grains. Distillers dried grains with solubles (DDGS) is a co-product resulting from the fermentation of cereal grains, mostly corn, for the production of ethanol. As a result of increase in ethanol production, there is an increase supply of DDGS as well [3]. America's corn farmers have improved their cultivation techniques significantly and increased their yield potential. In 1935, 82 million acres of corn were harvested in United States (U.S.) with an average yield of 24.2 bushels per acre; by 1950, the yield increased to 38.2 bushels per acre. Then in 1956, the problem with farms was the abundance of corn. Corn production continued increasing so that the yield was 149 bushels per acre by 2006. The increase in corn encouraged cattle feeding in the U.S, and with the growth of the ethanol industry, the demand for corn has improved [4]. Furthermore, researchers have identified the potential value of DDGS as a source of protein, which often ranges from 27% to 35%, fiber, minerals and vitamins [5]. As a result, scientists and engineers have been trying to find different ways of using DDGS in human foods, rather than solely as livestock feed. Researchers have explored incorporating DDGS in food products, especially cereal-based products. For instance, in a study done by Wu et al. [6], spaghetti was supplemented with corn distillers dried grains. Additionally, Finley and Hanamoto [7] used brewer's spent grain in bread, while Tsen et al. [8,9] used DDG flour in the production of bread and cookies and then evaluated the physical and chemical properties of final products. Corn distiller's grains have also been used in spaghetti [8]. Furthermore, the effect of DDGS on quality of cornbread has been investigated by Liu and colleagues [10].

Sodium Stearoyl-2-Lactilate (SSL) is an anionic emulsifier which is effective in increasing dough strength. Emulsifiers are mostly used in the baking industry to enhance baking quality. They can prevent mechanical damage to fermented dough, increase shelf life and improve the texture of baked products [11]. Hydrocolloids are often used in bread to improve the volume and texture, extend shelf life, and make softer bread crumbs [12]. SSL can function through interactions with flour protein which will improve the viscoelasticity of the dough [11]. Other protein-reactive softeners, such as DATEM (diacetyl tartaric ester of monoglycerides), can increase the strength of gluten protein matrix which will, in turn, improve loaf volume and tighten crumb structure [13].

Flat breads have a very short shelf life, usually a few hours. Because of that, many studies have been done to increase the shelf life of flat breads. For example, in a study by Qarooni [2], the anti-staling effect of ingredients such as shortening on Barbari bread's quality was investigated. The results from that study showed that adding 0.5% SSL and 0.3% shortening made the bread edible for up to 36 h, instead of the normal 16 h. Different Middle Eastern breads are made with various types of flours. For example, round shaped Baladi and Aish Meharha from Egypt and Bazlama, Pide and Yufca from Turkey are mainly made with wheat flour. Morocco has pan fried bread made with semolina flour. Afghanistan and Tajikistan have Bolani bread, which is flat bread stuffed with different vegetables. Although these breads are mainly made with wheat and other types of flours, each of them has its own physical and chemical characteristics. However, they may have deficiencies in certain nutrient components that can be remedied through fortification.

Among Middle Easterners, Iranians consume four major types of breads: Barbari, Lavash, Sangak and Taftoon, with Barbari being the most popular. On average, Barbari crust has a thickness of 1–2 mm, length of 67–75 cm, and width of 13.5–20 cm. Traditionally, this bread is made with all-purpose flour and the final product contains about 11% protein, 10% fiber and 0.5% fat. Barbari is thick and oval shaped, and is often topped with poppy seeds. The golden color of this bread comes from Romal, a mixture made from flour, baking soda, and boiling water which is brushed on the dough before baking. Barbari has a special aroma and its taste depends on the amount of sour dough and baking time.

In this study, three levels of DDGS (0%, 10% and 20%) and three levels of SSL (0%, 2% and 5%) were used for substitution of wheat flour in Barbari bread. The objectives of this study were to understand (1) the impact of substitution of three levels of DDGS and SSL on the physical and chemical attributes of final bread products, and (2) to study the changes in the physical properties of the dough with different levels of substitutions of DDGS and SSL.

2. Materials and Methods

2.1. Experimental Design

Distillers dried grains with solubles (DDGS) was obtained from a commercial fuel ethanol plant in South Dakota. All-purpose wheat flour and other ingredients were purchased from local markets. A control sample of Barbari bread was baked at 550 °C for 10 min. To fortify this bread three levels of DDGS substitution (0%, 10% and 20%) and three levels of SSL substitution (0%, 2% and 5%) were used, producing a two-factor design each with three levels, having a full factorial design. Two loaves of breads for each level of substitution were baked. All properties of each of these loaves were analyzed using three replications; thus, $n = 6$ measurements for each property, and for each treatment combination. In total, 54 samples were analyzed. Table 1 shows the amount of all-purpose flour, DDGS and SSL to be used in samples.

Table 1. Experimental design [1].

Treatment	Wheat [2] (%)	DDGS [3] (%)	SSL [4] (%)
0 (Control)	**100**	**0**	**0**
1	98	0	2
2	95	0	5
3	90	10	0
4	88	10	2
5	85	10	5
6	80	20	0
7	78	20	2
8	75	20	5

[1] Each treatment was replicated twice. [2] From market source, Hy-Vee bleached all-purpose flour. [3] DDGS is distillers dried grains with solubles, obtained from a commercial fuel ethanol plant. [4] SSL is sodium stearoyl-2-lactate.

2.2. Preparation

For the sour dough, 1 g of salt, 9 g of active dry yeast (Red Star Active Dry Yeast, purchased from local market), 400 g of flour (Gold Medal All-purpose Flour, purchased from local market) with 650 g of water were used and only 35 g of sour dough was used for each batch. Romal topping for the bread required 4.2 g of flour, 4.2 g of baking soda and 85 g of water.

For the control, bread was made with only wheat flour, 880 g of all-purpose flour (Gold Medal All-purpose Flour) was used; the rest of the ingredients were 4.2 g of sugar, 4.2 g of salt, and 689.76 g of water. For the other breads, the same ingredients were used, varying only the amount of flour.

2.3. Bread Production

Sour dough was prepared 18 h before bread preparation during which, the sour dough was covered and left at room temperature. In terms of bread preparation, first the yeast was dissolved in warm water and then sugar was added and put aside for 10 min. This was then mixed with salt and water and then flour was gradually added and sour dough from the previous day was added as well. The mixture was mixed until the dough was no longer sticky. The next step was proofing, where the dough was placed in a proofing chamber for an hour and half for further activity of the yeast. Then, 400 g of dough was weighed and kneaded to form a 20 inch (50.8 cm) by 20 inch (50.8 cm) square, using a square frame to assure consistency in dimension of all breads. The thickness of the dough was measured in three different areas at the edges, then the Romal was made and brushed on top of dough. The dough was put aside for 10 min. Next, bread was baked at 500 °C for 10 min on a pizza stone (14 inch by 16 inch) to make baking condition close to that of the traditional ovens used for Barbari in Iran.

The other breads were made the same way except for the amount of flour, DDGS and SSL which were incorporated accordingly in each bread sample (Table 1). In the breads other than control, the same procedure was used but with different proportions of all-purpose flour. The mixing time and other details of preparation were the same for control and all other breads.

2.4. Physical and Chemical Properties

A texture analyzer was used to study the firmness and extensibility of the bread samples using two different probes: SMS/Chen-Hoseney Dough stickiness RIG and Pizza Tensile RIG, (TX.XT-plus, Texture Technologies Corp., Scarsdale, NY, USA). For measurement of each of these variables, duplications were done for each loaf (n = 2), for a total of four samples for each type of bread, or 24 samples. The thickness at the edges and the center of the bread was measured using Vernier calipers (Digimatic Calipers w/Absolute Encoders, Series 500, Mitutoyo Corporation, Kawasaki, Kanagawa, Japan). For the center, because of the bubbles which were formed in the middle of breads, the thickness was measured three times. After that, breads were grinded and moisture content as well as water activity were determined. In order to determine the water activity, water activity meter for food quality was used (Aqua lab CX-2, Decagon Devices, Inc., Pullman, WA, USA). Color was measured by spectrophotometer (Minolta CM-508d, Ramsey, NJ, USA) in which L^* is the measure of lightness, a^* is the measure of greenness to redness, and b^* is the measure of blueness to yellowness. The color was determined for the baked products just like it was done for the dough, and L^*, a^* and b^* were measured to get the color values.

Protein content was measured using the American Association of Cereal Chemistry (AACC) method for combustion—AACC approved method 46-0 [14] with a CE Elantech instrument (Flash EA 1112, ThermoFinnigan Italia S.p.A., Rodano (MI) Italy). In this method, the amount of nitrogen which was determined by the machine was converted into protein using a conversion factor of 5.7. For the determination of neutral detergent fiber (NDF), AACC approved method 30-25 (2010) was used. Fat content was determined using AOAC method 920.39 (2003) with an automated extractor Soxhlet using petroleum ether (CH-9230, Buchi Laborotechnik AG, Flawil, Switzerland). Moisture content was determined using the AACC approved method 44-19 [15] convection oven drying at 135°C (Model Labline, Inc. Chicago, IL, USA).

The rheological properties of the dough were determined using a Mixolab (Tripette and Renaud Chopin, Villeneuve La Garenne cedex, France) and Rapid Visco Analyzer (RVA) (Newport Scientific Pty. Ltd., Warriewood, Australia). For the Mixolab, the minimum torque (C_2), peak torque (C_3), cooking stability (C_4), set back (C_5) and the α, β, and γ were evaluated. As for the RVA, peak viscosity, temperature at peak viscosity, time to peak viscosity, and breakdown were measured.

2.5. Data Analysis

All collected data were analyzed with Microsoft Excel v.2007 and SAS v.9.0 software (SAS Institute, Cary, NC, USA) using a Type I error rate (α) of 0.05, by analysis of variance (ANOVA) to identify significant differences among treatments. Post-hoc Fisher's Least Significant Differences LSD tests were used to determine where the differences occurred.

3. Results and Discussion

The results for each measurement are summarized in following tables: Table 2 shows the effect of adding DDGS or SSL on chemical properties of final breads; Table 3 shows the effect of adding both DDGS and SSL on chemical properties of final breads; Table 4 shows the main effect of adding DDGS or SSL on physical properties of final breads; and Table 5 describes the effect of adding both DDGS and SSL on physical attributes of final breads. The results from treatment effects on Mixolab and RVA are shown in Tables 6–10, respectively. Tables 11 and 12 show the results for the main effect and treatment effect of DDGS and SSL on bread quality, respectively.

Table 2. Main effects on chemical properties of baked breads [1].

Effect (% Substitution)	Protein (% db) [2]		Fiber (% db)		Fat (% db)		Moisture	
	Mean	SD [3]	Mean	SD	Mean	SD	Mean	SD
DDGS (%)								
0	11.10 a	0.23	0.45 c	0.37	1.22 c	0.84	0.43 ab	0.03
10	12.48 b	0.15	2.05 b	0.37	1.75 b	1.09	0.40 b	0.35
20	13.66 c	0.10	3.71 a	0.42	2.4 a	1.12	0.38 a	0.57
SSL (%)								
0	12.51 a	1.17	2.42 a	1.44	0.86 c	0.40	0.44 a	0.04
2	12.49 a	1.04	2.04 b	1.59	1.49 b	0.59	0.42 a	0.06
5	12.24 b	1.21	1.75 b	1.38	3.07 a	0.68	0.42 a	0.04

[1] Different letters for a given dependent variable denote significant differences ($\alpha = 0.05$) across treatment conditions for that independent variable. [2] All properties are reported as % dry basis (db). [3] SD is standard deviation.

Table 3. Treatment effects on chemical properties of baked breads [1].

DDGS (%)	SSL (%)	Protein (% db) [2]		Fiber (% db)		Fat (% db)		Moisture (% db)	
		Mean	SD [3]	Mean	SD	Mean	SD	Mean	SD
0	0	11.17 d	0.04	0.90 d	0.04	0.50 f	0.00	0.45 a	0.02
0	2	11.29 d	0.24	0.28 e	0.25	0.87 e	0.03	0.43 ab	0.03
0	5	10.86 e	0.12	0.17 e	0.05	2.29 c	0.10	0.40 ab	0.01
10	0	12.58 b	0.05	2.26 c	0.36	0.73 ef	0.05	0.41 ab	0.00
10	2	12.58 b	0.01	2.02 c	0.05	1.43 d	0.01	0.38 b	0.01
10	5	12.29 c	0.07	1.88 c	0.64	3.11 b	0.06	0.41 ab	0.07
20	0	13.79 a	0.05	4.09 a	0.21	1.35 d	0.20	0.47 a	0.05
20	2	13.62 a	0.02	3.84 a	0.00	2.19 c	0.13	0.46 a	0.08
20	5	13.57 a	0.056	3.20 b	0.07	3.82 a	0.15	0.46 a	0.03

[1] Different letters for a given dependent variable denote significant differences ($\alpha = 0.05$) across treatment conditions for that independent variable. [2] All properties are reported as % dry basis. [3] SD is standard deviation.

Table 4. Main effects on physical properties of baked breads [1].

Effect (% Substitution)	Firmness (N) [2]		Extensibility (N) [2]		Thickness (mm)		a_w		L^*		a^*		b^*	
	Mean	SD [3]	Mean	SD	Mean	SD	Mean	SD	Mean	SD	Mean	SD	Mean	SD
DDGS (%)														
0	31.28 ^{b}	8.98	19.06 ^{a}	8.08	13.97 ^{b}	3.24	0.93 ^{a}	0.01	61.6 ^{b}	5.88	9.78 ^{a}	3.32	20.02 ^{a}	4.67
10	42.52 ^{a}	8.13	13.15 ^{b}	6.14	14.80 ^{ab}	1.01	0.88 ^{a}	0.16	72.94 ^{a}	2.68	10.22 ^{a}	2.79	22.86 ^{a}	2.15
20	39.10 ^{a}	5.41	10.41 ^{b}	2.99	16.06 ^{a}	1.84	0.94 ^{a}	0.00	71.03 ^{a}	4.01	9.74 ^{a}	1.57	23.67 ^{a}	1.84
SSL (%)														
0	33.57 ^{b}	10.91	17.65 ^{a}	4.60	13.32 ^{b}	2.86	0.94 ^{a}	0.01	69.51 ^{a}	4.77	11.01 ^{a}	2.55	23.27 ^{a}	1.71
2	38.85 ^{ab}	5.12	15.55 ^{a}	9.32	15.67 ^{a}	1.46	0.89 ^{a}	0.17	67.95 ^{a}	9.39	8.63 ^{a}	2.35	20.60 ^{a}	4.85
5	40.57 ^{a}	8.68	9.42 ^{b}	2.56	15.85 ^{a}	1.64	0.93 ^{a}	0.013	68.13 ^{a}	5.78	10.11 ^{a}	2.43	22.68 ^{a}	2.73

[1] Different letters for a given dependent variable denote significant differences ($\alpha = 0.05$) across treatment conditions for that independent variable. [2] The force was measured over time for firmness, and over travel distance for extensibility. [3] SD is standard deviation. a_w is water activity; L^* is the measure of lightness; a^* is the measure of greenness to redness; and b^* is the measure of blueness to yellowness.

Table 5. Treatment effects on physical properties of baked breads [1].

DDGS (%)	SSL (%)	Firmness (N) [2]		Extensibility (N) [2]		Thickness (mm)		a_w		L^*		a^*		b^*	
		Mean	SD [3]	Mean	SD	Mean	SD	Mean	SD	Mean	SD	Mean	SD	Mean	SD
0	0	20.95 ^{d}	5.83	18.53 ^{b}	5.28	9.70 ^{d}	0.97	0.94 ^{a}	0.00	65.14 ^{cb}	6.56	13.54 ^{a}	2.02	25.13 ^{a}	1.27
0	2	38.75 ^{bc}	5.13	27.05 ^{a}	7.03	15.72 ^{abc}	0.69	0.94 ^{a}	0.00	55.97 ^{d}	2.34	6.70 ^{b}	1.71	14.99 ^{c}	2.19
0	5	34.15 ^{c}	2.83	11.59 ^{cd}	1.49	16.49 ^{ab}	0.56	0.92 ^{b}	0.00	63.74 ^{cd}	5.21	9.11 ^{ab}	0.28	19.95 ^{b}	0.11
10	0	42.36 ^{bc}	4.50	21.05 ^{b}	2.71	14.72 ^{bc}	0.98	0.93 ^{a}	0.00	70.97 ^{abc}	3.33	11.24 ^{ab}	0.26	23.02 ^{ab}	0.85
10	2	35.19 ^{bc}	3.89	9.18 ^{cd}	1.51	0.38 ^{c}	0.01	0.92 ^{b}	1.30	74.62 ^{a}	1.44	8.98 ^{ab}	3.18	22.21 ^{ab}	2.98
10	5	50.33 ^{a}	7.34	9.23 ^{cd}	1.97	15.24 ^{abc}	0.79	0.93 ^{a}	0.02	73.23 ^{ab}	3.04	10.45 ^{ab}	4.85	23.35 ^{ab}	3.50
20	0	37.42 ^{bc}	6.85	13.38 ^{c}	1.25	15.55 ^{abc}	1.22	0.95 ^{a}	0.00	72.41 ^{abc}	0.75	8.25 ^{b}	0.67	21.68 ^{ab}	0.57
20	2	42.63 ^{b}	4.20	10.43 ^{cd}	1.23	16.83 ^{a}	1.36	0.93 ^{a}	0.00	73.28 ^{ab}	1.01	10.21 ^{ab}	1.41	24.61 ^{a}	1.95
20	5	37.24 ^{bc}	4.21	7.44 ^{d}	2.51	15.80 ^{abc}	2.81	0.94 ^{a}	0.00	67.41 ^{abc}	6.24	10.76 ^{ab}	1.73	24.73 ^{a}	0.94

[1] Different letters for a given dependent variable denote significant differences ($\alpha = 0.05$) across treatment conditions for that independent variable. [2] The force was measured over time for firmness and over travel distance for extensibility. [3] SD is standard deviation. a_w is water activity; L^* is the measure of lightness; a^* is the measure of greenness to redness; and b^* is the measure of blueness to yellowness.

Table 6. Main effect of DDGS on Mixolab operational parameters [1].

Effect (% Substitution)	C1 Time (min)		C1 Torque (Nm)		C2 Torque (Nm)		C3 Torque (Nm)		C4 Torque (Nm)		C5 Torque (Nm)		α [4] (N-m/min)		β [4] (N-m/min)		γ [4] (N-m/min)		Water Abs [3] (%)		Stability (s)	
	Mean	SD [2]	Mean	SD	Mean	SD	Mean	SD	Mean	SD	Mean	SD	Mean	SD	Mean	SD	Mean	SD	Mean	SD	Mean	SD
0	2.15^{a}	2.23	1.09^{b}	0.03	0.37^{a}	0.06	1.49^{a}	0.52	1.66^{a}	0.35	2.34^{a}	0.49	-0.05^{a}	0.03	0.31^{ab}	0.26	-0.01^{a}	0.08	53.36^{a}	2.88	7.60^{a}	4.12
10	2.47^{a}	2.29	1.12^{ab}	0.03	0.36^{a}	0.05	1.16^{a}	0.46	1.29^{a}	0.75	2.23^{a}	0.95	-0.06^{a}	0.03	0.37^{a}	0.31	-0.01^{a}	0.06	53.13^{a}	2.05	5.77^{a}	3.90
20	3.90^{a}	3.48	1.16^{a}	0.07	0.39^{a}	0.06	0.69^{b}	0.15	1.01^{a}	0.67	2.20^{a}	0.94	-0.07^{a}	0.03	0.093^{b}	0.034	0.02^{a}	0.02	52.08^{a}	2.12	5.80^{a}	3.70

[1] Different letters for a given dependent variable denote significant differences ($\alpha = 0.05$) across treatment conditions for that independent variable. [2] SD is standard deviation. [3] Abs is absorption. [4] α shows protein breakdown, β shows gelatinization and γ shows cooking stability rate.

Table 7. Main effect of SSL on Mixolab operational parameters [1].

Effect (% Substitution)	C1 Time (Min)		C1 Torque (Nm)		C2 Torque (Nm)		C3 Torque (Nm)		C4 Torque (Nm)		C5 Torque (Nm)		α [4] (N-m/min)		β [4] (N-m/min)		γ 4 (N-m/min)		Water Abs [3] (%)		Stability (s)	
	Mean	SD [2]	Mean	SD	Mean	SD	Mean	SD	Mean	SD	Mean	SD	Mean	SD	Mean	SD	Mean	SD	Mean	SD	Mean	SD
0	4.33^{a}	2.34	1.13^{a}	0.08	0.35^{b}	0.03	1.31^{a}	0.54	1.52^{a}	0.11	2.27^{a}	0.30	-0.08^{b}	0.04	0.33^{a}	0.20	0.00^{a}	0.04	53.13^{a}	2.41	10.22^{a}	1.11
2	3.17^{ab}	3.48	1.11^{a}	0.05	0.42^{ab}	0.05	1.20^{ab}	0.52	1.51^{a}	0.54	2.61^{a}	0.43	-0.06^{ab}	0.02	0.37^{a}	0.32	0.00^{a}	0.06	53.45^{a}	2.71	5.74^{b}	3.49
5	1.02^{b}	0.14	1.13^{a}	0.03	0.35^{a}	0.06	0.83^{b}	0.41	0.93^{a}	0.90	1.89^{a}	1.20	-0.04^{a}	0.02	0.07^{b}	0.07	0.00^{a}	0.08	52.00^{a}	1.89	3.20^{b}	2.20

[1] Different letters for a given dependent variable denote significant differences ($\alpha = 0.05$) across treatment conditions for that independent variable. [2] SD is standard deviation. [3] Abs is absorption. [4] α shows protein breakdown, β shows gelatinization and γ shows cooking stability rate.

Table 8. Treatment effects on Mixolab operational parameters [1].

DDGS (%)	SSL (%)	C1 Time (Min)		C1 Torque (Nm)		C2 Torque (Nm)		C3 Torque (Nm)		C4 Torque (Nm)		C5 Torque (Nm)		α [3] (N-m/min)		β [3] (N-m/min)		γ [3] (N-m/min)		Water Abs [3] (%)		Stability (s)	
		Mean	SD [2]	Mean	SD	Mean	SD	Mean	SD	Mean	SD	Mean	SD	Mean	SD	Mean	SD	Mean	SD	Mean	SD	Mean	SD
0	0	1.43^{ab}	0.12	1.08^{a}	0.00	0.37^{ab}	0.04	1.73^{a}	0.14	1.44^{bc}	0.09	2.00^{ab}	0.13	-0.04^{abc}	0.04	0.50^{ab}	0.01	-0.05^{bc}	0.01	50.75^{b}	2.05	10.55^{a}	1.45
0	2	3.99^{ab}	3.83	1.06^{a}	0.01	0.37^{ab}	0.05	1.71^{a}	0.13	1.44^{bc}	0.16	2.13^{ab}	0.36	-0.08^{abc}	0.03	0.47^{abc}	0.04	-0.05^{bc}	0.07	56.05^{a}	1.48	9.81^{a}	0.04
0	5	1.05^{ab}	0.02	1.14^{a}	0.02	0.37^{ab}	0.13	1.04^{abc}	0.86	2.10^{a}	0.05	2.91^{ab}	0.33	-0.03^{ab}	0.01	-0.02^{d}	0.01	0.06^{a}	0.08	53.30^{ab}	2.68	2.46^{b}	1.75
10	0	5.42^{ab}	0.43	1.12^{a}	0.03	0.33^{b}	0.02	1.59^{ab}	0.15	1.53^{abc}	0.14	2.35^{ab}	0.39	-0.10^{bc}	0.02	0.42^{abc}	0.06	-0.01^{abc}	0.00	54.65^{ab}	2.33	10.21^{a}	1.18
10	2	0.93^{b}	0.02	1.11^{a}	0.00	0.43^{ab}	0.03	1.14^{abc}	0.59	1.99^{ab}	0.16	3.01^{a}	0.12	-0.04^{ab}	0.01	0.57^{a}	0.51	0.04^{a}	0.00	52.75^{ab}	2.47	3.70^{b}	2.44
10	5	1.07^{ab}	0.21	1.12^{a}	0.05	0.32^{b}	0.02	0.76^{bc}	0.02	0.37^{d}	0.00	1.34^{b}	1.25	-0.04^{ab}	0.04	0.12^{bcd}	0.01	-0.08^{c}	0.05	52.00^{ab}	1.41	3.40^{b}	3.08
20	0	6.15^{a}	1.24	1.18^{a}	0.16	0.34^{ab}	0.00	0.62^{c}	0.09	1.60^{abc}	0.09	2.46^{ab}	0.26	-0.11^{c}	0.04	0.07^{cd}	0.01	0.05^{a}	0.00	54.00^{ab}	1.41	9.92^{a}	1.52
20	2	4.59^{ab}	5.55	1.17^{a}	0.04	0.46^{a}	0.04	0.76^{c}	0.30	1.10^{c}	0.78	2.70^{ab}	0.04	-0.06^{abc}	0.00	0.09^{cd}	0.06	0.02^{ab}	0.03	51.55^{ab}	2.61	3.73^{b}	2.33
20	5	0.96^{b}	0.19	1.14^{a}	0.00	0.37^{ab}	0.00	0.69^{c}	0.06	0.33^{d}	0.09	1.44^{ab}	1.59	-0.03^{a}	0.00	0.11^{bcd}	0.00	0.00^{abc}	0.01	50.7^{b}	1.41	3.75^{b}	3.13

[1] Different letters for a given dependent variable denote significant differences ($\alpha = 0.05$) across all treatment conditions. [2] SD is standard deviation. [3] α shows protein breakdown, β shows gelatinization and γ shows cooking stability rate, Abs is Absorption.

Table 9. Main effects on RVA operational parameters [1].

Effects (% Substitution)	Peak 1 (cP)		Trough 1 (Nm)		Break Down		Final Visc [3] (cP)		Setback (cP)		Peak Time (min)		Pasting Temp (°C)	
	Mean	SD [2]	Mean	SD	Mean	SD	Mean	SD	Mean	SD	Mean	SD	Mean	SD
DDGS (%)														
0	1532.0 ^{a}	309.27	839.33 ^{a}	360.90	692.66 ^{a}	91.41	3243.83 ^{a}	1968.38	2404.50 ^{a}	1648.26	5.93 ^{a}	0.56	86.13 ^{a}	10.18
10	1208.17 ^{b}	133.12	613.33 ^{b}	181.97	594.83 ^{b}	56.79	2152.50 ^{b}	959.03	1539.17 ^{b}	785.28	5.53 ^{b}	0.29	85.21 ^{a}	8.59
20	1017.50 ^{b}	72.70	548.83 ^{b}	23.49	468.66 ^{c}	65.91	1561.00 ^{b}	322.52	1012.17 ^{b}	317.90	5.33 ^{b}	0.04	88.36 ^{a}	1.77
SSL (%)														
0	1121.67 ^{b}	71.48	474.33 ^{b}	59.53	647.33 ^{a}	98.98	993.50 ^{b}	250.70	519.16 ^{b}	233.97	5.25 ^{b}	0.05	79.15 ^{b}	8.99
2	1233.33 ^{ab}	221.02	661.33 ^{ab}	163.97	572.00 ^{b}	106.28	2676.50 ^{a}	1089.27	2015.17 ^{a}	935.38	5.65 ^{a}	0.35	89.30 ^{a}	0.75
5	1402.67 ^{a}	423.11	865.83 ^{a}	311.94	536.83 ^{b}	132.10	3287.33 ^{a}	1418.14	2421.50 ^{a}	1132.29	5.88 ^{a}	0.51	91.25 ^{a}	2.02

[1] Different letters for a given dependent variable denote significant differences ($\alpha = 0.05$) across treatment conditions for that independent variable. [2] SD is standard deviation. [3] Visc is viscosity. RVA is Rapid Visco Analyzer.

Table 10. Treatment effects on RVA operational parameters [1].

DDGS (%)	SSL (%)	Peak 1(cP)		Trough 1 (Nm)		Break Down		Final Visc [3] (cP)		Setback (cP)		Peak Time (min)		Pasting Temp (°C)	
		Mean	SD [2]	Mean	SD	Mean	SD	Mean	SD	Mean	SD	Mean	SD	Mean	SD
0	0	1205.50 ^{d}	16.26	455.50 ^{c}	0.70	750.00 ^{a}	15.55	802.50 ^{f}	427.79	347.00 ^{e}	428.50	5.26 ^{e}	0.00	75.00 ^{b}	11.31
0	2	1501.50 ^{b}	28.99	842.00 ^{b}	171.11	659.50 ^{ab}	142.12	3965.00 ^{b}	486.48	3123.00 ^{a}	315.36	6.06 ^{b}	0.18	89.65 ^{a}	0.91
0	5	1889.00 ^{a}	84.85	1220.50 ^{a}	191.62	668.50 ^{ab}	106.77	4964.00 ^{a}	272.94	3743.50 ^{a}	464.56	6.46 ^{a}	0.28	93.75 ^{a}	1.06
10	0	1082.00 ^{ef}	32.52	422.00 ^{c}	19.79	660.00 ^{ab}	12.72	1024.00 ^{f}	46.66	602.00 ^{ed}	26.87	5.19 ^{e}	0.00	76.12 ^{a}	10.92
10	2	1172.00 ^{ed}	11.31	595.00 ^{c}	57.98	577.00 ^{bc}	46.66	2363.00 ^{d}	523.25	1768.00 ^{cb}	465.27	5.56 ^{bc}	0.14	89.50 ^{a}	1.06
10	5	1370.50 ^{c}	16.26	823.00 ^{b}	2.82	547.50 ^{bc}	13.43	3070.50 ^{c}	3070.50	2247.50 ^{b}	5.00	5.83 ^{cd}	37.47	90.02 ^{a}	0.04
20	0	1077.50 ^{ef}	55.86	545.50 ^{c}	31.81	532.00 bcd	24.04	1154.00 ^{ef}	52.32	608.50 ^{ed}	20.50	5.29 ^{ed}	0.04	86.32 ^{ab}	1.16
20	2	1026.50 ^{fg}	79.90	547.00 ^{c}	39.59	479.50 ^{cd}	40.30	1701.50 ^{ed}	61.51	1154.50 ^{cd}	21.92	5.33 ^{ed}	0.00	88.77 ^{a}	0.03
20	5	948.50 ^{g}	6.36	554.00 ^{c}	9.89	394.50 ^{d}	16.26	1827.50 ^{d}	27.57	1273.50 ^{c}	37.47	5.36 ^{ed}	0.04	0.04 ^{a}	0.04

[1] Different letters for a given dependent variable denote significant differences ($\alpha = 0.05$) across treatment conditions for that independent variable. [2] SD is standard deviation. [3] Visc is viscosity. RVA is Rapid Visco Analyzer.

Table 11. Main effects on quality evaluation parameters [1].

Effect	Uniformity		Size		Thickness		Softness		Color	
	Mean	SD [2]	Mean	SD	Mean	SD	Mean	SD	Mean	SD
DDGS (%)										
0	7.96 [b]	0.66	7.30 [a]	0.74	7.10 [a]	0.99	8.36 [a]	0.99	8.30 [a]	0.74
10	8.60 [a]	0.77	5.66 [b]	1.34	6.23 [b]	1.30	4.86 [c]	1.27	7.70 [b]	0.53
20	8.50 [a]	0.93	7.20 [a]	0.84	6.90 [a]	1.24	6.93 [b]	1.25	6.93 [c]	0.78
SSL (%)										
0	8.56 [a]	1.04	6.50 [b]	1.50	6.96 [a]	0.96	6.53 [b]	1.96	7.50 [a]	0.820
2	8.40 [ab]	0.77	7.26 [a]	0.04	6.44 [a]	1.66	6.33 [b]	1.62	7.63 [a]	1.88
5	8.10 [b]	0.60	6.40 [b]	1.10	6.80 [a]	1.39	7.26 [a]	1.91	7.80 [a]	0.55

[1] Different letters for a given dependent variable denote significant differences ($\alpha = 0.05$) across treatment conditions for that independent variable. [2] SD is standard deviation.

Table 12. Treatment effects on quality evaluation parameters [1].

DDGS (%)	SSL (%)	Uniformity		Size		Thickness		Softness		Color	
		Mean	SD [2]	Mean	SD	Mean	SD	Mean	SD	Mean	SD
0	0	7.70 [d]	0.82	7.10 [ab]	0.87	7.00 [b]	0.94	8.50 [ab]	0.89	8.10 [b]	0.73
0	0	7.90 [d]	0.56	7.70 [a]	0.82	7.50 [ab]	1.26	7.80 [bc]	0.918	8.80 [a]	0.78
0	0	8.30 [bcd]	0.48	7.10 [ab]	0.31	6.80 [bc]	0.63	8.80 [a]	1.03	8.00 [bc]	0.41
10	2	9.10 [a]	0.87	4.90 [c]	1.97	7.00 [b]	1.05	4.20 [e]	0.42	7.70 [bc]	0.48
10	2	8.60 [abc]	0.51	6.70 [b]	1.05	6.10 [cd]	0.87	5.40 [d]	1.64	7.50 [c]	0.70
10	2	8.10 [cd]	0.56	5.4 [c]	1.17	5.60 [d]	1.57	5.00 [ed]	1.24	7.90 [bc]	0.31
20	5	8.90 [ab]	0.87	7.50 [ab]	0.84	6.90 [bc]	0.94	6.90 [c]	0.99	6.70 [d]	0.48
20	5	8.70 [abc]	0.94	7.40 [ab]	0.69	5.80 [d]	0.42	5.90 [d]	1.19	6.60 [d]	0.84
20	5	7.90 [d]	0.73	6.70 [b]	0.82	8.00 [a]	0.47	8.00 [ab]	0.47	7.50 [c]	0.70

[1] Different letters for a given dependent variable denote significant differences ($\alpha = 0.05$) across treatment conditions for that independent variable. [2] SD is standard deviation.

3.1. Chemical Properties

3.1.1. Protein

The protein content of bread can be influenced by the Maillard reaction and also the aggregation, which can happen due to the dehydration of the surface due to high temperature during baking. In this study, the results from the main effect of DDGS showed that the highest content of protein was obtained in the bread substituted with 20% DDGS, which was expected since DDGS is a rich source of protein. As for SSL, the highest protein value was for bread with 0% SSL, while the lowest was for the bread made with 5% SSL. Thus, in the treatment effects, the highest value for protein content was the bread made with 0% SSL and 20% DDGS; a significant difference was observed between breads made with this treatment and control. This result is in accordance with a study by Reddy et al. [16], which showed that addition of DDG in the production of muffins resulted in higher protein content compared to controls. Another study showed that the addition of DDGS to chocolate chip cookies resulted in an increased protein content by 30% [17]. The protein content of the bread can be the direct reflection of fermentation in dough, because fermentation is an important step for the protein solubilization [18].

3.1.2. Fiber

As expected, the highest value of fiber was in the bread made with 20% DDGS and 0% of SSL, with a significant difference from the control bread. Up to 5% addition of SSL reduced fiber in the bread. DDGS is a very good source of dietary fiber, which can increase the nutritional value and rheological properties of bread. Although fiber can increase the water absorption through hydrogen binding which is due to the hydroxyl groups in the fiber structure, it can reduce bread volume and affect the texture as well [19]. Since the non-enzymatic browning among peptides can produce fiber-like substances, fiber content of Barbari can increase as a result of baking [20]. Our result is consistent with other studies which also showed that incorporation of DDGS in other products had similar results for fiber content. For instance, addition of corn distillers (CDS) into spaghetti resulted in enhancement of fiber content up to 12–14% in comparison with the control sample [8]. In another study, it was shown that addition of DDGS in chocolate chip cookies and banana bread increased the fiber content of final products [17].

3.1.3. Fat

Addition of DDGS at level of 20% resulted in the highest value of fat for the DDGS main effect, and addition of 5% SSL resulted in the highest fat content for the SSL main effect. For the treatment effect combinations, addition of 20% DDGS and 5% SSL, resulted in a significantly higher value of fat content compared to the control bread. According to Rasco et al. [17], this increase can be due to the high fat content of DDGS. Addition of SSL to the bread formulation can help in evenly distribution of lipids, and generation of fatty acid-amylose complex which may remain in the starch granules [21]. Similar results can be observed in other studies. For example, in a study by Reddy et al. [16], the amount of lipid in soft wheat DDG increased up to 1.4–2.4 times when compared to whole grain wheat prior to fermentation; however, incorporation of 10% DDG into wheat muffin did not change the fat content significantly.

3.1.4. Moisture

In general, Barbari bread has the highest moisture content among Iranian breads [20]. However, in this study, the highest moisture content as a main effect of SSL was found in the bread without SSL, and for the main effect of DDGS, the highest value was for the bread made without any DDGS. Although in a study, it was shown that addition of DDGS to baked products resulted in an increase in the water absorption [22], in our study, no significant differences were seen between different treatments in moisture content, as they had almost the same amount of moisture.

3.2. *Physical Properties*

3.2.1. Thickness of Bread

Addition of 20% DDGS incorporated with 2% SSL resulted in the highest value of thickness, likely due to the use of SSL in the bread. The lowest value was for control, which was significantly lower compared to bread made with 20% DDGS and 2% SSL. Thickness can be affected by both the fiber content and the use of hydrocolloids. Dietary fiber, in general, reduces the volume of bread. In a study by Park et al. [23], incorporation of fiber into bread resulted in decrease of volume by 5–15% due to the poor gas retention in bread. Also, another study showed that supplementation of 15 and 25% DDGS reduced the average thickness of cookies [24]. On the other hand, using hydrocolloids in bread formulation, such as SSL, can improve the formations of gluten networks and increase the volume of the bread.

3.2.2. Texture

Texture has a direct impact on consumer acceptability and it has other effects through releasing flavor and its influence on appearance [9]. In this study, two textural attributes of final bread samples were measured; firmness and extensibility. The highest value of extensibility was found in bread made with 0% and 2% SSL, and increasing the value of SSL up to 5% resulted in the lowest amount of extensibility. Also, addition of DDGS up to 20% resulted in decreased extensibility which occurred due to the low amount of gluten content in bread. Thus, the highest value of extensibility was measured in the bread made with 0% DDGS and 2% SSL, and the lowest extensibility value was for the bread made with 20% DDGS and 5% SSL which were significantly different than each other. The most important factor which gives extensibility to bread is the gluten and SSL can help strengthen the gluten network and retain gas which is produced by yeast in the dough [21].

One important factor which can result in an increased firmness of bread is the amount of fiber in the flour. In one study, bread with 2% fiber-supplementation had significantly firmer crumb compared to control bread. This was due to the thickening of walls surrounding the air bubbles in the crumb [19]. The highest amount of firmness, for addition of DDGS was the bread made with 10% DDGS, but it was not significantly different from the 20% DDGS. As for the addition and main effect of SSL, the highest amount of firmness was determined in the bread made with 5% SSL. As for the treatment effect, the treatment with 10% DDGS and 5% SSL had the highest amount of firmness and was significantly different from the control bread. However, in a study by Marco and Rosell [25], addition of hydroxypropyl methylcellulose (HPMC) in bread resulted in a significant decrease in crumb hardness; but addition of protein increased the hardness. Thus, another factor, which can improve bread firmness, is the protein content. In a study by Ahlborn et al. [26] it was shown that the force required to compress bread was higher for the bread with protein added than standard wheat bread. The protein in bread is gluten, which provides unique functional properties in bread and is responsible for the protein-starch interaction, providing specific viscoelastic properties in bread dough [26]. Thus, with the high content of fiber and protein as well as the effect of SSL on gluten formation, it can be implied that both DDGS and SSL affected the firmness and texture of bread samples.

3.2.3. Water Activity

There were no significant differences in water activity between different treatments, but the treatment with 20% DDGS and 0% SSL was slightly higher compared to the other treatments. In a study by Marco and Rosell [25], addition of HPMC resulted in a significant decrease of moisture due to hydrocolloids retaining water. Water has an important role in the production of bread; it takes part in starch gelatinization, protein denaturation, flavor, and color development. Fiber plays a role in the water absorption; as the amount of fiber increases, the flour-water absorption increases as well [27].

3.2.4. Color

Color is a quality parameter which affects consumer acceptability of bread. The formation of the golden yellow color on Barbari bread is produced because of the Romal which is brushed on the bread. Romal is made from baking soda and wheat flour dissolved in warm water, which leads to the formation of dextrin during baking and finally the golden color. Thus, the type of flour and the browning reaction which are non-enzymatic reactions, play important roles. Since bread contains both reducing sugars and amino groups, when it is heated, caramelization and Maillard reaction may take place at the same time. One study showed that in order for browning reactions to take place, temperature greater than 120 °C and water activity less than 0.6 are required [28]. In this study, L^*, a^* and b^* were determined for bread samples. In terms of DDGS main effect, addition of 20% DDGS had the highest L^* value which is due to the natural dark color of DDGS. For SSL main effect, there were no significant differences between different values of SSL. Overall, bread made with 20% DDGS and 2% SSL had the highest value of L^* which was significantly different than breads made with 0% DDGS, 2 and 5% of SSL. This was due to the incorporation of SSL in the flour matrix and Maillard reactions during baking which contributes to the golden and brown color of breads. The a^* value was highest for the bread made with 10% DDGS, so it was more red than all others; however, there were really no significant differences for different amounts of DDGS in formulations. As for SSL, the highest value was for no addition of SSL. The treatment effect showed the highest value was for the control bread, but there were no significant differences between different treatments. The highest b^* value was in the bread made with 20% DDGS and 5% SSL, which resulted in yellower bread, while the b^* value for the control bread and breads made with 20% DDGS, 2 and 5% SSL had no significant differences. In a study by Rasco et al. [17], it was shown that 30% blends of all-purpose flour and DDGS had a darker color, more red and more yellow than control blends. Color also can be affected by the raw ingredients, especially flour. DDGS is an ingredient which can have a great impact on the final product's color. Different bakery products have been tested and made with DDGS. For example, adding 30% DDGS to muffins made them darker in comparison to control muffins, and adding up to 20% DDGS resulted in a darker color in hush puppies [29].

3.2.5. Quality

In this study, Barbari breads were also tested for quality attributes such as uniformity, thickness, softness, size and color by the test panelists. Bread made with 10% DDGS and 0% SSL had the highest uniformity, and was significantly different than control bread. Other studies show that adding up to 10% DDG to wheat muffins changed neither appearance nor texture; however, a grainy texture in muffins supplemented with 20% DDG was found [16]. In another study, adding 30% DDG to muffins made the muffins dry and more irregular in cell distribution compared to the control [29]. As for the size, the highest amount was related to the bread made with 0% of DDGS and 2% of SSL but it was not significantly different than the control; the lowest was determined for the bread made with 10% DDGS and 0% SSL. In evaluation of bread thickness, bread made with 20% DDGS and 5% SSL had the highest amount, while the one made with 10% DDGS and 5% SSL had the lowest thickness.

The results for softness of samples showed that bread made with 0% DDGS and 5% SSL was softest. Addition of emulsifiers to baked products can lead to crumb softening because of the interaction of emulsifiers with the starch. Also, by preventing amylose and amylopectin retrogradation, they can inhibit bread staling [27]. Finally, in evaluation of color (Figure 1), bread made with 0% DDGS and 2% SSL had a better color which was significantly different than the control (0% DDGS and 0% SSL). In general, as DDGS increased, color decreased.

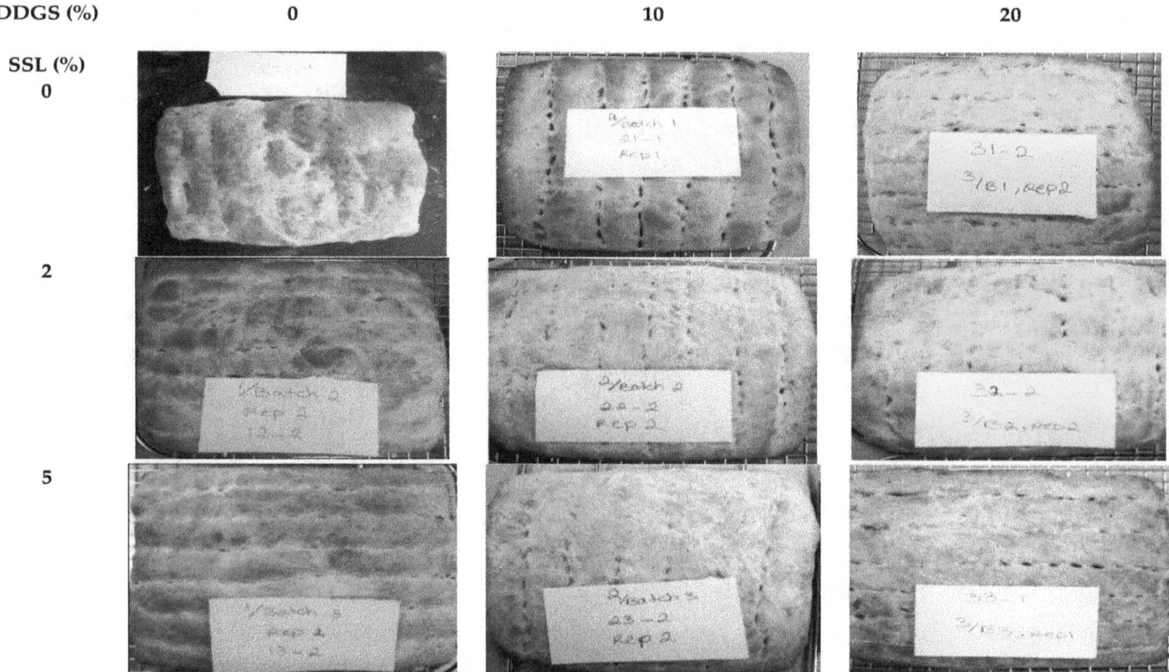

Figure 1. Final bread products baked with different blends of distillers dried grains with solubles (DDGS) and sodium stearoyl-2-lactate (SSL).

3.3. *Mixolab Results*

As shown in Table 8, different Mixolab parameters were measured in this study. Development time (C1) was a maximum value when 10% DDGS and 5% SSL were used, this part of the curve is where water is being added to the flour and the starch granules and proteins start to absorb water, making them swelled; C1 values were close to each other, and there were no significant differences between different levels of DDGS and SSL which indicates resistance of the dough in all treatments. The measurement of minimum torque (C2), which shows the protein behavior, also didn't show significant differences between different treatment effects. This part of the curve shows the protein behavior and how strong the protein can be in the dough network. Since addition of DDGS added to the protein value of the dough, it is reasonable to see insignificant differences in the C2 values. As for peak torque (C3), the highest value was for control sample, which indicates better quality of starch and shows a decrease as DDGS increased. The cooking stability (C4), which is the indication of amylastic activity, had the highest value for 0% DDGS and 5% SSL, and the lowest value was measured when 20% DDGS and 5% SSL were used, with significant differences between the two treatments. The set back (C5) had the highest value for 10% DDGS and 2% SSL, and it had a significant difference in treatment with lowest value of C5 in which 10% DDGS and 5% SSL were used; in this region retrogradation of starch happens, which caused an increase in the consistency as the temperature was decreasing.

Other parameters determined for Mixolab measurement were α, with the highest value for treatment with 20% DDGS and 5% SSL, which indicated that addition of DDGS to the wheat flour can help improving the protein network of the dough, as α shows the protein break down in the dough matrix. β, which is a good indicator of starch gelatinization, had the highest value for the treatment with 10% DDGS and 2% SSL, and lowest value for 0% of DDGS and 5% SSL, with significant differences between them; and γ, which shows the rate at which cooking stability is reached, had the highest value in the treatment with 0% DDGS and 5% SSL. Water absorption in the developing dough had its highest value for the treatment of 0% DDGS and 2% SSL, with significant difference from that of control dough. Also, the stability time had its highest value for the control sample, but the lowest value for the incorporation of 5% SSL and 0% DDGS. Stronger wheat flours have the ability to absorb and retain more water compared to weak flours (flours with lower protein content). Higher development time indicates stronger flour (flours with higher protein content) [12]. These results are in accordance with other studies; for instance, using an amylograph, it was determined that the addition of SSL to defatted soybean meal and defatted sesame meal caused slight delay of on-set of starch gelatinization and the flour with higher SSL had higher water absorption [30]. In another study, addition of surfactants decreased water absorption of flour by about 0.4–1.2%, and the dough development time decreased by 0.5 min with SSL and DATEM (mono and diacetyltartaric acid) combination [31]. In the study by Tsen et al. [9], replacement of flour by 10 to 20% DDG reduced dough development time.

3.4. *Rapid Visco Analyzer (RVA) Results*

RVA can be used to measure pasting properties. The RVA pasting curve can detect differences in flour viscosity with a small amount of sample and in a short period of time [32]. Because in our study, SSL was used, peak viscosity, pasting temperature and setback measured by the RVA can be useful in predicting the dough behavior during baking. Wheat chemistry is complex, involving interactions between gliadin and glutenin as well as starch and gluten network. Interactions between gliadin and glutenin are responsible for the initial RVA viscosity [33], and these interactions can affect bread quality. In our study, the highest peak value occurred for the treatment in which 0% DDGS and 5% SSL was used, which was significantly different from the sample made with 20% DDGS and 5% SSL. When starch granules start swelling, viscosity of the paste will increase until a maximum viscosity is reached at "peak viscosity" which is the reflection of water binding capacity of the starch [34]. The trough value was the highest when 0% of DDGS and 5% of SSL were used compared to the control sample which had the lowest value. When 20% DDGS and 5% of SSL were used, the break down had its lowest value compared to the control sample with highest value. In one study, the behavior of wheat flour subjected to shear stress was affected by adding hydrocolloids, causing an increase in water absorption and dough development time [12]. The final viscosity had the highest value with incorporation of 5% SSL and 0% DDGS which were significantly different from the control. As for the setback time, the highest value was measured when 0% DDGS were used and 5% SSL. The control sample had the lowest peak time, and the highest peak time value occurred when 0% DDGS and 5% SSL were used, with significant differences between these two treatments. The last parameter measured was pasting temperature, with the highest value when 0% DDGS and 5% SSL were used. This was expected because of the role of SSL in interaction between starch and gluten network. Changes in the gluten network, such as conformational modifications and loss of hydrogen bonds can decrease RVA viscosity during heating [33]. On the other hand, higher swelling capacity of starch will result in a higher peak viscosity, as the ability of the starch to withstand high temperatures and shear stresses is important [35].

4. Conclusions

Flat breads made from various types of flours, especially wheat flour, are the oldest type of food. Certain deficiencies and nutritional problems exist with cereal-based products, particularly breads. Because of the high demand for flat breads in most countries, fortification of breads can help providing additional nutrients to consumers. DDGS is a good source of protein as well as fiber and can be an inexpensive source for fortification of flat breads. In this study, three levels (0%, 10% and 20%) of DDGS were added to the wheat flour to study the changes in the physical and chemical properties of the final bread products. In addition to the DDGS, SSL was also added to the formulation at three levels (0%, 2% and 5%). The resulting breads were measured for their physical and chemical properties. Overall, the results of this study showed that addition of DDGS can increase fiber and protein values of Barbari bread significantly, while addition of 5% SSL can lead to a softer texture of bread. As the DDGS content increased in the bread formulations, the L^* increased because of the darkness in the DDGS. In addition to the physical and chemical properties of the final products, the rheological properties of the flours were also measured using Mixolab and RVA. The results showed that water absorption of the developing dough had its highest value for the treatment of 0% DDGS and 2% of SSL. For the RVA, highest amount of peak value was for the treatment in which 0% of DDGS and 5% of SSL. The final viscosity had the highest value with incorporation of 5% SSL and 0% of DDGS.

Acknowledgments: The authors would like to thank the USDA, ARS for providing funding, as well as South Dakota State University for use of facilities and equipment.

Author Contributions: K.A.R. and R.G.K conceived and designed the experiments; S.P. performed the experiments; S.P. and K.A.R. analyzed the data; S.P. and K.A.R. wrote the paper; K.A.R. and R.G.K edited the paper.

References

1. Mckevith, B. Nutritional aspects of Cereals. *Nutr. Bull.* **2004**, *29*, 111–142. [CrossRef]
2. Qarooni, J. *Flat Bread Technology*; Chapman and Hall: New York, NY, USA, 1996.
3. Schilling, M.W.; Battula, V.; Loar, R.E.; Jackson, V.; Kin, S.; Corzo, A. Dietary inclusion level effects of Distillers Dried Grains with Solubles on broiler meat quality. *Poult. Sci.* **2010**, *89*, 752–760. [CrossRef] [PubMed]
4. Bobcock, B.A.; Hayes, D.J.; Lawrence, J.D. *Using Distillers Grain in the US and International Livestock and Poultry Industry*; Midwest Agribusiness Trade Research and Information Center: Ames, IA, USA, 2008.
5. Belyea, R.L.; Rausch, K.D.; Tumbleson, M.E. Composition of corn and distillers dried grains with soluble from dry grind ethanol processing. *Bioresour. Technol.* **2004**, *94*, 293–298. [CrossRef] [PubMed]
6. Wu, Y.V.; Youngs, V.L.; Warner, K.; Bookwalter, G.N. Evaluation of spaghetti supplemented with corn distillers dried grains. *Cereal Chem.* **1987**, *64*, 434–436.
7. Finley, J.W.; Hanamoto, M.M. Milling and baking properties of dried brewer's spent grains. *Cereal Chem.* **1980**, *57*, 166–168.
8. Tsen, C.C.; Eyestone, W.; Weber, J. Evaluation of the quality of cookies supplemented with distillers dried grain flour. *J. Food Sci.* **1982**, *47*, 648–685. [CrossRef]
9. Tsen, C.C.; Weber, J.L.; Eyestone, W. Evaluation of DDG flour as a bread ingredient. *Cereal Chem.* **1983**, *60*, 295–297.
10. Liu, S.X.; Singh, M.; Inglett, G. Effect of incorporation of Distillers Dried Grain with Solubles (DDGS) on quality of cornbread. *Food Sci. Technol.* **2010**, *44*, 713–718. [CrossRef]
11. Caonkar, A.G.; Mcpherson, A. *Ingredient Interactions Effect on Food Quality*; Taylor and Francis Group: Boca Raton, FL, USA, 2006.
12. Rosell, C.M.; Collar, C.; Haros, M. Assessment of hydrocolloid effects on the thermo-mechanical properties of wheat using the Mixolab. *Food Hydrocoll.* **2007**, *21*, 452–462. [CrossRef]
13. Hebeda, R.E.; Zobel, H.F. *Baked Goods Freshness Technology, Evaluation and Inhibition of Staling*; CRC Press: New York, NY, USA; Marcel Dekker: New York, NY, USA, 1996.
14. AACC International. *Approved Methods of Analysis*, 11th ed.; Methods 08-03, 30-25, 44-19 and 46-30; AACCI: St. Paul, MN, USA, 2010.
15. AOAC International. *Official Methods of Analysis of the Association of Analytical Chemists*, 17th ed.; Method 920.39; The Association: Gaithersburg, MA, USA, 2003.
16. Reddy, N.R.; Pierson, M.D.; Cooler, F.W. Supplementation of wheat muffins with dried distillers grain flour. *J. Food Qual.* **1986**, *9*, 243–249. [CrossRef]
17. Rasco, B.A.; Dong, F.M.; Hashisaka, A.E.; Gazzaz, S.S.; Downey, S.E.; Buenarentura, M.S. Chemical composition of distillers dried grains with solubles from soft white wheat, hard red wheat and corn. *J. Food Sci.* **1987**, *52*, 236–237. [CrossRef]
18. Horszwald, A.; Troszynska, A.; Delcastillo, D.; Zielinski, H. Protein and sensorial properties of rye breads. *Eur. Food Res. Technol.* **2009**, *229*, 875–886. [CrossRef]
19. Gomez, M.; Ronda, F.; Banco, C.A.; Caballero, P.A.; Apestegulia, A. Effect of dietary fiber on dough rheology and bread quality. *Eur. Food Res. Technol.* **2003**, *216*, 51–56. [CrossRef]
20. Faridi, H.A.; Finney, P.L.; Rubenthaler, G.L.; Hubbard, J.D. Functional (bread making) and compositional characteristics of Iranian flat breads. *J. Food Sci.* **1982**, *47*, 926–929. [CrossRef]

21. Ghanbari, M.; Shahedi, M. Effect of shortening and SSL on the staling of Barbari bread. *J. Sci. Technol. Agric. Nat. Resour.* **2008**, *43*, 382–390.
22. Abbott, J.; O'Palka, J.; McGuire, C.F. DDGS: Particle size effect on volume and acceptability of baked products. *J. Food Sci.* **1991**, *5*, 1323–1326. [CrossRef]
23. Park, H.; Seib, P.A.; Chung, O.K. Fortifying bread with a mixture of wheat fiber and psyllium husk fiber plus three antioxidants. *Cereal Chem.* **1997**, *74*, 207–211. [CrossRef]
24. Sahlstrom, S.; Baevre, A.B.; Brathen, E. Impact of starch properties on hearth bread charactristics. *J. Cereal Sci.* **2002**, *37*, 275–284. [CrossRef]
25. Marco, C.; Rosell, C.M. Breadmaking performance of protein enriched, gluten free breads. *Eur. Food Res. Technol.* **2008**, *227*, 1205–1213. [CrossRef]
26. Ahlborn, G.J.; Pike, O.A.; Hendriz, S.B.; Hess, W.M.; Huber, C.S. Sensory, mechanical and microscopic evaluation of staling in low-protein and gluten free breads. *Cereal Chem.* **2005**, *82*, 328–335. [CrossRef]
27. Ribotta, P.D.; Perez, G.T.; Leon, A.E.; Anon, M.C. Effect of emulsifier and guar gum on micro structural, rheological and baking performance of frozen bread dough. *Food Hydrocoll.* **2004**, *18*, 305–313. [CrossRef]
28. Parlis, E.; Salvadori, V.O. Modeling the browning of bread during baking. *Food Res. Int.* **2009**, *42*, 865–870. [CrossRef]
29. Brochetti, D.; Penfield, M.P. Sensory characteristics of bakery products containing distillers dried grains form corn, barley and rye. *J. Food Qual.* **1989**, *12*, 413–426. [CrossRef]
30. Safdar, M.N.; Naseem, K.; Siddiqui, N.; Amjad, M.; Hameed, T.; Khalil, S. Quality evaluation of different wheat varieties for the production of unleavened flat bread (chapatti). *Pak. J. Nutr.* **2009**, *8*, 1773–1778. [CrossRef]
31. Azizi, M.H.; Rao, G.V. Effect of surfactant gel and gum combination on dough rheological characteristics and quality of bread. *J. Food Qual.* **2004**, *27*, 320–336. [CrossRef]
32. Sabanis, D.; Lebesi, D.; Tzia, C. Effect of dietary fiber enrichment on selected properties of gluten-free bread. *Food Sci. Technol.* **2009**, *42*, 1380–1389.
33. Lagrain, B.; Thewissen, B.G.; Brijs, K.; Delcour, J.A. Mechanism of glidin-glutenin cross-linkage during hydrothermal treatment. *Food Chem.* **2008**, *107*, 753–760. [CrossRef]
34. Farahnaki, A.; Majzoobi, M. Physiochemical properties of partbaked breads. *Int. J. Food Prop.* **2008**, *11*, 186–195. [CrossRef]
35. Ragaee, S.; Abdel-Aal, E.M. Pasting properties of starch and protein in selected cereals and quality of their products. *Food Chem.* **2006**, *95*, 9–18. [CrossRef]

11

Gluten-Free Alternative Grains: Nutritional Evaluation and Bioactive Compounds

Serena Niro [1], Annacristina D'Agostino [1], Alessandra Fratianni [1,*], Luciano Cinquanta [2] and Gianfranco Panfili [1]

[1] Dipartimento di Agricoltura, Ambiente e Alimenti, Università degli Studi del Molise, Via De Sanctis, 86100 Campobasso, Italy; serena.niro@unimol.it (S.N.); a.dagostino@studenti.unimol.it (A.D.A.); panfili@unimol.it (G.P.)

[2] Dipartimento Scienze Agrarie, Alimentari e Forestali, Università di Palermo, Viale delle Scienze 4, 90128 Palermo, Italy; luciano.cinquanta@unipa.it

* Correspondence: fratianni@unimol.it

Abstract: Interest in gluten-free grains is increasing, together with major incidences of celiac disease in the last years. Since to date, knowledge of the nutritional and bioactive compounds profile of alternative gluten-free grains is limited, we evaluated the content of water-soluble (thiamine and riboflavin) and liposoluble vitamins, such as carotenoids and tocols (tocopherols and tocotrienols), of gluten-free minor cereals and also of pseudocereals. The analysed samples showed a high content of bioactive compounds; in particular, amaranth, cañihua and quinoa are good sources of vitamin E, while millet, sorghum and teff (*Eragrostis tef*, or William's Lovegrass) are good sources of thiamine. Moreover, millet provides a fair amount of carotenoids, and in particular of lutein. These data can provide more information on bioactive compounds in gluten-free grains. The use of these grains can improve the nutritional quality of gluten-free cereal-based products, and could avoid the monotony of the celiac diet.

Keywords: minor cereal; pseudocereal; bioactive compound; gluten-free grain; tocols; carotenoids

---

1. Introduction

Celiac disease is a chronic systemic, autoimmune disorder in genetically-predisposed individuals, triggered by exposure to dietary gluten, and resulting in mucosal inflammation, villous atrophy and crypt hyperplasia [1]. It is characterised by an abnormal immune reaction consisting of an excessive response of the immune system to a group of cereal proteins, called prolamines (gliadin, hordein, sekalina, avenin), which are found in wheat, barley, rye and oats. Celiac disease affects approximately 1% of the world population, and it has significantly increased due to an underestimation, since it is often left undiagnosed [2]. The only treatment for people with the celiac problem is the adherence to gluten-free foods for their whole lifetime.

Several studies demonstrated that sticking to a gluten-free diet for a lifetime can lead to a nutritional imbalance in celiac subjects, such as a malabsorption of nutrients, and deficiencies of several vitamins and minerals. These deficiencies are due both to the phenomena of malabsorption at the intestinal level, and to the monotony of a diet based mainly on rice and maize [3–6].

Recently, more attention has been given to gluten-free minor cereals and pseudocereals as alternatives to those conventionally used for celiacs. Many of them have been defined as "orphan crops" or "underutilised crops"; they are indigenous crops scarcely documented and rarely used by food industries [7]. Many underutilised crops are relatively more drought-tolerant than most major cereals; they play a significant role in many developing countries, providing food security and income to resource-poor farmers [8].

Gluten-free alternative sources studied in this work include minor cereals (sorghum, teff, millet and wild rice), and pseudocereals (quinoa, cañihua, chia, and amaranth). These grains are mainly consumed as flours and seeds, which can be added to preparations such as soups, yogurt, cakes, breads and others cereal-based products; nevertheless, any commercialisation of these products is still quite limited in the Italian market. Some of these are a source of nutrients and bioactive compounds that could improve the nutritional quality of gluten-free products.

Carotenoids are a significant group of bioactive compounds with health promoting properties [9,10] and are responsible for the colour of a wide variety of grains [11]. Some carotenoids are the precursors of retinol (vitamin A), and are very strong natural antioxidants. Carotenoids are known to be efficient physical and chemical quenchers of singlet oxygen, as well as potent scavengers of other reactive oxygen species [9]. Vitamin E is a natural antioxidant comprising two groups of vitamers, tocopherols and tocotrienols, occurring in eight forms: α-tocopherol (α-T), β-tocopherol (β-T), γ-tocopherol (γ-T), and δ-tocopherol (δ-T) and α-tocotrienol (α-T3), β-tocotrienol (β-T3), γ-tocotrienol (γ-T3), and δ-tocotrienol (δ-T3). Vegetable oils are the main tocol sources, however, substantial amounts of these compounds are also reported in most cereal grains [12–14]. The potential health benefits of tocols include the prevention of certain types of cancer, heart diseases and other chronic diseases [15,16]. Thiamine (B1) is one of the major water-soluble vitamins, as it plays an important role as a co-factor of several key enzymes involved in the carbohydrate metabolism and defence mechanism [17]. It can be found in moderate amounts in all foods: Nuts and seeds, legumes, wholegrain/enriched cereals and breads, as well as pork [18]. Thiamine deficiency is rare in healthy individuals in food-secure settings, where access to thiamine-rich foods ensures adequate intakes [19]. Riboflavin (B2) is a precursor of the co-enzymes flavin mononucleotide (FMN; riboflavin phosphate) and flavin adenine dinucleotide (FAD), which are components of oxidases and dehydrogenases. It is also important for skin health and normal vision, and can be found in whole cereals, breads, leafy green vegetables and milk products [18].

To date, the evaluation of nutritional and bioactive compound profiles of alternative gluten-free grains is limited, if not lacking [20–23]. These researches are of a great importance in order to formulate gluten-free cereal-based products with a higher nutritional value. Thus, in this work, samples of minor cereals and pseudocereals commercialised in Italy have been characterised for their nutritional value, with a particular focus on some bioactive compounds, such as carotenoids, tocols, thiamine and riboflavin, in order to increase the awareness of their nutritional profile. Moreover, data coming from this study may be included in food nutrient databases.

2. Material and Methods

2.1. Sample Collection and Preparation

Thirty one different minor cereals and pseudocereals were bought in Italian specialised shops (Table 1). Different brands were considered for each grain. Grains were grounded with a refrigerated IKA A10 laboratory mill (Staufen, Germany), then carefully mixed and stored at −20 °C until analysis. Each sample was analysed in triplicate.

Table 1. List of analysed gluten-free grains.

Minor Cereals	Samples (*n*)
Millet (*Panicum miliaceum* L.)	6
White Sorghum (*Sorghum bicolor* L.)	3
Teff (*Eragrostis tef* (Zucc.) Trotter)	4
Wild rice (*Zizania aquatica* L.)	2

Table 1. *Cont.*

Pseudocereals	
White quinoa (*Chenopodium quinoa* Willd.)	3
Pigmented quinoas (red and black) (*Chenopodium quinoa* Willd.)	4
Cañihua (*Chenopodium pallidicaule*)	3
Amaranth (*Amaranthus* spp.)	3
Chia (*Salvia hispanica* L.)	3

2.2. *Chemical Analysis*

2.2.1. Proximate Analysis

Moisture, ash, fat, and protein contents were determined using an ICC standard procedure [24]. Briefly, moisture was determined using an oven set at 130 °C, and ash was quantified using a muffle furnace set at 525 °C. The protein content was determined though the Kjeldhal method (N × 6.25), and lipids were determined by the Soxhlet method. Carbohydrates plus fibre were calculated as a difference, using the following equation: (100 − (% moisture + % lipids + % proteins + % ash)).

2.2.2. Carotenoid Analysis

Carotenoid extraction was carried out using the saponification method reported by Panfili et al. [14]. About 0.2 g of milled sample was weighed and placed in a screw-capped tube. Then, 5 mL of ethanolic pyrogallol (60 g/L) was added as an antioxidant, followed by 2 ml of absolute ethanol, 2 mL of sodium chloride (10 g/L) and 2 mL of potassium hydroxide (600 g/L). The tubes were placed in a 70 °C water bath and mixed every 5–10 min during saponification. After alkaline digestion at 70 °C for 45 min, the tubes were cooled in an ice bath, and 15 mL of sodium chloride (10 g/L) were added. The suspension was then extracted twice with 15 mL portions of n-hexane/ethyl acetate (9:1, *v*/*v*). The organic layers, containing carotenoids, were collected and evaporated to dryness; the dry residue was dissolved in 2 mL of isopropyl alcohol (10%) in *n*-hexane. A HPLC Dionex (Sunnyvale, CA) analytical system, consisting of a U6000 pump system and a 50 µL injector loop (Rheodyne, Cotati) was used. The chromatographic separation of the compounds was achieved by means of a 250 mm × 4.6 mm i.d., 5 µm particle size, Kromasil Phenomenex Si column (Torrance, CA, USA). The mobile phase was *n*-hexane/isopropyl alcohol (5%) at a flow rate of 1.5 mL/min. Spectrophotometric detection was achieved by means of a diode array detector set in the range of 350–500 nm. Peaks were detected at 450 nm. Carotenoids were identified through their spectral characteristic, and comparison of their retention times with known standard solutions. Data were stored and processed by a Dionex Chromeleon Version 6.6 chromatography system (Sunnyvale, CA, USA). All-trans-β-carotene and lutein were obtained from Sigma Chemicals (St. Louis, MO, USA); zeaxanthin and β-cryptoxanthin were obtained from Extrasynthese (Z.I. Lyon-Nord, Genay, France).

2.2.3. Tocol Analysis

Tocols were determined after the same saponification method described for carotenoids. An aliquot of the carotenoid extract was collected and evaporated to dryness, and the dry residue was dissolved in 2 mL of isopropyl alcohol (1%) in *n*-hexane, and was analysed by HPLC, under normal phase conditions, using a 250 × 4.6 mm i.d., 5 mm particle size Kromasil Phenomenex Si column (Torrance, CA, USA) [14]. Fluorometric detection of all compounds was performed at an excitation wavelength of 290 nm and an emission wavelength of 330 nm by means of an RF 2000 spectrofluorimeter (Dionex, Sunnyvale, CA, USA). The mobile phase was *n*-hexane/ethylacetate/acetic acid (97.3:1.8:0.9 *v*/*v*/*v*), at a flow rate of 1.6 mL/min [14,25]. Compounds were identified by a comparison of their retention times with those of known available standard solutions, and quantified through the calibration curves of the standard solutions. The concentration range was 5–25 µg/mL for every tocol standard. Vitamin E activity was expressed as Tocopherol Equivalent (T.E.) (mg/100 g of fresh weight f.w.), calculated as reported by Sheppard et al. [26].

2.2.4. Thiamine and Riboflavin Analysis

Thiamine and riboflavin were extracted as in Hasselman et al. [27]. Briefly, samples were placed in 100 mL volumetric flasks containing 20 mL of 0.1 N HCl and heated in a water bath at 100 °C for 30 min. After cooling at room temperature, the pH of the samples was adjusted to 4.5 with 2.5 M NaOAc. Following the addition of 0.2 mL of aqueous Clara-Diastase (50 mg/mL), these samples were incubated for 3 h at 37 °C. After cooling, the samples were brought up to 25 mL with distilled water. Then these same samples were centrifuged and filtered through a 0.45 µm filter. Thiamine was converted to thiochrome by adding 1.25 mL of 1% potassium ferricyanide in 15% aqueous NaOH to 2.5 mL of filtered extract. After 1 min for oxidation, 0.25 mL of 85% H_3PO4 was added. The extract was purified on a Sep-Pak C18 cartridge. The cartridge was washed with 5 mL MeOH, followed by 5 ml of 0.05 M NH_4OAc (adjusted to pH 5.0 (acidic) with HOAc). The sample (5 mL) was loaded into a Sep-Pak C18 cartridge, and then the cartridge was washed with 0.05 M NH_4OAc and, finally, the vitamins were eluted with 5 mL mobile phase. Extracts were separated by a HPLC Dionex (Sunnyvale, CA, USA), with a U3000 pump and an injector loop (Rheodyne, Cotati). Separation was made at a flow rate of 0.8 mL/min with Methanol: NaOAc (40:60 *v*/*v*) as a mobile phase, by using a 5 µm C18 Luna, Phenomenex (Torrance, CA, USA) stainless steel column (250 × 4.6 mm i.d.). Fluorometric detection was performed at an excitation wavelength of 366 nm and an emission wavelength of 453 nm for thiamine, and an excitation wavelength of 453 nm and an emission wavelength of 580 nm for riboflavin, by means of an RF 2000 spectrofluorimeter (Dionex, Sunnyvale, CA, USA). Data were processed by a Dionex Chromeleon Version 6.6 chromatography system (Sunnyvale, CA, USA). Thiamine and riboflavin were compared with known available standards, and identified considering their retention times and relative elution order. Thiamine and riboflavin standards were obtained from Sigma Chemicals (St. Louis, MO, USA).

3. Results and Discussion

3.1. Nutritional Composition

The nutritional composition of analysed minor cereals and pseudocereals is shown below in Table 2.

Table 2. Nutritional composition of gluten-free grains (g/100 g).

	Minor Cereals				Pseudocereals			
	Millet	**Sorghum**	**Teff**	**Wild Rice**	**Quinoa (White and Pigmented)**	**Cañihua**	**Amaranth**	**Chia**
Moisture	12.7 (2.0) [a]	12.5 (6.9)	11.5 (1.4)	10.5 (0.4)	11.5 (9.8)	8.6 (5.7)	11.0 (1.0)	8.4 (6.7)
Ash	1.0 (63.0)	1.4 (8.6)	2.3 (5.6)	1.8 (7.2)	2.2 (3.0)	2.4 (6.6)	2.3 (8.7)	4.5 (2.7)
Protein	11.7 (3.3)	9.0 (0.1)	11.7 (1.7)	12.4 (6.1)	12.9 (1.5)	14.1 (2.6)	13.8 (3.4)	21.5 (7.6)
Fat	4.4 (0.4)	2.6 (26.9)	2.4 (4.1)	1.2 (4.5)	5.8 (12.0)	8.4 (1.1)	6.1 (5.7)	35.4 (2.1)
Carbohydrate + Fibre *	70.2	74.5	72.1	74.1	67.6	66.8	66.8	30.2

* Calculated by difference; [a]: coefficient of variability.

The composition of the chia seeds notably differs from all the other cereal and pseudocereal samples, showing high concentrations of fats (35.4 g/100 g), proteins (21.5 g/100 g) and ash (4.5 g/100 g). These values are similar to those observed by other authors for the chia seeds [28]. In general, wild rice and pseudocereals are a good source of protein. Taking European law into account [29], wild rice, all quinoa seeds, cañihua and amaranth can be declared in a label with the claim "source of protein", since they contain at least 12 g of protein per 100 g. Chia seeds can be declared with a "high protein content", since they contain at least 20 g of protein per 100 g. The fat content was significantly higher for pseudocereals, if compared to minor cereals. Wild rice shows the lower fat content (1.2 g/100 g).

3.2. *Carotenoids*

Table 3 shows the carotenoid amounts of analysed samples. Carotenoids content (μg/100 g dry weight d.w.) varied significantly from 22 μg/100 g in amaranth to 763 μg/100 g in millet. In all gluten-free grains the main compounds are lutein and zeaxanthin. A comparison with the literature related to the HPLC analysis of carotenoids is very difficult, since the available few data are obtained by different methods, and these pigments may vary depending on genotype and location. The total carotenoid content of millet, wild rice, quinoas and cañihua is comparable with that of wheat (about 305 μg/100 g for durum and about 150 μg/100 g for soft wheat) [12,30], and of pigmented rice (460–50 μg/100 g) [31], but it is significantly lower than that of maize (about 1110 μg/100 g) [30,32]. Among minor cereals, literature data are reported only for sorghum [33], where the authors found an average amount of 20 μg/100 g as the sum of lutein and zeaxanthin, with a high variability among the different genotypes.

Table 3. Carotenoid composition in gluten-free grains (μg/100 g d.w.).

Carotenoids	Minor Cereals				Pseudocereals				
	Millet	Sorghum	Teff	Wild Rice	White Quinoa	Pigmented Quinoas	Cañihua	Amaranth	Chia
β-Carotene	19.8 (15.0) [a]	9.86 (10.0)	7.8 (20.0)	6.23 (10.0)	12.3 (10.0)	23.6 (23.0)	20.2 (28.0)	tr	12.4 (10.0)
β-Criptoxanthin	20.0 (30.0)	nd	tr	tr	tr	tr	tr	nd	nd
Lutein	535.5 (3.4)	11.2 (64.0)	36.45 (30.0)	196.2 (36.6)	85.6 (1.3)	265.2 (33.0)	325.3 (0.1)	19.8 (5.0)	tr
Zeaxanthin	188.3 (10.0)	28.9 (10.0)	18.4 (40.0)	9.7 (10.0)	11.2 (11.0)	13.2 (30.0)	40.2 (4.2)	2.2 (11.3)	33.5 (10.0)
Total Carotenoid	763.1 (4.0)	50.46 (8.0)	62.6 (28.0)	212.3 (8.0)	109.1 (11.0)	302.0 (26.0)	385.7 (10.0)	22.0 (10.0)	45.9 (8.0)

[a]: Coefficient of variability; nd: not detectable; tr: traces.

In the present study, the variability of the total carotenoid content within the same cereal (expressed by the coefficient of variability, CV%), is from 4% in millet to 26% in pigmented quinoa. This variability may be due to genetic, pedoclimatic and varietal factors [34]. Regarding pseudocereals, results for chia are similar to those obtained in the work of da Silva et al. [28]. Significant differences between white and pigmented quinoas were found for total carotenoids, due to the different lutein amounts, as also observed by Tang et al. [35], who indicate a direct correlation between the higher total carotenoid content and the darkness of the seed coat.

3.3. *Tocols*

The characterisation of tocols in minor cereals and pseudocereals is reported in Table 4. Except for wild rice, which shows a minor content of total tocols (TC) (about 0.4 mg/100 g), the TC of minor cereals and amaranth are comparable with that of wheat, maize and rice (about 3.5–7.0, 6.0–7.0 and 2.3–2.7 mg/100g, respectively) [12,14,36] while, for the remaining pseudocereals, these values are significantly higher. Among minor cereals, teff shows the highest amount of total tocols (6 mg/100g d.w.), followed by millet and sorghum with about 4 and 3 mg/100g respectively.

Table 4. Tocol composition in gluten-free grains (mg/100g d.w.)

Tocols	Minor Cereals				Pseudocereals			
	Millet	Sorghum	Teff	Wild Rice	Quinoa (White and Pigmented)	Cañihua	Amaranth	Chia
α-T	0.16 (6.2) [a]	0.60 (83.0)	0.11 (18.2)	0.13 (11.5)	2.86 (9.58)	4.2 (35.7)	1.28 (44.5)	0.33 (33.3)
β-T	0.06 (16.6)	0.08 (62.5)	0.06 (20.0)	0.10 (13.0)	0.11 (23.0)	0.28 (21.0)	3.43 (46.0)	nd [b]
γ-T	2.73 (47.2)	2.32 (41.4)	5.52 (8.3)	0.10 (1.0)	5.9 (8.3)	12.50 (4.3)	0.30 (36.7)	13.59 (21.5)
δ-T	0.45 (29.0)	0.03 (33.0)	0.14 (14.0)	nd	0.22 (1.0)	0.40 (5.0)	1.28 (35.0)	0.38 (34.0)
α-T3	nd	nd	nd	nd	nd	nd	nd	nd
β-T3	0.12 (50.0)	nd	nd	0.03 (16.6)	tr	nd	nd	nd
γ-T3	0.04 (25.0)	nd	0.15 (73.0)	nd	tr	nd	nd	0.13 (23.0)
δ-T3	0.24 (45.8)	nd	nd	nd	nd	nd	nd	nd
Total tocols	3.80 (45.0)	3.09 (51.0)	5.99 (5.0)	0.36 (1.0)	9.10 (8.0)	18.06 (3.9)	6.31 (42.0)	14.43 (22.0)
T.E.	0.43 (28.0)	0.78 (82.0)	0.56 (21.0)	0.17 (5.9)	3.62 (1.0)	4.5 (2.0)	2.7 (33.0)	1.6 (24.0)

[a]: Coefficient of variability; [b]: Not detectable; tr: traces; T.E.: Tocopherol equivalent (mg/100g f.w.).

Except for wild rice, where α-tocopherol is the prevalent isomer, the main tocopherol isomer is γ-tocopherol, which represents the 92%, 72% and 75% of the total content in teff, millet and sorghum, respectively. For pseudocereals, the highest content of total tocols was found in cañihua (about 18 mg/100 g), followed by chia seeds (about 14 mg/100 g d.w.) and quinoas, with an average of 9.1 mg/100 g d.w. Contrarily to carotenoids, among all analysed quinoa seeds, all of the found vitamers did not show significant qualitative and quantitative differences. Amaranth is the pseudocereal with the lowest total tocol amounts (about 6 mg/100g). For chia, cañihua and quinoa the predominant isomer is γ-tocopherol (94%, 69% and 64% of total tocols), while for amaranth the prevalent isomer is β-tocopherol, which represents 54% of the total tocols.

γ-Tocopherol has also been found as the main vitamer in quinoa and chia in other works [28,35,37]. References for tocols are not available for all analysed gluten-free grains and, where present, they show similar results in millet and sorghum [3,23]. Moreover a comparison with the literature data related to tocol analysis is very difficult, for the same reasons already explained for carotenoids.

Table 4 also reports values of vitamin E activity provided by 100 g of product, expressed as Tocopherol Equivalent (T.E.) (mg/100 g product) [26]. Taking into account the Recommended Daily Allowance (RDA) for vitamin E, which is of 12 mg/day [38], 100 g of amaranth contribute to 22% of the RDA, while quinoas and cañihua approximately to 35% of the RDA, so as to be declared in a label as a "source of vitamin E". A portion of these pseudocereals (70 g) contributes approximately to 15% of the RDA for amaranth and to 25% of the RDA for quinoas and cañihua.

3.4. *Thiamine and Riboflavin*

Table 5 reports the values of the thiamine and riboflavin of analysed grains. The concentrations of thiamine are different between minor cereals and pseudocereals, except for wild rice. In whole wheat grains about 0.40 mg/100g are found in the literature [39,40]. Low values of riboflavin were found for all samples, except for wild rice, with values comparable to those of whole wheat grains and maize (0.15 and 0.20 mg/100g, respectively) [39,40].

Table 5. Thiamine and riboflavin content in gluten-free grains (mg/100g d.w.).

	Thiamine (mg/100g d.w.)	CV%	%RDA (1.1 mg/100g f.w.)	Riboflavin (mg/100g d.w.)	CV%	%RDA (1.4 mg/100g f.w.)
Minor Cereals						
Millet	0.28	49	23	0.02	25	1
Sorghum	0.28	61	23	tr	75	-
Teff	0.22	35	17	0.02	15	1
Wild rice	0.08	28	6	0.17	3	11
Pseudocereals						
Quinoa (white and pigmented)	0.13	50	9	0.02	32	1
Cañihua	0.04	6	3	0.09	8	6
Amaranth	0.03	23	3	0.01	20	1
Chia	0.06	2	5	0.02	20	1

tr: traces.

Taking into account the Recommended Daily Allowance (RDA) for thiamine, which is of 1.1 mg/day [38], 100 g of teff would contribute to approximately 17% of the RDA, while 100 g of millet and sorghum to 23% of the RDA, so as to be declared in a label as a "source of thiamine". A portion of 80 g contributes approximately to 16% of the RDA for teff and to 20% of the RDA for millet and sorghum.

4. Conclusion

Naturally gluten-free products are corn, rice, potatoes, soybean, millet, buckwheat, tapioca, amaranth, cassava, lentils, beans, sago, sorghum, nuts, as well as meat, fruit and vegetables. Among these, cereals and pseudocereals are becoming increasingly important. This work confirms that minor cereals and pseudocereals are an important source of bioactive compounds. In particular, wild rice and all analysed pseudocereals are good sources of protein. Taking into account the Recommended Daily Allowance (RDA) for vitamins established by the Commission of the European Communities, amaranth, cañihua and quinoa can be declared on the label as a source of vitamin E, the main antioxidant found in cells involved in the prevention of several diseases. Moreover, millet, sorghum and teff can be declared on the label as a potential source of thiamine. Millet also provides a fair amount of lutein. In the light of these results, it is possible to use the combined mix of these flours in order to improve the nutritional value of cereal-based gluten-free products.

Author Contributions: Conceptualization, writing-review and editing, G.P; investigation and writing-original draft preparation, S.N. and A.D.A.; data curation, writing-review and editing A.F; writing-review and editing, L.C.

References

1. Nasr, I.; Nasr, I.; Al Shekeili, L.; Al Wahshi, H.A.; Nasr, M.H.; Ciclitira, P.J. Celiac disease, wheat allergy and non celiac gluten sensitivity. *Integr. Food Nutr. Metab.* **2016**, *3*, 336–340. [CrossRef]
2. Rubio-Tapia, A.; Kyle, R.A.; Kaplan, E.L.; Johnson, D.R.; Page, W.; Erdtmann, F.; Brantner, T.L.; Kim, W.R.; Phelps, T.K.; Lahr, B.D.; et al. Increased prevalence and mortality in undiagnosed celiac disease. *Gastroenterology* **2009**, *137*, 88–93. [CrossRef] [PubMed]
3. Saturni, L.; Ferretti, G.; Bacchetti, T. The gluten-free diet: Safety and nutritional quality. *Nutrients* **2010**, *2*, 16. [CrossRef] [PubMed]
4. Vici, G.; Belli, L.; Biondi, M.; Polzonetti, V. Gluten free diet and nutrient deficiencies: A review. *Clin. Nutr.* **2016**, *35*, 1236–1241. [CrossRef] [PubMed]
5. Gobbetti, M.; Pontonio, E.; Filannino, P.; Rizzello, C.G.; De Angelis, M.; Di Cagno, R. How to improve the gluten-free diet: The state of the art from a food science perspective. *Food Res. Int.* **2018**, *110*, 22–32. [CrossRef] [PubMed]

6. De Lourdes Moreno, M.; Comino, I.; Sousa, C. Update on nutritional aspects of gluten-free diet in celiac patients. *J. Nutr.* **2014**, *1*, 7–18.
7. Cheng, A.; Mayes, S.; Dalle, G.; Demissew, S.; Massawe, F. Diversifying crops for food and nutrition security-a case of teff. *Biol. Rev.* **2017**, *92*, 188–198. [CrossRef]
8. Cheng, A. Review: Shaping a sustainable food future by rediscovering long-forgotten ancient grains. *Plant Sci.* **2018**, *269*, 136–142. [CrossRef]
9. Fiedor, J.; Burda, K. Potential role of carotenoids as antioxidants in human health and disease. *Nutrients* **2014**, *6*, 466. [CrossRef]
10. Eggersdorfer, M.; Wyss, A. Carotenoids in human nutrition and health. *Arch. Biochem. Biophys.* **2018**, *652*, 18–26. [CrossRef]
11. Fratianni, A.; Mignogna, R.; Niro, S.; Panfili, G. Determination of lutein from fruit and vegetables through an alkaline hydrolysis extraction method and HPLC analysis. *J. Food Sci.* **2015**, *80*, 2686–2691. [CrossRef] [PubMed]
12. Fratianni, A.; Giuzio, L.; Di Criscio, T.; Zina, F.; Panfili, G. Response of carotenoids and tocols of durum wheat in relation to water stress and sulfur fertilization. *J. Agric. Food Chem.* **2013**, *61*, 2583–2590. [CrossRef] [PubMed]
13. Mignogna, R.; Fratianni, A.; Niro, S.; Panfili, G. Tocopherol and tocotrienol analysis as a tool to discriminate different fat ingredients in bakery products. *Food Control.* **2015**, *54*, 31–38. [CrossRef]
14. Panfili, G.; Fratianni, A.; Irano, M. Normal phase high-performance liquid chromatography method for the determination of tocopherols and tocotrienols in cereals. *J. Agric. Food Chem.* **2003**, *51*, 3940–3944. [CrossRef] [PubMed]
15. Tiwari, U.; Cummins, E. Nutritional importance and effect of processing on tocols in cereals. *Trends Food Sci. Technol.* **2009**, *20*, 511–520. [CrossRef]
16. Shahidi, F.; de Camargo, A.C. Tocopherols and tocotrienols in common and emerging dietary sources: Occurrence, applications, and health benefits. *Int. J. Mol. Sci.* **2016**, *17*, 1745. [CrossRef] [PubMed]
17. Martin, P.R.; Singleton, C.K.; Hiller-Sturmhöfel, S. The role of thiamine deficiency in alcoholic brain disease. *Alcohol. Res. Health* **2003**, *27*, 134–142. [PubMed]
18. Zhang, Y.; Zhou, W.; Yan, J.; Liu, M.; Zhou, Y.; Shen, X.; Ma, Y.; Feng, X.; Yang, J.; Li, G. A review of the extraction and determination methods of thirteen essential vitamins to the human body: An update from 2010. *Molecules* **2018**, *23*, 1484. [CrossRef] [PubMed]
19. Thurnham, D.I. Thiamin: Physiology. *Encycl. Hum. Nutr.* **2013**, *4*, 274–279.
20. Vilacundo, R.; Hernández-Ledesma, B. Nutritional and biological value of quinoa (*Chenopodium quinoa* Willd). *Curr. Opin. Food Sci.* **2017**, *14*, 1–6. [CrossRef]
21. Zhu, F. Chemical composition and food uses of teff (Eragrostis tef). *Food Chem.* **2018**, *239*, 402–415. [CrossRef] [PubMed]
22. Alvarez-Jubete, L.; Arendt, E.K.; Gallagher, E. Nutritive value of pseudocereals and their increasing use as functional gluten free ingredients. *Trends Food Sci. Technol.* **2010**, *21*, 106–113. [CrossRef]
23. Asharani, V.T.; Jayadeep, A.; Malleshi, N.G. Natural antioxidants in edible flours of selected small millets. *Int. J. Food Prop.* **2010**, *13*, 41–50. [CrossRef]
24. ICC. *International Association for Cereal Science and Technology*; ICC: Vienna, Austria, 1995.
25. Fratianni, A.; Caboni, M.F.; Irano, M.; Panfili, G. A critical comparison between traditional methods and supercritical carbon dioxide extraction for the determination of tocochromanols in cereals. *Eur. Food Res. Technol.* **2002**, *215*, 353–358. [CrossRef]
26. Sheppard, A.J.; Pennington, J.A.T.; Weihrauch, J.L. Analysis and distribution of vitamin E in vegetable oil and foods. In *Vitamin E in Health and Disease*; Packer, L., Fuchs, J., Eds.; Marcel—Dekker: New York, NY, USA, 1993.
27. Hasselmann, C.; Franck, D.; Grimm, P.; Diop, P.A.; Soulrs, C. High performance liquid chromatographic analysis of thiamin and riboflavin in dietetic foods. *J. Micronutr. Anal.* **1989**, *5*, 269–279.
28. Da Silva, B.P.; Anunciação, P.C.; Matyelka, J.C.D.S.; Della Lucia, C.M.; Martino, H.S.D.; Pinheiro-Sant'Ana, H.M. Chemical composition of Brazilian chia seeds grown in different places. *Food Chem.* **2017**, *221*, 1709–1716. [CrossRef] [PubMed]
29. Regulation, E.C. No 1924/2006 of the European Parliament and of the Council of 20 December 2006 on nutrition and health claims made on foods. *Off. J. Eur. Union* **2007**, *12*, 3–18.

30. Panfili, G.; Fratianni, A.; Irano, M. Improved normal-phase high-performance liquid chromatography procedure for the determination of carotenoids in cereals. *J. Agric. Food Chem.* **2004**, *52*, 6373–6377. [CrossRef]
31. Melini, V.; Panfili, G.; Fratianni, A.; Acquistucci, R. Bioactive compounds in rice on Italian market: Pigmented varieties as a source of carotenoids, total phenolic compounds and anthocyanins, before and after cooking. *Food Chem.* **2019**, *277*, 119–127. [CrossRef]
32. Alfieri, M.; Hidalgo, A.; Berardo, N.; Redaelli, R. Carotenoid composition and heterotic effect in selected Italian maize Germplasm. *J. Cereal Sci.* **2014**, *59*, 181–188. [CrossRef]
33. De Morais Cardoso, L.; Pinheiro, S.S.; Da Silva, L.L.; de Menezes, C.B.; de Carvalho, C.W.P.; Tardin, F.D.; Queiroz, V.A.V.; Martino, H.S.D.; Pinheiro-Sant'Ana, H.M. Tocochromanols and carotenoids in sorghum (*Sorghum bicolor* L.): Diversity and stability to the heat treatment. *Food Chem.* **2015**, *172*, 900–908. [CrossRef] [PubMed]
34. Abdel-Aal, E.; Wood, P. *Specialty Grains for Food and Feed*; American Association of Cereal Chemists: Paul, MN, USA, 2005.
35. Tang, Y.; Li, X.; Chen, P.X.; Zhang, B.; Hernandez, M.; Zhang, H.; Marcone, M.F.; Liu, R.; Tsao, R. Characterisation of fatty acid, carotenoid, tocopherol/tocotrienol compositions and antioxidant activities in seeds of three Chenopodium quinoa Willd. genotypes. *Food Chem.* **2015**, *174*, 502–508. [CrossRef] [PubMed]
36. Irakli, M.N.; Samanidou, V.F.; Katsantonis, D.N.; Biliaderis, C.G.; Papadoyannis, I.N. Phytochemical profiles and antioxidant capacity of pigmented and non-pigmented genotypes of rice (*Oryza sativa* L.). *Cereal Res. Commun.* **2016**, *44*, 98–110. [CrossRef]
37. Pereira, E.; Encina-Zeladaa, C.; Barrosa, L.; Gonzales-Barrona, U.; Cadaveza, V.; Ferreira, I.C.F.R. Chemical and nutritional characterization of Chenopodium quinoa Willd (quinoa) grains: A good alternative to nutritious food. *Food Chem.* **2019**, *280*, 110–114. [CrossRef] [PubMed]
38. Regulation, E.U. No 1169/2011 of the European Parliament and of the Council of 25 October 2011 on the provision of food information to consumers. *Off. J. Eur. Union* **2011**, *50*, 18–63.
39. Călinoiu, L.F.; Vodnar, D.C. Whole grains and phenolic acids: A review on bioactivity, functionality, health benefits and bioavailability. *Nutrients* **2018**, *10*, 1615. [CrossRef] [PubMed]
40. Gwirtz, J.A.; Garcia-Casal, M.N. Processing maize flour and corn meal food products. *Ann. N. Y. Acad. Sci.* **2014**, *1312*, 66–75. [CrossRef]

12

Sodium Chloride and its Influence on the Aroma Profile of Yeasted Bread

Markus C. E. Belz [1], Claudia Axel [1], Jonathan Beauchamp [2], Emanuele Zannini [1], Elke K. Arendt [1,*] and Michael Czerny [2]

[1] School of Food and Nutritional Sciences, University College Cork, National University of Ireland, College Road, T12 Y337 Cork, Ireland; belz.markus@web.de (M.C.E.B.); c.axel@umail.ucc.ie (C.A.); e.zannini@ucc.ie (E.Z.)

[2] Department of Sensory Analytics, Fraunhofer Institute for Process Engineering and Packaging IVV, 85354 Freising, Germany; jonathan.beauchamp@ivv.fraunhofer.de (J.B.); michael.czerny@ivv.fraunhofer.de (M.C.)

* Correspondence: e.arendt@ucc.ie

Academic Editor: Anthony Fardet

Abstract: The impact of sodium chloride (NaCl) concentration on the yeast activity in bread dough and its influence on the aroma profile of the baked bread was investigated. Key aroma compounds in the bread samples were analysed by two-dimensional high-resolution gas chromatography-mass spectrometry in combination with solvent-assisted flavour evaporation distillation. High-sensitivity proton-transfer-reaction mass spectrometry was used to detect and quantify 2-phenylethanol in the headspace of the bread dough during fermentation. The analyses revealed significant ($p < 0.05$) changes in the aroma compounds 2-phenylethanol, (E)-2-nonenal, and 2,4-(E,E)-decadienal. Descriptive sensory analysis and discriminating triangle tests revealed that significant differences were only determinable in samples with different yeast levels but not samples with different NaCl concentrations. This indicates that a reduction in NaCl does not significantly influence the aroma profile of yeasted bread at levels above the odour thresholds of the relevant compounds, thus consumers in general cannot detect an altered odour profile of low-salt bread crumb.

Keywords: descriptive sensory; PTR-MS; GC-MS; Ehrlich pathway; bread aroma; salt reduction chemical compounds: 2-phenylethanol (PubChem CID: 6054); (E)-2-nonenal (PubChem CID: 5283335); 2,4-(E,E)-decadienal (PubChem CID: 5283349)

---

1. Introduction

Sodium chloride (NaCl), or salt, is a major taste contributor to food. A reduction of salt in food products generally leads to less intense taste and flavour. The impact of salt reduction on taste profiles has been demonstrated for numerous foods, amongst them white yeasted bread. An early investigation on white yeasted, rye and rye-sourdough breads indicated a low consumer preference for the reduced-salt breads [1]. In contrast, however, Wyatt [2] observed no significant difference in consumer preference for white bread containing 50% less NaCl than a reference bread. The current challenge for food producers is to develop products with a reduced salt content but an unimpaired and consistent taste. This has been investigated with the use of salt replacers such as potassium chloride, magnesium chloride, ammonium chloride, calcium chloride and calcium carbonate [3,4], the use of sourdough [5], the inclusion of flavour-enhancing acids and other potent aroma compounds [6,7], or by changes to the bread crumb texture that influence the saltiness perception [8–10]. In contrast to taste, less is known about the influence of salt reduction on the volatile aroma profile of food. Volatile aroma compounds impart flavour to food, and the volatile fraction of bread is highly complex with about 600 volatile compounds reported to be present in bread crumb [11]. In particular, the yeast metabolism plays a key role in the development of the aroma profile of bread, and salt, primarily its sodium ions, have a direct impact on yeast activity. In addition to ethanol and carbon dioxide, many low-molecular-weight flavour compounds such as further alcohols, aldehydes, acids, esters, sulphides and carbonyl compounds are produced by the yeast metabolism. These volatile compounds are essential contributors to the flavour of fermented foods and beverages [12,13]. The Ehrlich pathway is one of several routes responsible for the generation of aroma compounds by yeast in bread. In particular it leads to the formation of potent compounds such as fusel alcohols and acids. The efficacy of the Ehrlich pathway in converting amino acids into alcoholic odorants was investigated, amongst others, by Czerny and Schieberle [14], who used stable isotope dilution assays (SIDAs) to demonstrate the conversion of ^{13}C (6)-leucine to the metabolite 3-methylbutanol.

The reducing activity of yeast during bread dough fermentation also has a critical impact on bread aroma, as has been similarly observed during beer wort fermentation [15]. Unsaturated aldehydes such as (E)-2-nonenal and 2,4-(E,E)-decadienal are derived from the oxidation of linoleic acid and are well-known for their contribution to fatty odours in wheat bread [11]. The reduction of these unsaturated volatile compounds by yeast to their corresponding alcohols has an impact on bread aroma; as such, a variation in yeast activity results in an altered aroma of the bread. Notably, it has been observed that *Saccharomyces cerevisiae* fully reduces unsaturated aldehydes to the corresponding alcohols [16].

The present work aimed at determining the impact of NaCl on the yeast metabolism in bread dough during fermentation and its influence on the overall aroma of the bread. More specifically, the unsaturated aldehydes (E)-2-nonenal (fatty) and 2,4-(E,E)-decadienal (fatty), and the alcoholic compound 2-phenylethanol (rose-like) were investigated as the key aroma compounds in bread based on preliminary analyses and supported by reports in the literature [11,17,18]. Recently Martins et al., 2015 evaluated the impact of bread fortification with dry spent yeast from brewing industry on physical, chemical and sensorial characteristics of home-made bread with the goal of increasing its β-glucan content. The sensory analysis showed how only the key odour hexanal was presented a significant increase in fortified bread [19]. A complementary analytical approach using two-dimensional high-resolution gas chromatography-mass spectrometry (2D-HRGC-MS) and proton-transfer-reaction mass spectrometry (PTR-MS) was used to quantify and monitor the generation of the selected aroma compounds in bread crumb samples containing different levels of NaCl and yeast. Sensory analysis was performed on the bread crumb samples to determine their odour characteristics and assess the impact of salt reduction on bread crumb based on a discrimination triangle test.

2. Materials and Methods

2.1. Microbiology

Instant active dry yeast consisting of living cells of *Saccharomyces cerevisiae* (Panté; Puratos, Belgium) was diluted in Ringer solution at a concentration of 10^{-5} g mL^{-1}. An aliquot of 10 μL of the yeast solution was grown as a centre colony on yeast-selective potato dextrose agar plates (Fluka Chemie AG, Buchs, Switzerland) containing different amounts of sodium chloride (NaCl) (0, 0.3%, 1.2%, 2.0%, 3.0%, and 4.0% w/w) at 30 °C for 8 days. The growth rate was recorded every day by measuring the diameter of the visible colonies with an electronic calliper.

2.2. Baking Procedure and Loaf Analyses

Wheat bread was prepared by mixing (spiral mixer, Kenwood KM020, Kenwood Manufacturing Co., Ltd., Hampshire, UK) Baker's flour (Odlums, Dublin, Ireland), yeast, NaCl (Glacia British Salt Limited, Middlewich, UK) at levels of 0, 0.26%, 1.04%, 1.73%, 2.60% and 3.46% (w/w) and tap water (water levels set to 500 Brabender units, BU, depending on the amount of NaCl by using a farinograph, Brabender OHG, Duisburg, Germany). Considering an average bake loss of 13.5% the

NaCl concentrations in the final bread loaves resulted in 0, 0.3%, 1.2%, 2.0%, 3.0% and 4.0% (Table 1). For each of the 10 different batches 6 loaves were prepared. For dough samples with varying amounts of yeast (1.5%, 0.9%, 0.6%, 0.3%), the concentrations of water and NaCl relative to the mass of flour were kept constant at 61.75% and 0.26% (w/w), respectively (Table 1). After bulk fermentation for 15 min at 30 °C and 85% relative humidity, bread loaves (450 ± 1 g) were formed using a molding machine (Machinefabriek Holtkamp B.V., Almelo, The Netherlands). The loaves were then placed into non-stick baking tins (180 mm × 120 mm × 60 mm), fermented for 75 min at 30 °C and 85% relative humidity, and then baked for 35 min at 230 °C (top and bottom heating). The ovens were pre-steamed (0.3 L water) and then steamed when loaded (0.7 L water). After baking, the loaves were removed from the tins and left to cool on cooling racks for 120 min at room temperature. Bake loss and specific volume were measured for all of the baked loaves. The bake loss was determined as the difference in mass between the dough and baked loaf. The specific volume was determined by a 3D laser scan using a VolScan Profiler 300 (Stable Micro Systems, Godalming, UK).

Table 1. Ingredient quantities in the breads containing varying amounts of NaCl at constant yeast (1.2% w/w) and varying amounts of yeast at constant NaCl (0.3% w/w) *.

Ingredient	Ingredient Quantity for Each Type of Bread (% w/w flour)									
	Variable NaCl (% w/w) at 1.2% w/w Yeast						Variable Yeast (% w/w) at 0.3% w/w NaCl			
	0	0.26	1.04	1.73	2.60	3.46	1.5	0.9	0.6	0.3
Wheat flour	100.00	100.00	100.00	100.00	100.00	100.00	100.00	100.00	100.00	100.00
Yeast	2.00	2.00	2.00	2.00	2.00	2.00	2.47	1.48	0.98	0.48
Tap water (30°)	62.95	61.75	61.00	60.90	59.75	59.75	61.75	61.75	61.75	61.75
NaCl	0.00	0.43	1.72	2.87	4.36	5.80	0.43	0.43	0.43	0.43

* The 0.3% NaCl concentration was used in accordance to the Directive 80/777/EEC to claim a bread low in salt.

2.3. *Rheofermentometer*

A rheofermentometer (RheoF3, Chopin Technologies, Villeneuve-la-Garenne, Paris, France) was used to evaluate carbon dioxide (CO_2) release and dough development of the different dough samples. Samples of 300 g of each dough were prepared in the same manner as described above for baking trials. The tests were performed at 30 °C over a 90 min period. As common practice for wheat dough, a cylindrical weight of 1.5 kg was applied onto the fermentation chamber. The total volume of CO_2, the volume of retention for each sample, the lost volume of CO_2, and the retention coefficient (capability of a dough to retain gas) were determined. Results are presented as the average of triplicate measurements.

2.4. *Extraction of Volatile Aroma Compounds*

Samples were prepared by cutting the bread crumb into 1 cm^3 cubes, freezing these in liquid nitrogen, and then grinding them using a standard blender. Isotope-labelled standard solutions ([$^2H_2$]-(E)-2-nonenal 0.24 μg/mL; [$^2H_2$]-2,4-(E,E)-decadienal 0.50 μg/mL; [$^2H_{4-5}$]-2-phenylethanol 10.30 μg/mL) were added as internal standard to 50 ± 1 g of the ground crumb and the aroma compounds were extracted with 150 mL dichloromethane that was stirred at 120 rpm for 60 min at room temperature and then filtered to remove the suspension. This extraction step was repeated twice for each 50-g crumb sample and the filtrates were combined. The extracts were purified using solvent-assisted flavour evaporation (SAFE) distillation [20]. The distillates were concentrated down to a volume of 0.1 mL and these were subsequently stored at −20 °C prior to the analysis.

2.5. *Two-Dimensional High-Resolution Gas Chromatography-Mass Spectrometry (2D-HRGC-MS)*

Quantification of the selected aroma compounds was made using a two-dimensional high-resolution gas chromatography-mass spectrometer (2D-HRGC-MS), with a cryogenic trapping system (CryoTrap; Gerstel, Stadt, Germany) connecting the first GC system (Type 3800, Varian, Darmstadt, Germany) with a preparative DB-5 column to the second GC with a DB-FFAP column (each 30 m × 0.32 mm, 0.25 μm film thickness). The helium carrier gas flow was set to 1.5 mL min^{-1}. The initial temperature of the first GC oven was 40 °C, which was subsequently heated at a rate of 8 °C min^{-1} to 230 °C. The eluting aroma compounds were transferred at defined retention times onto the cryo-trap, which was cooled to −100 °C. The volatiles were then flushed onto the column in the second GC oven by thermal desorption at 250 °C. The temperature of this second oven was increased from 40 °C to 250 °C at a rate of 6 °C min^{-1} and then held for 5 min at 250 °C. The eluting compounds were analysed with a Saturn 2200 mass spectrometer (Varian, Darmstadt, Germany) by chemical ionisation (CI) using methanol as the reagent gas.

2.6. Proton-Transfer-Reaction Mass Spectrometry (PTR-MS)

A high sensitivity proton-transfer-reaction mass spectrometer (hs-PTR-MS; IONICON Analytik GmbH, Innsbruck, Austria) was used to analyse the release of selected aroma compounds from the breads during fermentation. The instrument was operated at an electric field to buffer gas number density ratio (E/N) of 132 Td, which was established with drift tube settings of 600 V, 2.2 mbar and 60 °C. The PTR-MS was set to measure in mass scan mode in the range m/z 20–130 at a dwell time of 500 ms per m/z. Five individual scans of 51 s duration were made per sampling period, resulting in a complete analysis time of 255 s. A 1-m long, 1/16″ OD, 0.04″ ID Silcosteel™ (Restek GmbH, Bad Homburg, Germany) sample inlet line, heated to 65 °C and with a flow of 500 mL min^{-1}, was used to transfer the sample gas to the instrument reaction chamber.

Dough samples of 300 g were placed in 1-L perfluoroalkoxy (PFA) containers (AHF Analysentechnik GmbH, Darmstadt, Germany) for the on-line measurement of volatiles in the headspace of the dough during fermentation at 30 °C and 85% RH over 75 min. Five scan cycles of zero-air—i.e., air free of volatile organic compounds (VOCs)—in the empty sample container were made at the beginning of each analysis to determine the background noise and the limit of detection of the system. The mean signals from these scans were subtracted from the sample signals to correct for this background.

The intensities of the m/z relating to the abundance of the selected aroma compounds in the headspace gas of the sample chamber were converted to approximate concentrations (with an estimated accuracy of ± 30%) using a standard reaction rate (k) of 2.0×10^{-9} cm^3/s [21]. The data were screened for m/z 105 specific to 2-phenylethanol, which is ionised to a cation by dehydroxylation and protonation. For the unsaturated aldehydes, the respective molecular ions at m/z 141 for (E)-2-nonenal and m/z 153 for 2,4-(E,E)-decadienal were outside the m/z scan range and thus could not be detected. It might be noted that a certain degree of fragmentation of these two compounds is expected to occur, thus their potential detection at m/z values within the scanned range might have been achievable, but this was hindered by a lack of knowledge of the exact fragments or their potential overlap with other compounds, and instrumental problems that impaired the sensitivity to m/z in the higher range. Thus only 2-phenylethanol will be reported for the PTR-MS data here.

2.7. Sensory Analysis

Sensory analyses of the samples were performed via the aroma profile analysis (APA) technique. Descriptive analyses were performed using a trained panel of 15 members, with at least ten assessors participating in each individual sensory session. The panellists were trained in weekly sessions to recognise the selected aroma compounds according to their odour qualities by smelling reference aqueous aroma solutions at different odorant concentrations. Training was performed over a period of at least six months prior to participation in the actual sensory experiments and the performance of each panellist was assessed via standard procedures.

Bread loaves were cut into 2 cm-thick slices and the crust was removed. The yeasted dough and wheat flour bread samples were presented to the sensory panel for orthonasal assessment after storage in a closed glass beaker for 30 min at room temperature. The perceived odour qualities of the bread crumbs were described as being yeast/dough-like and flour-like based on a comparison to aqueous reference solutions. The panel agreed on the characteristic odour attributes of each sample in a group discussion. The pure compounds used for the reference solutions were purchased from Sigma-Aldrich (Taufkirchen, Germany), Acros (Geel, Belgium) and AromaLab (Freising, Germany). Crumb samples were then presented again to the panel in a second sensory session to evaluate the intensities of the aforementioned odour attributes on a scale from 0 (not detectable) over 1 (weak intensity), 2 (medium intensity) to 3 (high intensity). The sensory score of each attribute was calculated as an arithmetic mean. The assessors were trained immediately prior to the analysis with aqueous odorant solutions at defined super-threshold concentrations (factor 100 above the odour threshold) [18,22].

Sensory triangle tests were additionally performed on selected sample pairs by the panel to determine whether potential odour changes are detectable by consumers. The sample pairs, namely 0.3% and 1.5% yeast, 0.3% and 1.2% NaCl, and 1.2% and 3.0% NaCl were chosen based on a 'standard-salt' level of 1.2% w/w NaCl [23], a "low-salt" level of 0.3% w/w NaCl, and an "high-salt" level of 3.0% w/w NaCl. The bread loaves were sliced and uniform round pieces were punched-out for presentation. The panellists were required to smell the samples and identify which of the three samples differed (forced-choice test). The tests were repeated for all combinations of each sample pair during each of the three independent sessions.

2.8. Statistical Analysis

Statistical analyses were performed on the sensory assessment results using Minitab for Windows statistical analysis software package (Systat Software, Inc., Chicago, IL, USA). The data were subjected to one-way analysis of variance (ANOVA). A Fisher's least significant difference (LSD) test was performed for multiple comparisons for cases when an F-test showed significant differences ($p < 0.05$). Mean values of the three separate experiments with three independent samples from each batch were then calculated and are presented here, unless otherwise stated. The significance level was set to $p < 0.05$ throughout, unless otherwise stated.

3. Results and Discussion

3.1. Microbiology and Rheofermentometer

Initial assessments of the impact of NaCl on the activity and proliferation of the yeast showed an exponential inhibition of yeast proliferation with increasing amounts of NaCl. These results reflect previously reported effects of NaCl on yeast. Increased amounts of NaCl in the growth environment reduce the number of viable yeast cells as well as the biomass of the culture, while the length of the lag phase is increased [24–27]. The most important metabolite of yeast in bread dough is CO_2, which leavens the dough and increases the volume of the bread loaf; thus, CO_2 can also be used to monitor the yeast activity in dough. Table 2 lists the parameters relating to the yeast performance in wheat dough during fermentation; as can be seen, the total volume of CO_2 produced decreased with increasing amounts of NaCl. The higher the amount of NaCl, the higher the osmotic pressure on the yeast cells, leading to growth inhibition and an inhibitory impact on the yeast metabolism [24,25]. The non-significant difference between bread dough containing 0% and 0.26% NaCl is due to the NaCl threshold concentration required before conditions act to have an inhibitory influence on yeast [27,28]. The higher the NaCl level, the higher the retention coefficient, which leads to a higher retention of CO_2 by the dough, as previously reported [23]. A lower CO_2 production results in a lower pressure on the membranes of the gluten network. In addition, there are several reports that gluten networks are strengthened by NaCl and can thereby retain more CO_2 [23,29,30].

Table 2. Yeast performance in wheat dough with different NaCl concentrations during 3 h fermentation.

NaCl Concentration (% w/w)	Total Volume of Dough (mL)	Volume of Retention (mL)	Volume of CO_2 Lost (mL)	Retention Coefficient
0.00	2241 ± 54 [a]	1435 ± 23 [a]	806 ± 75 [a]	64.1 ± 2.4 [a]
0.26	2108 ± 40 [a]	1459 ± 11 [a]	649 ± 49 [b]	69.2 ± 1.8 [d]
1.04	1581 ± 126 [b]	1337 ± 54 [b]	243 ± 78 [c]	84.8 ± 3.7 [c]
1.73	982 ± 28 [c]	953 ± 22 [c]	30 ± 8 [d]	97.0 ± 0.7 [b]
2.60	573 ± 15 [d]	569 ± 14 [d]	4.0 ± 1.7 [e]	99.4 ± 0.2 [a]
3.46	313 ± 11 [e]	311 ± 11 [e]	2.0 ± 0.0 [f]	99.4 ± 0.1 [a]

Values in one column followed by the same superscript letter are not significantly different ($p < 0.05$).

3.2. *Specific Bread Loaf Volume and Bake Loss*

The specific volume and bake loss of the baked bread loaves were determined as a standard quality parameter (Table 3). The specific loaf volume decreased significantly for increasing amounts of NaCl at a yeast level of 1.2%. The bread containing no NaCl did not show a significantly larger volume than the bread with 0.3% NaCl, despite its water level being the highest at 62.95% (Table 1).

Table 3. Specific volume and bake loss of bread loaves with different NaCl concentrations and standard yeast level of 1.2% w/w and with different yeast concentrations and standard NaCl concentration of 0.3% w/w.

Bread Type		Specific Bread Volume (mL/g)	Bake Loss *	
			(% w/w)	(% of Water Level)
Varying NaCl (% w/w) at 1.2% w/w yeast	0.0	3.85 ± 0.13 [a]	14.9 ± 0.5 [a,b]	39.1 ± 1.2 [a,b,c]
	0.3	3.81 ± 0.08 [a]	15.3 ± 0.3 [a]	40.6 ± 0.8 [a]
	1.2	3.49 ± 0.09 [b]	14.4 ± 0.4 [b]	38.6 ± 0.9 [b]
	2.0	3.11 ± 0.05 [c]	13.4 ± 0.5 [c]	37.4 ± 0.6 [c]
	3.0	2.52 ± 0.02 [d]	12.3 ± 0.4 [d]	32.7 ± 1.0 [d]
	4.0	1.93 ± 0.03 [e]	10.6 ± 0.3 [e]	28.6 ± 0.8 [e]
Varying yeast (% w/w) at 0.3% w/w NaCl	0.3	3.02 ± 0.02 [i]	13.4 ± 0.2 [g]	36.2 ± 0.5 [g]
	0.6	3.70 ± 0.05 [f]	14.7 ± 0.2 [f]	39.8 ± 0.7 [f]
	0.9	3.62 ± 0.19 [f,g]	14.7 ± 0.2 [f]	39.7 ± 0.6 [f]
	1.2	3.49 ± 0.09 [g,h]	14.4 ± 0.4 [f]	38.6 ± 0.9 [f]
	1.5	3.37 ± 0.10 [h]	13.9 ± 0.5 [f,g]	38.2 ± 0.9 [f]

* The bake loss is shown as a percentage of the dough mass as well as a percentage of the water level. Values in one column followed by the same superscript letter are not significantly different ($p < 0.05$).

Although the dough was mixed to a standard consistency of 500 BU, this observation might be explained by a weaker gluten network in the absence of NaCl [23,29,30]. The data from the rheofermentometer corroborate this hypothesis; the generation of a non-significant higher amount of CO_2 did not lead to a greater bread volume. The higher the NaCl concentration, the smaller was the bread volume and surface area, and less water could evaporate, which again is supported by the rheofermentometer data. The bake loss expressed as a percentage of the water level for each of the individual bread loaves showed that small adjustments of the water level to achieve a dough consistency of 500 BU did not significantly influence the bake loss (Table 3). The breads with yeast levels ranging from 0.3% to 1.5% at a constant NaCl level of 0.3% w/w had the highest specific volume at 0.6%. At lower yeast concentrations, the amount of yeast did not produce sufficient CO_2 to stretch the gluten network to its maximum. At yeast concentrations, higher than 0.6% the specific volume decreased with increasing amounts of yeast. Similarly, increasing amounts of yeast led to excessive fermentation and a resulting expansion of the gluten network, thereby increasing the loss of CO_2 [23,25,27].

3.3. Analyses of Volatile Aroma Compounds in Bread Crumb

Three key aroma compounds in wheat bread crumb are the alcoholic compound 2-phenylethanol [14,31] and the unsaturated aldehydes (E)-2-nonenal and 2,4-(E,E)-decadienal [16,32]. These three compounds were analysed in the aroma extracts of bread crumb by 2D-HRGC-MS (Table 4). The 2-phenylethanol decreased in concentration exponentially with increasing amounts of NaCl, but increased significantly with increasing amounts of yeast, albeit not for the highest yeast concentrations (0.9%, 1.2% and 1.5% w/w).

Table 4. Concentration of 2-phenylethanol, (E)-2-nonenal and 2,4-(E,E)-decadienal in bread-crumb samples as determined by 2D-HRGC-MS.

Bread Type		Concentration (μg/kg)		
		2-Phenylethanol	**(E)-2-Nonenal**	**2,4-(E,E)-Decadienal**
Varying NaCl (% w/w) at 1.2% w/w yeast	0.0	4441 ± 686 [a]	12.9 ± 1.7 [c,d]	12.7 ± 1.1 [a]
	0.3	3055 ± 549 [a]	13.5 ± 1.2 [c,d]	11.1 ± 0.7 [a]
	1.2	1582 ± 6 [b]	12.1 ± 0.3 [d]	8.5 ± 0.8 [b]
	2.0	1685 ± 88 [c]	15.9 ± 2.6 [b,c]	9.2 ± 1.3 [a,b]
	3.0	1189 ± 9 [d]	16.4 ± 1.2 [b]	10.6 ± 2.0 [a,b]
	4.0	845 ± 58 [e]	20.8 ± 2.7 [a]	9.3 ± 0.7 [a,b]
Varying yeast (% w/w) at 0.3% w/w NaCl	0.3	1164 ± 64 [i]	19.7 ± 0.0 [e]	20.2 ± 1.8 [c]
	0.6	1773 ± 40 [h]	16.5 ± 1.9 [f]	17.9 ± 3.1 [c]
	0.9	2607 ± 165 [g]	10.2 ± 2.2 [g,h]	11.4 ± 0.7 [d]
	1.2	3056 ± 549 [f,g]	13.5 ± 1.2 [f,g]	11.1 ± 0.7 [d]
	1.5	3288 ± 315 [f]	8.0 ± 2.3 [h]	8.6 ± 0.1 [e]

Values in one column followed by the same superscript letter are not significantly different ($p < 0.05$).

The concentrations of (E)-2-nonenal differed significantly for 3% and 4% NaCl compared to the lowest NaCl concentrations of 0%–0.6%. Increasing the yeast content led to a significant decrease in (E)-2-nonenal for the samples containing 0.3% and 0.6% yeast compared to the samples containing 0.9% and 1.5% yeast. Here, 2,4-(E,E)-decadienal did not show any significant change for the different NaCl concentrations, but decreased with increasing yeast content. These changes can be explained by the reducing activity of the baker's yeast. Decreasing the yeast concentration or inhibiting the yeast with more salt lowers the overall yeast activity during the fermentation process, thereby resulting in a lower production of the unsaturated aldehydes. The reducing activity of yeast has been previously investigated [33]. Furthermore, Saison et al., 2010 demonstrated a change in beer aroma production based on the reducing activity of (E)-2-nonenal by *S. cerevisiae*, suggesting that the reducing activity metabolism of yeast is not affected by increased concentrations of NaCl in the same manner as the Ehrlich pathway or other parts of the yeast metabolism. Correlations ($R^2 \geq 0.75$) were found between CO_2 and 2-phenylethanol or (E)-2-nonenal, indicating that these compounds must arise during yeast metabolism and are influenced by the amount of NaCl in bread dough. A negative correlation for the unsaturated aldehyde (E)-2-nonenal indicates that the reduction capacity of yeast increased with increasing yeast activity, thus an increased amount of (E)-2-nonenal was reduced to the corresponding alcohol.

3.4. PTR-MS Analyses of Bread Dough during Fermentation

The PTR-MS data for the rose-like aroma compound 2-phenylethanol at m/z 105 in the headspace of the dough showed that its concentration increased for increasing amounts of yeast (0.3%–1.5%), albeit with the regressions between 0.6 and 1.2% being similar (Figure 1a). The more NaCl that was added to the bread samples, the less 2-phenylethanol was present due to the inhibiting effect of NaCl on yeast (Figure 1b). The headspace concentrations of 2-phenylethanol correlate with the concentration of this compound in the respective bread crumb samples, as measured by 2D-HRGC-MS.

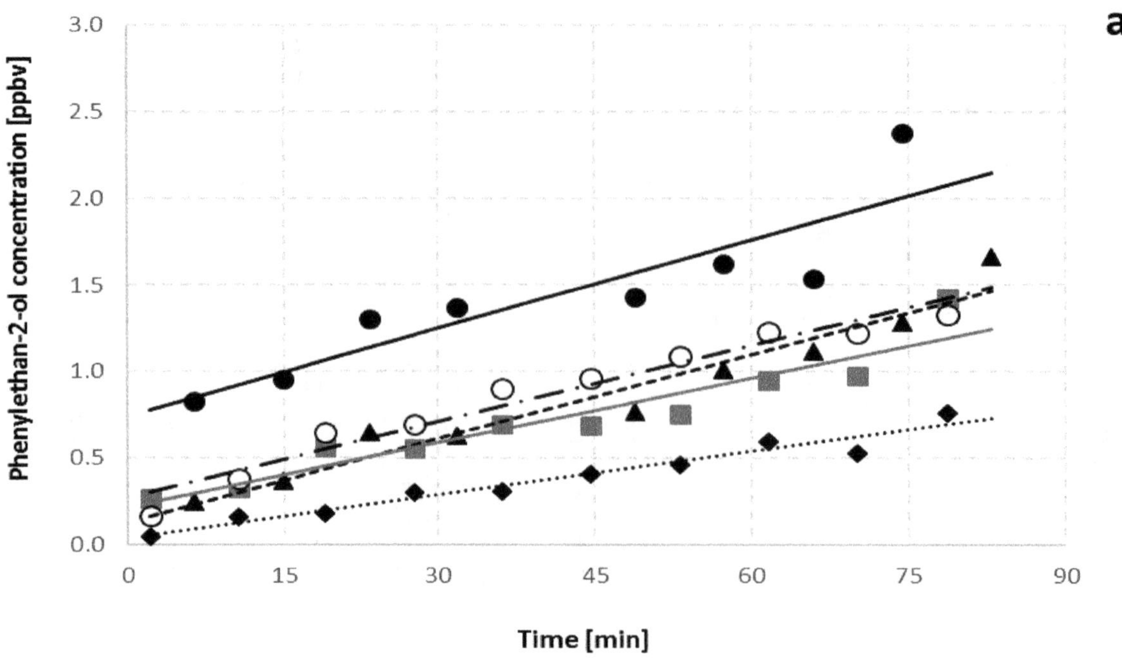

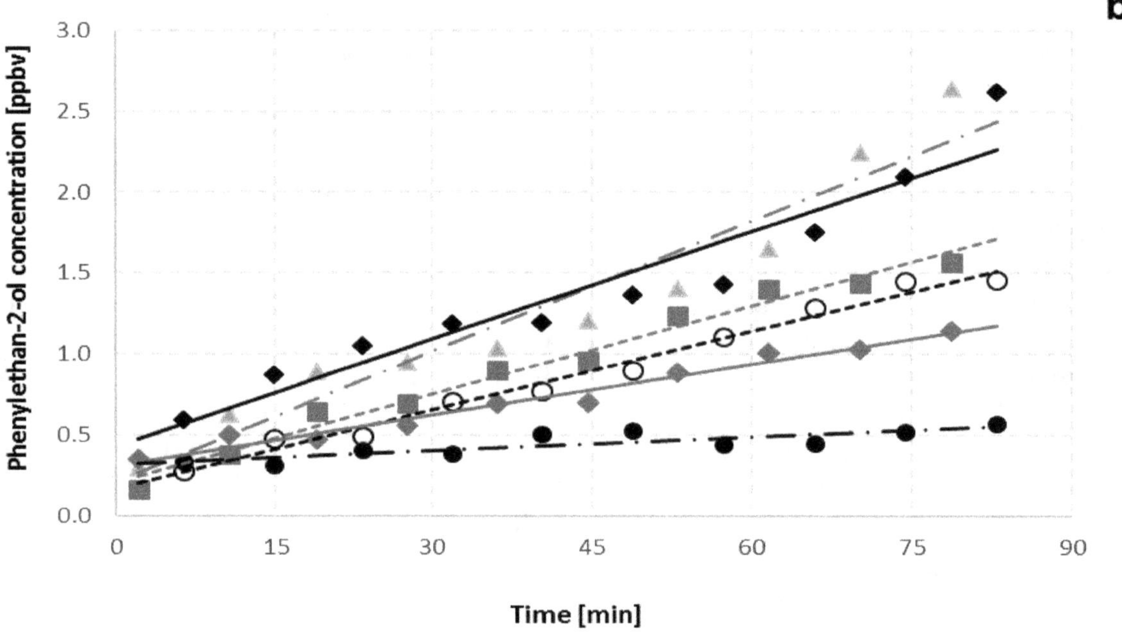

Figure 1. Volume mixing ratios of 2-phenylethanol in the headspace of bread dough containing (**a**) different yeast concentrations (w/w) of 1.5% (filled circles with solid regression line), 1.2% (open circles with black dot-dashed regression line), 0.9% (filled squares with grey regression line), 0.6% (filled triangles with dashed regression line), 0.3% (filled diamonds with dotted regression line) and (**b**) different NaCl concentrations (w/w) of 0.0% (filled triangles with grey dot-dashed regression line), 0.3% (filled diamonds with solid regression line), 1.2% (filled squares with grey dashed regression line), 2.0% (open circles with black dashed regression line), 3.0% (filled diamonds with grey regression line) and 4% (filled circles with dot-dashed regression line) over 90 min of incubation under fermentation conditions (30 °C, 85% RH).

3.5. Descriptive Sensory Evaluation

Ten sensory attributes were collected for the bread-crumb samples, whereby the dominating attributes were roasty, yeasty, malty, flour like, buttery, cheesy and fatty. The APAs of the bread-crumb samples revealed significant differences only for the attributes *cheesy* and rose-like (Figure 2).

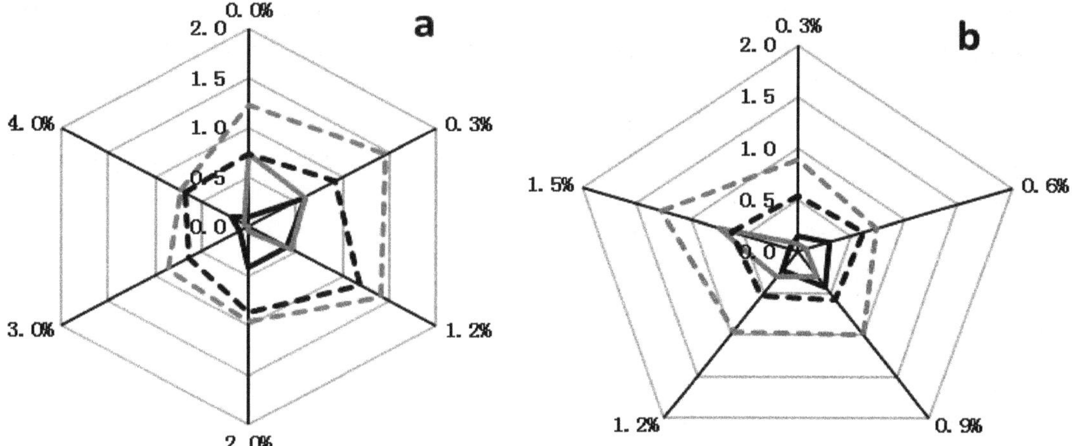

Figure 2. Aroma profiles of bread crumbs for the attributes *cheesy* (grey line), *rose-like* (black line), *fatty* (black dashed line) and *buttery* (grey dashed line) at (**a**) different NaCl concentrations (0.0%, 0.3%, 1.2%, 2.0%, 3.0% and 4% w/w) and (**b**) different yeast levels (0.3%, 0.6%, 0.9%, 1.2% and 1.5% w/w) on a scale from 0 (not detectable) over 1 (weak intensity) to 2 (medium intensity), as determined by sensory panel.

The *cheesy* aroma was significantly different between the samples with the three highest NaCl levels (2%, 3%, and 4% w/w) and the three lowest levels (0.0%, 0.3%, and 1.2% w/w NaCl) (Figure 2a). In the samples with varying yeast levels only the highest (1.5% w/w yeast) and lowest (0.3% w/w yeast) levels differed significantly with respect to the *cheesy* odour impression (Figure 2b). Butanoic acid is well-known as a volatile metabolic compound of yeast with a *cheesy* odour note, and is listed in the Yeast Metabolic Database (YMDB) ID 01392 [34]. The results of these APAs correlate with the yeast activity during fermentation. Increased amounts of yeast as well as decreasing NaCl levels result in higher yeast activities and hence, a higher metabolism rate, including production of the metabolite butanoic acid, which results in a more intense cheesy odour.

The attribute rose-like determined by the sensory panel (Figure 2) correlated directly with the concentration of 2-phenylethanol in the bread crumb samples (Table 4) and hence, with the yeast activity. Increasing yeast activity during dough fermentation led to higher concentrations of 2-phenylethanol. The lower the NaCl level or the higher the yeast level, the more intense was the rose-like odour, as determined by the sensory panel (Figure 2). At 0.0% w/w NaCl the panel did not perceive a rose-like odour, which might reflect a totally excessive and uncontrolled yeast activity in the complete absence of NaCl. Odour impressions described as cheesy and buttery dominated the overall odour characteristic and covered the rose-like impression (Figure 2). The same effect is shown for an increased amount of yeast above 0.9% w/w. The rose-like compounds, namely 2-phenylethanol and 2-phenylacetic acid, have higher odour thresholds compared to the other aroma compounds considered here, therefore the rose-like odour fraction can easily be dominated by other volatile aroma compounds or influence their recognition [22].The fatty impression in the samples with differing NaCl content did not vary significantly, as confirmed by 2D-HRGC-MS analyses of the unsaturated aldehydes (E)-2-nonenal and 2,4-(E,E)-decadienal, both of which have characteristic fatty odour impressions. By contrast, significantly different concentrations of both aldehydes were found in the samples of varying yeast content (Table 4), although the sensory panel could not differentiate between these samples. This might be due to an increasing yeast activity, which predominantly produces other volatile aroma compounds such as butanoic acid and Ehrlich pathway metabolites, which results in an increase in the buttery odour, as observed here (Figure 2).

3.6. Sensory Triangle Test

Sensory triangle test analyses of the two sample pairs with different NaCl levels indicated that there was no significant difference between the pairs ($p > 0.2$). The sample pair with 0.3% and 1.5% w/w yeast was significantly distinguishable ($p < 0.1$). These findings show that NaCl reduction has no significant influence on the overall volatile aroma fraction of the bread crumb recognisable by a human panellist. On the contrary, a 5-fold increase of yeast led to a distinguishable difference based on a 5-fold increase of the yeast metabolism activity in the dough system. The descriptive sensory results show several changes for isolated attributes and compounds in particular based on the determined attributes rose-like and cheesy. However, the aroma profile as a whole did not change to an extent that would be recognisable by consumers.

4. Conclusions

The influence of yeast activity on the generation of volatile aroma compounds in bread crumb was investigated using sensory assessments in combination with two-dimensional high-resolution gas chromatography-mass spectrometry (2D-HRGC-MS) and proton-transfer-reaction mass spectrometry (PTR-MS). A correlation between different yeast metabolites was shown. The metabolic pathways in yeast cells seem to correlate with the reducing activity, independently of the amount of yeast present or the concentration of NaCl. Bread samples with a 5-fold increase in yeast concentration (from 0.3% to 1.5% w/w) were distinguishable by a trained sensory panel. Indeed, when the concentration of NaCl was kept at 0.3%, yeast cells were metabolically over-performing due to the lack of the inhibiting effect normally carried out by the presence of NaCl in the dough system. This related to an increased yeast metabolic activity during the fermentation process, which showed to have a significant impact on the final bread crumb aroma [17]. A reduction in NaCl from the standard concentration of 1.2% w/w to 0.3% w/w increased the yeast activity but the increase in volatile aroma components, as determined by 2D-HRGC-MS and PTR-MS, could not be detected by the sensory panel. These observations suggest that NaCl reduction does not influence the volatile aroma of bread significantly and consumers in general are not able to recognise any reduced amounts of salt in the odour of bread crumb. While salt reduction in bread impacts on the quality characteristics of taste, shelf-life and texture [22,35], the aroma quality remains unchanged.

Acknowledgments: The authors would like to thank Franziska Wiegand and Tom Hannon for their support. The authors wish to acknowledge that this project was funded under the Irish National Development Plan, through the Food Institutional Research Measure, administered by the Department of Agriculture, Fisheries and Food, Ireland.

Author Contributions: All authors participated in the experimental design of the study. Emanuele Zannini and Elke Arendt coordinated the execution of the study. Jonathan Beauchamp and Michael Czerny contributed their knowledge, expertise and support in the 2D-HRGC-MS, PTR-MS and sensory analysis. Markus Belz performed the experiments, data processing and drafted the manuscript. Claudia Axel, Emanuele Zannini and Jonathan Beauchamp corrected and revised the manuscript to its final version.

References

1. Tuorila-Ollikainen, H.; Lahteenmaki, L.; Salovaara, H. Attitudes, norms, intentions and hedonic responses in the selection of low salt bread in a longitudinal choice experiment. *Appetite* **1986**, *7*, 127–139. [CrossRef]
2. Wyatt, C. Acceptability of Reduced Sodium in Breads, Cottage Cheese, and Pickles. *J. Food Sci.* **1983**, *48*, 1300–1302.
3. Bassett, M.N.; Pérez-Palacios, T.; Cipriano, I.; Cardoso, P.; Ferreira, I.M.P.L.V.O.; Samman, N.; Pinho, O. Development of Bread with NaCl Reduction and Calcium Fortification: Study of Its Quality Characteristics. *J. Food Qual.* **2014**, *37*, 107–116. [CrossRef]

4. Charlton, K.E.; MacGregor, E.; Vorster, N.H.; Levitt, N.S.; Steyn, K. Partial replacement of NaCl can be achieved with potassium, magnesium and calcium salts in brown bread. *Int. J. Food Sci. Nutr.* **2007**, *58*, 508–521. [CrossRef] [PubMed]
5. Rizzello, C.G.; Nionelli, L.; Coda, R.; Di Cagno, R.; Gobbetti, M. Use of sourdough fermented wheat germ for enhancing the nutritional, texture and sensory characteristics of the white bread. *Eur. Food Res. Technol.* **2010**, *230*, 645–654. [CrossRef]
6. Ghawi, S.K.; Rowland, I.; Methven, L. Enhancing consumer liking of low salt tomato soup over repeated exposure by herb and spice seasonings. *Appetite* **2014**, *81*, 20–29. [CrossRef] [PubMed]
7. Jimenez-Maroto, L.A.; Sato, T.; Rankin, S.A. Saltiness potentiation in white bread by substituting sodium chloride with a fermented soy ingredient. *J. Cereal Sci.* **2013**, *58*, 313–317. [CrossRef]
8. Kuo, W.-Y.; Lee, Y. Effect of Food Matrix on Saltiness Perception—Implications for Sodium Reduction. *Compr. Rev. Food Sci. Food Saf.* **2014**, *13*, 906–923. [CrossRef]
9. Pflaum, T.; Konitzer, K.; Hofmann, T.; Koehler, P. Influence of Texture on the Perception of Saltiness in Wheat Bread. *J. Agric. Food Chem.* **2013**, *61*, 10649–10658. [CrossRef] [PubMed]
10. Noort, M.W.J.; Bult, J.H.F.; Stieger, M. Saltiness enhancement by taste contrast in bread prepared with encapsulated salt. *J. Cereal Sci.* **2012**, *55*, 218–225. [CrossRef]
11. Schieberle, P.; Grosch, W. Potent odorants of the wheat bread crumb differences to the crust and effect of a longer dough fermentation. *Z. Lebensm.-Unters. Forsch.* **1991**, *192*, 130–135. [CrossRef]
12. Suomalainen, H.; Lehtonen, M. The production of aroma compounds by yeast. *J. Inst. Brew.* **1979**, *85*, 149–156. [CrossRef]
13. Whiting, G.C. Organic acid metabolism of yeasts during fermentation of alcoholic beverages—A review. *J. Inst. Brew.* **1976**, *82*, 84–92. [CrossRef]
14. Czerny, M.; Schieberle, P. Labelling studies on pathways of amino acid related odorant generation by *Saccharomyces cerevisiae* in wheat bread dough. In *Flavour Science: Recent Advances and Trends*; Bredie, W.L.P., Petersen, M.A., Eds.; Elsevier: Amsterdam, The Netherland, 2006; pp. 89–92.
15. Saison, D.; De Schutter, D.P.; Vanbeneden, N.; Daenen, L.; Delvaux, F.; Delvaux, F.R. Decrease of aged beer aroma by the reducing activity of brewing yeast. *J. Agric. Food Chem.* **2010**, *58*, 3107–3115. [CrossRef] [PubMed]
16. Vermeulen, N.; Czerny, M.; Gänzle, M.G.; Schieberle, P.; Vogel, R.F. Reduction of (E)-2-nonenal and (E,E)-2,4-decadienal during sourdough fermentation. *J. Cereal Sci.* **2007**, *45*, 78–87. [CrossRef]
17. Birch, A.N.; Petersen, M.A.; Arneborg, N.; Hansen, Å.S. Influence of commercial baker's yeasts on bread aroma profiles. *Food Res. Int.* **2013**, *52*, 160–166. [CrossRef]
18. Birch, A.N.; Petersen, M.A.; Hansen, Å.S. The aroma profile of wheat bread crumb influenced by yeast concentration and fermentation temperature. *LWT Food Sci. Technol.* **2013**, *50*, 480–488. [CrossRef]
19. Martins, Z.E.; Erben, M.; Gallardo, A.E.; Barbosa, I.; Pinho, O.; Ferreira, I.M.P.L.V.O. Effect of spent yeast fortification on physical parameters, volatiles and sensorial characteristics of home-made bread. *Int. J. Food Sci. Technol.* **2015**, *50*, 1855–1863. [CrossRef]
20. Engel, W.; Bahr, W.; Schieberle, P. Solvent assisted flavour evaporation—A new and versatile technique for the careful and direct isolation of aroma compounds from complex food matrices. *Eur. Food Res. Technol.* **1999**, *209*, 237–241. [CrossRef]
21. Lindinger, W.; Hansel, A.; Jordan, A. Proton-transfer-reaction mass spectrometry (PTR-MS): On-line monitoring of volatile organic compounds at pptv levels. *Chem. Soc. Rev.* **1998**, *27*, 347–375. [CrossRef]
22. Czerny, M.; Christlbauer, M.; Christlbauer, M.; Fischer, A.; Granvogl, M.; Hammer, M.; Hartl, C.; Hernandez, N.M.; Schieberle, P. Re-investigation on odour thresholds of key food aroma compounds and development of an aroma language based on odour qualities of defined aqueous odorant solutions. *Eur. Food Res. Technol.* **2008**, *228*, 265–273. [CrossRef]
23. Lynch, E.J.; Dal Bello, F.; Sheehan, E.M.; Cashman, K.D.; Arendt, E.K. Fundamental studies on the reduction of salt on dough and bread characteristics. *Food Res. Int.* **2009**, *42*, 885–891. [CrossRef]
24. Almagro, A.; Prista, C.; Castro, S.; Quintas, C.; Madeira-Lopes, A.; Ramos, J.; Loureiro-Dias, M.C. Effects of salts on *Debaryomyces hansenii* and *Saccharomyces cerevisiae* under stress conditions. *Int. J. Food Microbiol.* **2000**, *56*, 191–197. [CrossRef]
25. Watson, T.G. Effects of sodium chloride on steady-state growth and metabolism of *Saccharomyces cerevisiae*. *J. Gen. Microbiol.* **1970**, *64*, 91–99. [CrossRef] [PubMed]

26. Wei, C.-J.; Tanner, R.D.; Malaney, G.W. Effect of Sodium Chloride on Bakers' Yeast Growing in Gelatin. *Appl. Environ. Microbiol.* **1982**, *43*, 757–763. [PubMed]
27. Oda, Y.; Tonomura, K. Sodium chloride enhances the potential leavening ability of yeast in dough. *Food Microbiol.* **1993**, *10*, 249–254. [CrossRef]
28. Kawai, H.; Bagum, N.; Teramoto, I.; Isobe, U.; Yokoigawa, K. Effect of sodium chloride on the growth and fermentation activity of Saccharomyces yeasts. *Res. J. Living Sci.* **1999**, *45*, 55–61.
29. Dal Bello, F.; Clarke, C.I.; Ryan, L.A.M.; Ulmer, H.; Schober, T.J.; Ström, K.; Sjögren, J.; van Sinderen, D.; Schnürer, J.; Arendt, E.K.; et al. Improvement of the quality and shelf life of wheat bread by fermentation with the antifungal strain *Lactobacillus plantarum* FST 1.7. *J. Cereal Sci.* **2007**, *45*, 309–318. [CrossRef]
30. Beck, M.; Jekle, M.; Becker, T. Sodium chloride—Sensory, preserving and technological impact on yeast-leavened products. *Int. J. Food Sci. Technol.* **2012**, *47*, 1798–1807. [CrossRef]
31. Ehrlich, F. Über die Bedingungen der Fuselölbildung und über ihren Zusammenhang mit dem Eiweißaufbau der Hefe. *Ber. Deutsch. Chem. Ges.* **1907**, *40*, 1027–1047. [CrossRef]
32. Frasse, P.; Lambert, S.; Levesque, C.; Melcion, D.; Richard-Molard, D.; Chiron, H. The influence of fermentation on volatile compounds in French bread crumb. *Food Sci. Technol.—Lebensm.-Wiss. Technol.* **1992**, *25*, 66–70.
33. Chwastowski, J.; Koloczek, H. The kinetic reduction of Cr (VI) by yeast *Saccharomyces cerevisiae, Phaffia rhodozyma* and their protoplasts. *Acta Biochim. Pol.* **2013**, *60*, 829–834. [PubMed]
34. Jewison, T.; Knox, C.; Neveu, V.; Djoumbou, Y.; Guo, A.C.; Lee, J.; Liu, P.; Mandal, R.; Krishnamurthy, R.; Sinelnikov, I.; et al. YMDB: The Yeast Metabolome Database. *Nucl. Acids Res.* **2012**, *40*, D815–D820. [CrossRef] [PubMed]
35. Belz, M.C.E.; Mairinger, R.; Zannini, E.; Ryan, L.A.M.; Cashman, K.D.; Arendt, E.K. The effect of sourdough and calcium propionate on the microbial shelf-life of salt reduced bread. *Appl. Microbiol. Biotechnol.* **2012**, *96*, 493–501. [CrossRef] [PubMed]

13

Bread for the Aging Population: The Effect of a Functional Wheat–Lentil Bread on the Immune Function of Aged Mice

Marina Carcea *, Valeria Turfani, Valentina Narducci, Alessandra Durazzo, Alberto Finamore, Marianna Roselli and Rita Rami

Research Centre for Food and Nutrition, Council for Agricultural Research and Economics (CREA), via Ardeatina 546, 00178 Roma, Italy; valeria.turfani@crea.gov.it (V.T.); valentina.narducci@crea.gov.it (V.N.); alessandra.durazzo@crea.gov.it (A.D.); alberto.finamore@crea.gov.it (A.F.); marianna.roselli@crea.gov.it (M.R.); rita.rami@crea.gov.it (R.R.)

* Correspondence: marina.carcea@crea.gov.it

Abstract: A functional bread tailored for the needs of the aging population was baked by substituting 24% of wheat flour with red lentil flour and compared with wheat bread. Its nutritional profile was assessed by analysing proteins, amino acids, lipids, soluble and insoluble dietary fibre, resistant starch, total polyphenols, lignans and the antioxidant capacity (FRAP assay). The wheat–lentil bread had 30% more proteins than wheat bread (8.3%, as is), a more balanced amino acids composition, an almost double mineral (0.63%, as is) as well as total dietary fibre content (4.6%, as is), double the amount of polyphenols (939.1 mg GAE/100g on dry matter, d.m.), higher amounts and variety of lignans, and more than double the antioxidant capacity (71.6 µmoL/g d.m.). The in vivo effect of 60 days bread consumption on the immune response was studied by means of a murine model of elderly mice. Serum cytokines and intraepithelial lymphocyte immunophenotype from the mice intestine were analysed as markers of systemic and intestinal inflammatory status, respectively. Analysis of immune parameters in intraepithelial lymphocytes showed significant differences among the two types of bread indicating a positive effect of the wheat–lentil bread on the intestinal immune system, whereas both breads induced a reduction in serum IL-10.

Keywords: wheat bread; lentil bread; bread composition; aged mice; immune function; intraepithelial lymphocytes; gut health

---

1. Introduction

According to recent statistics [1], the European population in particular is an aging one: In fact, the proportion of the population over 65 has steadily increased over the past decade. Aging is a condition that brings about a number of factors contributing to the risk of malnutrition which are related to physiological changes and medical and social conditions [2,3]. Current data for mean nutrient intakes suggest that, as a group, older adults are at risk of not meeting the recommended dietary allowance (RDA) or adequate intake (AI) values for calcium, vitamins, minerals, fibre [4] and protein [5]. It is well known that increased thresholds for taste and smell resulting in bland and uninteresting food tasting, coupled with impaired masticatory efficiency and swallowing difficulties can lead to consumption of a narrow, nutritionally imbalanced diet in the aged population [6–8]. Moreover, older adults have less money to spend on food.

All the above mentioned factors impact on the nutritional status of older adults, contributing to age-associated disorders including dysregulation of the immune system [9,10]. In fact, aging is associated with a declined immune function, a process known as immunosenescence, that negatively impacts on the capacity to properly respond to immune challenges thus contributing to the increased susceptibility of older persons to infections, poor vaccine efficacy and progressive development of low-grade, chronic inflammatory status [10–12].

Since a variety of bioactive dietary components have been shown to affect the immune system, an appropriate nutritional intervention may be a promising approach to counteract the impaired immune function occurring with aging [13,14]. Enriching staple or widely consumed foods can be a simple strategy to increase the intake of such components. Bread is an important food in the daily diet of several populations around the world. It is generally produced from refined white flour that lacks the nutrients, fibre and bioactive components present in the bran, but other ingredients can be added to increase the nutritional value of bread without altering its appearance and nature.

Lentils have been gaining increasing interest in the development of healthy and functional foods, due to the fact of their nutritional properties [15–20]. The existing varieties of lentils vary in colour, size and texture, but they all have a low level of antinutrients and a mild taste [21]. Lentils contain 28.7%–31.5% protein, which is considerable among legumes, and provide the essential amino acids lysine and leucine [22]. They are a valuable source of dietary fibre, mainly the insoluble component, but also the soluble one [19]. Dietary fibres provide many health benefits, such as lowering serum levels of LDL cholesterol, glucose and blood pressure, reducing constipation and other intestinal disorders and preventing intestinal cancer [23]. Moreover, the soluble fibres of lentils contain nutritionally significant amounts of prebiotic molecules, such as galacto-oligosaccharides (GOS) and fructo-oligosaccharides (FOS), that are known to selectively stimulate the growth and/or activity of some beneficial bacteria in the colon, having the potential to improve host health, such as several *Bifidobacteria* and lactobacilli strains [24–26]. Finally, lentils are reported to have a high content of phenolic compounds and to show a high antioxidant activity [27]. Actually, phytochemicals, and among them phenolic compounds, are known to have a major impact on health, since they can provide therapeutic benefits including prevention and/or treatment of diseases and physiological disorders [28]. Amongst the lentil varieties, red lentils distinguish themselves for being an important source of proteins, fibre and particularly of bioactive substances [29,30].

A recent study from our laboratory showed that red lentil flour can be blended with wheat flour up to 24% to produce bread with good volume, pleasant texture and taste [31]. We thus engaged in further studies, which are reported in the present paper, to describe the nutritional profile of our 24% red lentil bread and to get some insight into the in vivo effect of its consumption, with particular regard to the aging condition. The bread nutritional profile was described by analysing proteins, amino acids, lipids, soluble and insoluble dietary fibre, resistant starch, total polyphenols and specifically lignans, which is an interesting group of polyphenols present in pulses; in addition, its antioxidant power was measured by the ferric reducing antioxidant power (FRAP) assay.

The same bread was chosen for an in vivo experiment with aged mice, used as a vulnerable animal model, to evaluate if a substitution of common wheat bread with this special wheat–legume bread could counteract the immune decline typical of older adults. The immune response was mainly assessed at the intestinal level, since the mucosal immune system, which is known to be also impaired in the older adults [32], represents the first line of contact with ingested antigens and molecules reaching the intestinal lumen. Some parameters, namely, serum cytokines and intraepithelial lymphocyte immunophenotype were analysed, as they represent markers of systemic and intestinal inflammatory status, respectively.

2. Materials and Methods

2.1. Flours and Bread Preparation

Commercial wheat flour ("0" type according to the Italian flour classification, Horeca brand) and commercial dehulled red lentils (Select, San Giuseppe Vesuviano, Napoli, Italy) were purchased from the market.

The wheat flour had a moisture level of 12.8% (International Association for Cereal Science and Technology (ICC) standard 110/1 [33]), ash 0.63% d.m. (indicated on the product label), total protein of 10.5% d.m. (product label), lipids of 0.8% d.m. (product label) and total dietary fibre of 3.2% d.m. of which 2.1% was insoluble and 1.1% soluble (measured according to Lee et al. [34] using a reagent kit (K-TDFR, Megazyme Int., Wicklow, Ireland)).

Red lentils were ground in a refrigerated laboratory mill (M20, Janke and Kunkel Ika Labortechnik, Staufen, Germany) (a cutting/impact mill with no sieve, operating at a speed of 20,000 rpm for 2 min) to produce a very homogeneous flour that had a moisture level of 10.3% (ICC standard 110/1 [33]), ash content of 2.39% dry matter (d.m.) (ICC standard 104/1 [33]), total protein of 24.6% d.m. (product label), lipids of 1.3% d.m. (product label) and total dietary fibre content of 17.1% d.m. of which 15.2% was insoluble and 1.9% soluble (measured according to Lee et al. [34] using a reagent kit (K-TDFR, Megazyme Int., Wicklow, Ireland)).

A blend was prepared by mixing wheat flour with red lentil flour in the proportions of 76% and 24%, respectively. These proportions were chosen according to the results of Turfani et al. [31], who determined the maximum amount of red lentil flour that could be added to wheat flour in order to avoid technical problems during bread making, such as excessive dough sticking, poor dough rheological properties and bread with unacceptably low volume, poor texture and excessive legume flavour.

The bread formulation was kept simple in order to study the nutritional properties of bread produced from the flour blend without additives. Loaves of bread were produced from wheat flour (wheat bread) and from a wheat–lentil flour blend by adapting the ICC standard method No. 131 [33] because solution 1 was not used, thus reducing sugar and eliminating ascorbic acid from the ingredients (the same adapted method was used in References [20,31]). Thus, 1000 g of flour blend were weighted at 14% m.b. and mixed with 15 g salt in the mixer bowl; the optimum water amount (previously determined by the Brabender Farinograph according to ICC Standard 151/1 [33]) was added to the flour blend, except for the small amount required to activate yeast; compressed baker's yeast (18 g) was activated in 72 g of 5% sucrose solution (containing 68.4 g water and 3.6 g sucrose) at 35 °C for 10 min, then added to the flour blend. The dough was mixed for 10 min in a planetary bread mixer (Quick 20 by Sottoriva, Marano, Italy), then the dough temperature was checked (27 ± 1 °C) and the dough was fermented for 30 min in a fermentation cabinet at 30 °C with 85% relative humidity. After fermentation, the dough was scaled in four equal pieces, which were placed in baking tins and proofed for 50 min at 30 °C with 85% relative humidity, then baked for 30 ± 2 min at 220 °C in a convection/steam oven. The bread volume was determined within 20 ± 4 h by the rapeseed displacement method (AACCI Method 10-05.01) [35].

Bread for mouse feeding was baked all together at the beginning of the experiment to prevent variability due to the different preparation conditions, divided in aliquots sufficient for weekly diet preparation and frozen. Bread aliquots were thawed at room temperature at the moment of diet preparation.

2.2. *Chemicals and Standards for Bread Analysis*

The solvents used (i.e., acetone, diethyl ether, ethanol, ethyl acetate, methanol, n-hexane) were of HPLC or analytical grade and were purchased from Carlo Erba (Milan, Italy). Reagents were of the highest available purity. Hydrochloric acid 35%, formic acid 99%, glacial acetic acid, sulphuric acid 96%, tartaric acid, boric acid, sodium hydroxide, sodium hydroxide 32% solution, tris(hydroxymethyl)-aminomethane (TRIS), Folin–Ciocalteu reagent, sodium carbonate 20% solution, iron (II) sulphate heptahydrate (99%) and iron (III) chloride hexahydrate (97%–102%) were purchased from Carlo Erba. Kjieltabs (CuSO4/K2SO4), sulphuric acid solution 0.1 N and hydrogen peroxide 30% were purchased from VWR International PBI (Milan, Italy). Sodium citrate dihydrate, sodium acetate trihydrate, sodium chloride, glacial acetic acid, 2-metoxyethanol, ninhydrin were purchased from Merck-BDI (Darmstadt, Germany). Tin (II) chloride dehydrate, sodium acetate trihydrate 99%, MES (2(N-morpholino)-ethanesulpohonic acid), trolox

(6-hydroxy-2,5,7,8-tetramethylchroman-2-carboxylic acid), TPTZ (2,4,6-Tris(2-pyridyl)-s-triazine) and Helix Pomatia μ-glucuronidase/sulphatase S9626–10KU Type H-1, 0.7 G solid, 14,200 units/g solid were purchased from Sigma–Aldrich (Milan, Italy). Standards were of the highest available grade: Amino acids standards and gallic acid monohydrate were purchased from Sigma–Aldrich, whereas isolariciresinol, secoisolariciresinol, lariciresinol and pinoresinol were from Chemical Research (Rome, Italy). Ultra-pure water was produced by using in sequence a Millipore Elix 5 system and a Millipore Synergy 185 system (Millipore, Molsheim, France).

2.3. Proximate Composition, Amino Acids, Total Polyphenols, Lignans and Antioxidant Properties of Bread

Moisture, proteins (conversion factor 6.25 for legume flours and 5.70 for wheat flour), lipids and ash were determined by standard ICC methods 110/1, 105/2, 136, 104/1, respectively [33]. Soluble (SDFs), insoluble (IDFs) and total (TDFs) dietary fibres were determined according to Lee et al. [32] using a reagent kit (K-TDFR, Megazyme Int., Wicklow, Ireland). Available carbohydrates were calculated by difference. Resistant starch was determined according to AACC Method 32-40.01 [31] by means of a reagent kit (RSTAR, Megazyme); however, the results of all determinations were below the limit of detection (2%) and they are not shown in the tables.

Amino acids were determined according to Spackman, Stein and Moore [36] using a Beckman System Gold 126 amino acid analyser (Beckman Coulter Inc., Brea, CA, USA) equipped with a Beckman Spherogel IEX High-Performance Sodium column P/N 727450 and a Beckman UV detector with ninhydrin reactor. The samples were hydrolysed in hydrochloric acid 6 M under vacuum in sealed tubes at 105 °C for 24 h. For the determination of valine and isoleucine, the hydrolysis lasted 72 h. For cysteine and methionine, the samples were oxidised by oxygen peroxide and formic acid (88%) at 0 °C for 4 h at first, then the reagents were removed by evaporation under vacuum and the residue was hydrolysed in hydrochloric acid 6 M at 105 °C for 22 h. After hydrolysis and removal of the excess HCl, residues were re-dissolved in citrate buffer 0.2 M and injected.

Total polyphenols (TPCs) were extracted from samples as described by Durazzo et al. [30] in two separate fractions. Free polyphenols were extracted in methanol/water 1:1 and acetone/water 3:7. The residue was treated with hot sulphuric acid in methanol in order to free the hydrolysable polyphenols. The polyphenol content in the aqueous–organic extract and in the hydrolysed residue was determined by means of the Folin–Ciocalteau reagent [37], by measuring absorbance at 760 nm and using gallic acid as a standard.

For the analysis of lignans, samples were preliminarily defatted with hexane and diethyl ether for 8 h in a Soxhlet apparatus. The lignans were extracted and analysed by High Performance Liquid Chromatography (HPLC) as in Durazzo et al. [30]. The HPLC analyses were performed with a 50 μL extract using an ESA-HPLC system (ESA, Chelmsford, MA, USA) consisting of an ESA Model 540 autoinjector, an ESA Model 580 solvent delivery module with two pumps, an ESA 5600 eight channels coulometric electrode array detector and the ESA CoulArray operating software which controlled all the equipment and carried out data processing. A SUPELCOSIL LC-18 column (25 cm × 4.6 mm, 5 μm) with a Perisorb Supelguard LC-18 (Supelco, Milan, Italy) was used. Isolariciresinol, lariciresinol, secoisolariciresinol and pinoresinol were detected and quantified.

The antioxidant properties were determined by means of the FRAP assay according to Durazzo et al. [30].

2.4. In Vivo Experiments: Experimental Design, Animals and Diets

The Balb/c aged mice (20 months old) were kept at 23 °C with a 12 h light–dark cycle and fed ad libitum with standard laboratory diets. Mice had free access to food and water. Body weight and food intake were recorded every week and every other day, respectively. After one week of adaptation, animals were randomly divided into three groups (6 animals per group), receiving three different diets for two months (60 days): One group was fed a standard control diet (control group, 20% casein, Laboratorio Dottori Piccioni, Gessate, Milan, Italy), one group was fed the wheat bread containing diet (wheat bread group), and a third group was fed the wheat–lentil bread containing diet (wheat–lentil bread group). The standard control diet was prepared using as reference the AIN-93M formulation [38]. The bread containing diets were appropriately balanced and were isocaloric in respect to the control diet. At the end of the experimental periods, animals were fasted for 16 h, anesthetised with intraperitoneal injection of pentobarbital (10 mg/kg) and sacrificed. Blood was drawn via cardiac puncture, whereas small intestine and colon were excised and immediately placed in cold phosphate buffered saline (PBS). The animal experiments were carried out in strict accordance with the recommendation of the European Guidelines for the Care and Use of Animals for Research Purposes. All experimental procedures complied with the Animal Care and Use Committee of the CREA—Research Centre for Food and Nutrition—and were approved by the National Health Ministry, General Direction of Animal Health and Veterinary Drugs (agreement number 0006828/03/02/2014). All efforts were made to minimise the suffering of the animals.

2.5. Intraepithelial Lymphocytes (IELs) Preparation

The intraepithelial lymphocytes (IELs) were prepared from jejunum and colon. Briefly, intestines were placed on ice in 10 mL RPMI-1640 medium (Sigma–Aldrich, Milan, Italy), washed twice with cold PBS, longitudinally opened and cut into small size pieces. Intestinal pieces were washed in Hank's balanced salt solution (HBSS) and stirred twice for 45 min at 37 °C in an orbital shaker in HBSS added with 100 g/L foetal calf serum (FCS, Euroclone, Milan, Italy), 1 × 105 U/L penicillin, 100 mg/L streptomycin, 1 mM ethylendiamin-tetraacetic acid (EDTA), 5 mM Hepes, 1 mM dithiothreitol. The solution was passed through 100 and 40 μm nylon cell strainers (BD Falcon, Milan, Italy) and centrifuged at 650× *g*. The IELs were isolated from enterocytes by discontinuous 440/670 g/L Percoll gradient (PercollTM, GE Healthcare, Milan, Italy) in RPMI-1640 medium, and centrifuged at 650× *g* for 25 min.

2.6. Flow Cytometry Analysis of IELs Subpopulations

The following monoclonal antibodies were used for lymphocyte surface staining: Fluorescein isothiocyanate (FITC) anti-CD3 (clone 17.12), phycoerythrin (PE) anti-CD4 (clone GK1.5), phycoerythrin–cyanine 5 (PE-Cy5) anti-CD8 (clone 53-67), PE anti-CD19 (clone ID3), peridinin–chlorophyll-protein (PerCP) anti-CD45 (clone 30-F11), PE anti-TCR $\gamma\delta$ (clone GL3), PE-Cy5 anti-TCR $\alpha\beta$ (clone H57-597) and anti-CD16/CD32 (clone 2.4G2) (BD Pharmingen, Milan, Italy). Each antibody was previously titrated to determine the optimal concentration for maximal staining. The IELs (1 × 106 cells) were pre-incubated for 20 min with anti-CD16/CD32 to block Fc receptors. Cells were then washed and labelled with the appropriate mixture of antibodies for 30 min, centrifuged at 650× *g* and resuspended in FacsFlow (BD Biosciences, Milan, Italy). Flow cytometry analysis was performed using a FACSCalibur instrument (BD Biosciences). To exclude dead/dying cells and, therefore, non-specific antibody-binding cells, lymphocytes were gated according to forward and side scatter. The percentage of B and T lymphocytes was calculated on leukocyte (CD45+) gate, whereas the CD4+, CD8+ and CD4+CD8+ subsets, as well as $\alpha\beta$ and $\gamma\delta$ lymphocytes, were calculated on T lymphocyte (CD3+) gate. At least 10,000 events were acquired. Data were analysed using CellQuest software (BD Biosciences).

2.7. Analysis of Inflammatory Status in Mice Intestine

Small parts of jejunum and colon (1 cm) were immediately washed in cold PBS to remove stools and frozen in liquid nitrogen. To evaluate the inflammatory status of intestine, frozen tissues were weighted and homogenised in cold radioimmunoprotein (RIPA: 20 mM Tris-HCl pH 7.5, 150 mM NaCl, 0.1% Sodium Dodecyl Sulfate (SDS), 1% Na deoxycholate, 1% Triton X- 100) assay buffer supplemented with 1 mM phenylmethylsulphonyl fluoride, protease inhibitor cocktail (Complete Mini,

Roche, Milan, Italy) and phosphatase inhibitor cocktail (PhosSTOP, Roche). Protein concentration was measured by the Lowry assay. Intestinal homogenates (50 μg total proteins) were dissolved in sample buffer (50 mM Tris-HCl, pH 6.8, 2% SDS, 10% glycerol, 100 g/L bromophenol blue, 10 mM beta-mercaptoethanol), heated for 5 min, fractionated by SDS-polyacrylamide gel (4–20% gradient) electrophoresis and transferred to 0.2 μm nitrocellulose filters (Trans-Blot Turbo, Biorad, Milan, Italy). Membranes were incubated with the following primary antibodies: Rabbit polyclonal anti-mouse NF-kB p65 and P-p65. Proteins were detected with horseradish peroxidase conjugated secondary antibodies (Cell Signaling Technology, Danvers, MA) and enhanced chemiluminescence reagent (ECL kit LiteAblot Extend, Euroclone, Milan, Italy), followed by analysis of chemiluminescence with the charge-coupled device camera detection system Las4000 Image Quant (GE Health Care Europe GmbH, Milan, Italy). The expression of the P-p65 proteins was normalised to their corresponding unphosphorylated forms.

2.8. Cytokine Secretion in Mice Serum

Blood samples were collected in test tubes, centrifuged (2000× g for 10 min at 4 °C) and the supernatant (serum) was stored at −80 °C until further analysis. The levels of cytokines and chemokines were analysed using Bio-plex/Luminex technology (mouse magnetic Luminex screening assay, Labospace, Milan, Italy). Briefly, Luminex multi-analyte profiling is a multiplexing technology allowing simultaneous analysis of up to 500 bioassays from a small sample volume. The following cytokines and chemokines were simultaneously detected in 50 μL undiluted samples: Tumour necrosis factor (TNF)-alpha, granulocyte macrophage-colony stimulating factor (GM-CSF), regulated upon activation normal T cell expressed and secreted (RANTES), interleukin (IL)-23, IL-17, IL-10, IL-12 and IL-6.

2.9. Presentation of Results and Statistics

Proximate composition, dietary fibre and lignan analyses were performed in triplicate whereas four replicates were used for polyphenols and FRAP. Mean values and percent coefficient of variation (%CV) are reported, together with the significance level of Student's t-test between wheat bread and wheat–lentil bread. Amino acids were analysed by a single determination without replicates. Calculations were performed by means of Microsoft Excel and PAST statistical package, version 2.17c [39].

For the results of in vivo experiments, values in graphs and tables represent means and %CV. Statistical significance was evaluated by one-way ANOVA followed by post-hoc Tukey's honestly significant difference (HSD) test. Normal distribution and homogeneity of variance of data were previously verified with appropriate statistical tests. Differences with p-values < 0.05 were considered significant. Statistical analysis was performed with the PAST statistical package.

3. Results

Table 1 shows the proximate composition of wheat bread and of the wheat–lentil bread. The two breads did not significantly differ in their moisture content (38.9% as is basis and 40.0% as is basis for the wheat bread and the wheat–lentil bread, respectively), whereas significant differences were observed for protein (6.4% as is basis and 8.3% as is basis for the wheat and the wheat–lentil bread, respectively), ash (0.39% as is basis and 0.63% as is basis for the wheat and the wheat-lentil bread, respectively) and IDF (1.6% as is basis and 3.1% as is basis for the wheat and the wheat-lentil bread, respectively).

Table 1. Proximate composition of wheat and wheat–lentil bread (76% wheat flour/24% red lentil) #.

Bread	Moisture%		Protein%		Fat%		Ash%		IDF §%		SDF §%		TDF §%		Available Carbohydrates (by Difference)%	
	Mean ns	CV	Mean **	CV	Mean ns	CV	Mean **	CV	Mean *	CV	Mean ns	CV	Mean ns	CV	Mean ns	CV
Wheat bread	38.9	0.8%	6.4	1.6%	1.0	0%	0.39	0%	1.6	13%	1.0	20%	2.6	15%	50.8	1.6%
Wheat–lentil bread	40.0	0.8%	8.3	1.2%	0.9	3%	0.63	0.02%	3.1	16%	1.5	60%	4.6	28%	45.5	4.0%

Values are the mean of three replicates, on wet basis; § IDF—insoluble dietary fibre; SDF—soluble dietary fibre; TDF—total dietary fibre; *, **, ns significance (*t*-test) of difference among the two samples: * significant at $p < 0.05$; significant ** at $p < 0.01$; ns not significant.

The content of 17 amino acids in mg/100 g proteins (eight essentials, tryptophan was not determined, plus alanine, arginine, aspartic acid, cysteine, glutamic acid, glycine, proline, serine and tyrosine) in both wheat and wheat–lentil bread is reported in Table 2. The main differences observed were aspartic acid (4.20 and 6.05 for the wheat and the wheat–lentil bread, respectively), glutamic acid (39.75 and 34.36 for the wheat and the wheat–lentil bread, respectively), proline (9.90 and 8.39 for the wheat and the wheat–lentil bread, respectively), lysine (2.18 and 3.30 for the wheat and the wheat–lentil bread, respectively) and arginine (3.89% and 4.91% for the wheat and the wheat–lentil bread, respectively).

Table 2. Amino acid composition of wheat and wheat–lentil bread (mg/100 g proteins) [#, §].

Sample	Aspartic Acid	Threonine	Serine	Glutamic Acid	Proline	Glycine	Alanine	Cystine	Valine
Wheat bread	4.20	2.82	4.98	39.75	9.90	3.67	3.03	1.89	4.53
Wheat–lentil bread	6.05	3.01	5.04	34.36	8.39	3.79	3.27	1.60	4.84
Sample	**Methionine**	**Isoleucine**	**Leucine**	**Tyrosine**	**Phenylalanine**	**Histidine**	**Lysine**	**Arginine**	**NH_4**
Wheat bread	1.36	4.07	7.08	2.77	4.88	2.28	2.18	3.89	5.12
Wheat–lentil bread	1.13	4.27	7.21	2.76	4.92	2.41	3.30	4.91	4.42

[#] Amino acids were analysed as a single determination without replicates. [§] Tryptophan was not analysed.

Data on total polyphenols content (TPC) (both in the aqueous organic extract and in the hydrolysable residue), four lignans content—namely, isolariciresinol, lariciresinol, secoisolariciresinol, pinoresinol—and the antioxidant power measured by the FRAP (both in the aqueous organic extract and hydrolysable residue) in our experimental wheat and wheat–lentil bread are reported in Table 3.

With regards to TPC, significant differences were observed between the wheat bread and the wheat–lentil bread both in the aqueous organic extract and the hydrolysable residue with values of 59.4 and 250.0 mg GAE/100 g d.m. in the aqueous organic extract of wheat and wheat–lentil bread, respectively, and higher values of 411.8 and 689.1 in the hydrolysable residue of the same samples.

With regards to the content of the four determined lignans, lariciresinol and pinoresinol were not detectable in the wheat bread whereas they reached 45.2. and 27.3 μg/100g d.m., respectively, in wheat–lentil bread. Significant differences between the two types of bread were observed for isolariciresinol (2.4 and 66.5 μg/100g d.m. for wheat and wheat–lentil bread, respectively) and for secoisolariciresinol (4.5 and 7.0 μg/100 g d.m. for wheat and wheat–lentil bread, respectively). Significant differences were also observed in the FRAP values of the aqueous organic extract and the hydrolysable residue of both types of bread which were higher for lentil bread in both cases (21.9 versus 6.4 and 49.7 versus 21.1 μmoL/g d.m., respectively).

Table 3. Total polyphenols, lignans and FRAP of wheat and wheat–lentil bread #.

Bread	TPC (mg GAE/100 g d.m.)				Lignans (µg/100 g d.m.)								FRAP (µmol/g d.m.)			
	Aqueous–Organic Extract		Hydrolysable Residue		Isolariciresinol		Lariciresinol		Secoisolariciresinol		Pinoresinol		Aqueous–Organic Extract		Hydrolysable Residue	
	Mean **	CV	Mean **	CV	Mean *	CV	Mean	CV	Mean **	CV	Mean	CV	Mean **	CV	Mean **	CV
Wheat bread	59.4	1.5%	411.8	0.3%	2.4	8.3%	n.d.		4.5	4.4%	n.d.		6.4	3.1%	21.1	12.3%
Wheat–lentil bread	250.0	2.0%	689.1	4.9%	66.5	18.6%	45.2	12.2%	7.0	4.3%	27.3	18%	21.9	12.8%	49.7	7.8%

Values are means of four to seven replicates; GAE—gallic acid equivalent; d.m.—dry matter; TPC—total phenols content; FRAP—ferric reducing antioxidant power; n.d.—not detectable. *, ** Significance (*t*-test) of differences among the two samples: Significant ** at $p < 0.01$ and * at $p < 0.05$.

Data on the composition of the diets which were given to the aged mice are reported in Table 4.

Table 4. Diets composition.

Component	Control (g/kg)	Wheat Bread (g/kg)	Wheat–Lentil Bread (g/kg)
Bread		465.7	465.7
Maize starch	465.7	66.4	92.6
Casein	140.0	88.8	74.8
Maltodextrins	155.0	155.0	155.0
Sucrose	100.0	100.0	100.0
Soya oil	40.0	35.6	35.4
Cellulose	50.0	39.2	27.2
Saline mix	35.0	35.0	35.0
Vitamin mix	10.0	10.0	10.0
L-cystine	1.8	1.8	1.8
Choline chloride	2.5	2.5	2.5
TBHQ #	0.008	0.008	0.008

tert-Butylhydroquinone.

Table 5 reports the data relative to mice initial (i.e., at the beginning of treatment) and final (i.e., at the end of treatment) body weight, as well as daily food intake. No significant differences were observed among the three groups in body weight nor in food intake.

Table 5. Body weight and daily food intake of control, wheat bread and wheat–lentil bread fed mice *.

Diet	Initial Body Weight (g)		Final Body Weight (g)		Food Intake (g/day)	
	Mean	CV	Mean	CV	Mean	CV
Control	24.0	8.3%	25.0	9.6%	3.6	22.2%
Wheat bread	25.5	8.2%	25.5	12.9%	3.4	23.5%
Wheat–lentil bread	24.0	15.0%	25.7	5.8%	3.7	24.3%

* Data represent means and %CV of 6 mice per group.

Among all the analysed cytokines and chemokines in serum, only three resulted at detectable levels: The anti-inflammatory IL-10, the pro-inflammatory IL-17 and the GM-CSF chemokine. Interleukin-10 significantly decreased in the wheat and wheat–lentil bread-treated animals as compared to control, whereas no significant differences were observed in IL-17 and GM-CSF levels among the three groups (Table 6).

Table 6. Cytokine serum secretion #.

Diet	Cytokine (pg/mL)					
	IL-17		IL-10		GM-CSF	
	Mean	CV	Mean	CV	Mean	CV
Control	25.79	4.96%	13.49	55.75%	3.02	10.26%
Wheat bread	23.01	10.30%	4.81 *	64.66%	2.50	22.40%
Wheat–lentil bread	23.52	1.0%	6.73 *	26.60%	2.65	3.77%

Data represent means and %CV of 6 mice per group; * $p < 0.05$ versus control.

The IELs subpopulation percentages in jejunum (panel A) and colon (panel B) of mice fed control, wheat bread or wheat–lentil bread diets are presented in Figure 1. Histograms show a significant increase of cytotoxic T cell (CD3+CD8+) percentages in the jejunum of mice fed both types of bread compared to the control diet, whereas the percentage of total T cells (CD3+CD45+) were reduced in mice fed wheat bread compared to control and wheat–lentil bread. In the colon, only a significant increase of B cell (CD19+CD45+) percentages was observed in mice fed wheat–lentil bread. No differences in the percentages of other lymphocyte subpopulations were observed among the groups.

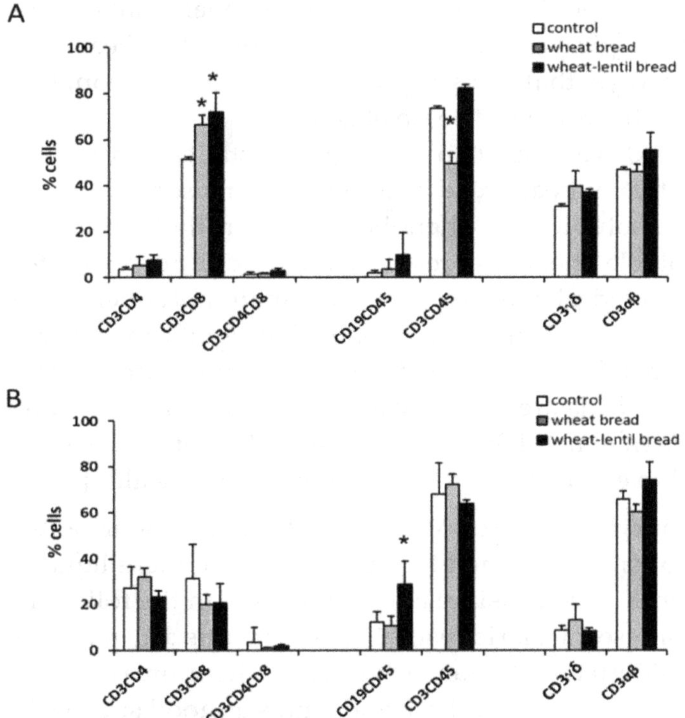

Figure 1. Intraepithelial lymphocyte (IEL) subpopulations in the jejunum (**A**) and colon (**B**) of mice fed a control, a wheat bread and a wheat–lentil diet measured by flow cytometry. (The percentage of B and T lymphocytes was calculated on leukocyte (CD45+) gate, whereas the CD4+, CD8+ and CD4+CD8+ subsets, as well as αβ and γδ lymphocytes, were calculated on T lymphocyte (CD3+) gate). Data represent the means ± SD of 6 mice. * $p < 0.05$ versus control.

Western blot analysis of the phosphorylated form of the p65 subunit of NF-kB in the jejunum and colon of mice did not show any significant difference among groups, indicating that the treatment with wheat and wheat–lentil bread did not induce an inflammatory status in the mice intestine (data not shown).

4. Discussion

As expected, the proximate composition of the wheat and the wheat–lentil bread mirrored the proximate composition of the flours of origin (see the Materials and Methods section and Table 1). In fact, the wheat–lentil bread contained 30% more proteins than wheat bread, it had an almost double ash content, therefore a higher level of minerals in general, together with an almost double amount of total dietary fibre, especially the insoluble component. Moreover, the lentil–wheat bread contained a lower amount of available carbohydrates than wheat bread.

Besides having a higher protein content, wheat–lentil bread had a more balanced amino acid profile than wheat bread (Table 2). Indeed, the amino acid profiles of wheat and lentils are complementary. For example, lysine is abundant in lentils, whereas sulphur amino acids are present in higher amounts in wheat. Lentil proteins are, in fact, mainly constituted by globulins and albumins [40] and, thus, have a different composition from wheat proteins, which are mainly constituted of prolamins and glutelins. The presence of the lentil flour increases the level of almost all the essential amino acids in bread (Table 2).

The lower amount of available carbohydrates in wheat–lentil bread is due to the fact that lentils contain less starch than wheat (about 40–45%, [18]); it is also reported that legume starch has a higher fraction of amylose than wheat (about 35%, [41]).

Regarding dietary fibre, both wheat and wheat–lentil breads contain only a small amount of the soluble component, around 1%; however, the soluble fibre of lentils is reported to contain beta glucans [18]. Beta-glucans are very interesting from a functional point of view, because they are known to induce a variety of physiological effects with a positive impact on health, acting in particular through immunomodulatory pathways, that can suppress cancer proliferation, lower cholesterol levels and thus reduce the risk for cardiovascular disease [42,43].

The wheat–lentil bread was richer in phenolic substances, in particular those present in the aqueous organic extract, than wheat bread and this is the reason why it also had better antioxidant properties (Table 3). The soluble free phenolics found in the extract come mainly from cellular vacuoles whereas the insoluble phenolics present in the residue are bound to other components mainly fibre. The hydrolysable bound phenols represent the main polyphenol fraction in both bread types (between 73% and 87% of TPC). The literature reports that significant amounts of phenolic compounds remain in the extraction residues, associated with the food matrix [44]. The phenolic molecules most frequently found in cereals are phenolic acids and flavonoids whereas in pulses we also find tannins [45]. Polyphenols in general, both the free and the bound ones, thanks to their antioxidant properties are considered to exert a protective effect on human health [46].

The lignans, secoisolariciresinol and isolariciresinol, were found in both breads (Table 3). However, the wheat–lentil bread not only contained higher amounts of these lignans, but also had additional lignan types and, in particular, lariciresinol and pinoresinol in the following order: Isolariciresinol > lariciresinol > pinoresinol > secoisolariciresinol. These results are in agreement with data on lignan content in legume flours reported by Durazzo et al. [30]. Literature data indicate flaxseed and sesame as major alimentary sources of lignans and rye and lentils as good sources [30,47]. Lignans are a large group of polyphenols of increasing interest because their intake has been related to beneficial health effects, including cancer and cardiovascular disease prevention [48]. In this regard it is interesting to report that in 2012 the research group of During et al. [49] published a paper to report on their investigation of whether plant lignans are taken up by intestinal cells and modulate the intestinal inflammatory response using the Caco-2 cell model. Their findings suggest that plant lignans can be absorbed and metabolised in the small intestine and, among the plants lignans tested, pinoresinol exhibited the strongest anti-inflammatory properties.

The antioxidant power as measured by FRAP was significantly higher in wheat–lentil bread than in wheat bread. The FRAP assay is a quick and sensitive way to measure the antioxidant capacity of biological samples. In both cases, the hydrolysable residue had a higher FRAP value than the aqueous–organic extract thus providing the major contribution to the total antioxidant power (from 69% to 77%); this matches the results of the total polyphenols content. Thus, a bread recipe where about one-quarter of the wheat flour is substituted by red lentil flour more than doubles the antioxidant capacity of bread (Table 3).

Concerning animal experiments, our first consideration was that no significant differences were observed in body weight and food intake among the groups of mice fed the control and the two types of bread diets; this indicates that the different diets had the same palatability for the mice, and that they did not impact on eating behaviour and appetite; and that all the differences observed in our sets of data were due to differences in the composition of the diets.

Analysis of the immune parameters in IELs isolated from jejunum showed an increase of cytotoxic T lymphocytes (CD3+CD8+) percentages in both wheat and wheat–lentil bread-treated animals, as compared to the control. Moreover, total T lymphocytes (CD3+CD45+) were significantly reduced in the wheat bread group and increased in the wheat–lentil bread group, compared to the control (Figure 1A). The IEL subpopulation's analysis in colon showed a significant increase of the B lymphocytes (CD19+CD45+) percentage in lentil bread-treated animals as compared to wheat bread and the control (Figure 1B). In this regard, we could hypothesise a role of the higher amount of β-glucans in the lentil bread while not ignoring that such compounds can increase the percentage of activated B lymphocytes and stimulate immune response [50,51].

We can say that the results of our study indicate a positive effect of wheat–lentil bread supplementation on the intestinal immune system of aged mice, as this supplementation was able to counteract some of the immune alterations typical of the older adults. In fact, aging is characterised by intrinsic changes in hematopoietic precursors that affect their proliferative potential, and this represents a key factor contributing to age-related decline in B- and T-cell production [52]. Thus, the increase of total T lymphocytes indicates a better immune response, and the increase of cytotoxic T lymphocytes suggests an improved capacity to respond to toxic agents and/or pathogens, that is known to be reduced in older adults. We can also hypothesise that the increase of B lymphocytes in the colon indicates a more efficient antibody response. In fact, it is well known that the antibody response is impaired in the older adults [53]. Moreover, it has been largely demonstrated that an antioxidants-containing diet may ameliorate lymphocyte response and protect immune cells from oxidative stress-induced apoptosis [54]. Besides polyphenols in general, the positive effects on the immune system in our specific case could also be ascribed to the significantly higher amount of the lignan isolariciresinol (27 times higher) and the presence of the lignan pinoresinol in wheat–lentil bread compared to wheat bread; these two lignans in particular have been shown to exert immunomodulatory and anti-inflammatory effects [49,55].

No significant differences were observed in the other analysed IELs subpopulations (Figure 1A,B).

Among all the analysed cytokines in serum, only IL-10 was significantly decreased in the wheat and wheat–lentil bread treated animals as compared to the control (Table 6). The role of IL-10 in older adults is controversial; while some studies report that IL-10 increased the inflammatory status, others indicate that this cytokine plays a key role as an anti-inflammatory factor [56,57]. It has also been reported that aging is associated with an increase of IL-10 that, together with other cytokines, could be considered as a marker of frailty [58,59].

5. Conclusions

It is increasingly coming to general attention that the aging population needs to eat appropriately to prevent and reduce all the health risks associated with this phase of human life. In other words, there is a need for tailored foods for aging people. Enriching staple or widely consumed foods can be a simple strategy to guaranty the intake of key nutrients able to have a beneficial effect on the negative aspects associated with aging such as the decline of the immune function. Based on previous studies done in our laboratory, we identified bread as a target food and red lentil flour as a raw material useful to add functionality to bread. We also identified technological constraints that allowed a maximum addition of 24% lentil flour.

For the purpose of this study, we baked two kinds of bread: A common wheat bread and a wheat–24% lentil flour bread. The chemical analysis of the bread components showed that the wheat–lentil bread had 30% more proteins than wheat bread coupled with a more balanced amino acid composition; it had an almost double mineral as well as total dietary fibre content, especially the insoluble component, double the amount of polyphenols, an interesting lignans content and more than double the antioxidant capacity. Thus, this wheat–lentil bread proved to be nutritionally richer and more functional than common wheat bread.

The in vivo effect of the consumption of wheat–lentil bread versus wheat bread on the immune response was studied by means of a murine model of aged mice. Analysis of the immune parameters in intraepithelial lymphocytes isolated from the mice intestine showed significant differences between the two types of bread indicating a positive effect of the lentil–wheat bread on the intestinal immune system. Cytokines in serum were also analysed. Considering that IL-10 is indicated as a frailty marker, we suppose that wheat and wheat–lentil breads in diets could have a positive effect on inflammatory status and improve the health status of aged mice.

This study clearly demonstrates that this is possible by substituting wheat flour with another suitable flour to manufacture a simple and well-accepted food, such as bread, which shows more functionality and is more tailored for the aging population than traditional, common bread with soft wheat only.

Author Contributions: M.C. planned and supervised the research, acquired funds and wrote the final manuscript, V.N. and V.T. performed all the bread analyses but the lignans which were performed by A.D. A.F. and M.R. designed the animal experimental setup and performed the experiments and analysed and interpreted the data. R.R. prepared the experimental diets and took care of the animals.

Acknowledgments: Grateful acknowledgements are due to Luigi Bartoli and Francesco Mellara for technical help in the bread preparation.

References

1. EUROSTAT. Your Key to European Statistics. 2019. Available online: https://ec.europa.eu/eurostat/data/database (accessed on 25 July 2019).
2. Morley, J.E. Undernutrition in older adults. *Fam. Pract.* **2012**, *29*, i89–i93. [CrossRef] [PubMed]
3. Starr, K.N.P.; McDonald, S.R.; Bales, C.W. Nutritional vulnerability in older adults: A continuum of concerns. *Curr. Nutr. Rep.* **2015**, *4*, 176–184. [CrossRef]
4. Lichtenstein, A.H.; Rasmussen, H.; Yu, W.W.; Epstein, S.R.; Russell, R.M. Modified MyPyramid for older adults. *J. Nutr.* **2008**, *138*, 5–11. [CrossRef] [PubMed]
5. Ziylan, C.; Haveman-Nies, A.; Kremer, S.; de Groot, L.C. Protein-enriched bread and readymade meals increase community-dwelling older adults' protein intake in a double-blind randomized controlled trial. *J. Am. Med. Dir. Assoc.* **2016**, *18*, 145–151. [CrossRef] [PubMed]
6. Boyce, J.M.; Shone, G.R. Effects of ageing on smell and taste. *Postgrad. Med. J.* **2006**, *82*, 239–241. [CrossRef] [PubMed]
7. Ney, D.M.; Weiss, J.M.; Kind, A.J.; Robbins, J. Senescent swallowing: Impact, strategies, and interventions. *Nutr. Clin. Pract.* **2009**, *24*, 395–413. [CrossRef] [PubMed]
8. Rémond, D.; Shahar, D.R.; Gille, D.; Pinto, P.; Kachal, J.; Peyron, M.A.; Dos Santos, C.N.; Walther, B.; Bordoni, A.; Dupont, D.; et al. Understanding the gastrointestinal tract of the elderly to develop dietary solutions that prevent malnutrition. *Oncotarget* **2015**, *6*, 13858–13898. [CrossRef]
9. Chandra, R.K. Nutrition and the immune system from birth to old age. *Eur. J. Clin. Nutr.* **2002**, *56*, S73–S76. [CrossRef]
10. Fülöp, T.; Dupuis, G.; Witkowski, J.M.; Larbi, A. The role of immunosenescence in the development of age-related diseases. *Rev. Investig. Clín.* **2016**, *68*, 84–91.
11. Castelo-Branco, C.; Soveral, I. The immune system and aging: A review. *Gynecol. Endocrinol.* **2014**, *30*, 16–22. [CrossRef]
12. Pera, A.; Campos, C.; López, N.; Hassouneh, F.; Alonso, C.; Tarazona, R.; Solana, R. Immunosenescence: Implications for response to infection and vaccination in older people. *Maturitas* **2015**, *82*, 50–55. [CrossRef] [PubMed]
13. Pae, M.; Meydani, S.N.; Wu, D. The Role of nutrition in enhancing immunity in aging. *Aging Dis.* **2012**, *3*, 91–129. [PubMed]
14. Vulevic, J.; Juric, A.; Walton, G.E.; Claus, S.P.; Tzortzis, G.; Toward, R.E.; Gibson, G.R. Influence of galacto-oligosaccharide mixture (B-GOS) on gut microbiota, immune parameters and metabonomics in elderly persons. *Br. J. Nutr.* **2015**, *114*, 586–595. [CrossRef] [PubMed]
15. Dalgetty, D.D.; Baik, B.K. Fortification of bread with hulls and cotyledon fibers isolated from peas, lentils and chickpeas. *Cereal Chem.* **2006**, *83*, 269–274. [CrossRef]
16. Borsuk, Y.; Arntfield, S.; Lukow, O.M.; Swallow, K.; Malcolmson, L. Incorporation of pulse flours of different particle size in relation to pita bread quality. *J. Sci. Food Agric.* **2012**, *92*, 2055–2061. [CrossRef] [PubMed]
17. Baik, B.K.; Han, I.H. Cooking, roasting and fermentation of chickpeas, lentils, peas and soybeans for fortification of leavened bread. *Cereal Chem.* **2012**, *89*, 269–275. [CrossRef]
18. Faris, M.A.I.E.; Takruri, H.R.; Issa, A.Y. Role of lentils (Lens culinaris L.) in human health and nutrition: A review. *Med. J. Nutr. Metab.* **2012**, *6*, 3–16. [CrossRef]
19. Aslani, Z.; Alipour, B.; Mirmiran, P.; Bahadoran, Z. Lentil's (Lens culinaris L.) functional properties in prevention and treatment of non-communicable chronic diseases: A review. *Int. J. Nutr. Food Sci.* **2015**, *4*, 15–20. [CrossRef]
20. Turfani, V.; Narducci, V.; Durazzo, A.; Galli, V.; Carcea, M. Technological, nutritional and functional properties of wheat bread enriched with lentil or carob flours. *LWT-Food Sci. Technol.* **2017**, *78*, 361–366. [CrossRef]

21. Nienke, M.; Lindeboom, T.; Baga, M.; Vandenberg, A.; Chibbar, R.N. Composition and correlation between major seed constituents in selected lentil (Lens culinaris. Medik) genotypes. *Can. J. Plant Sci.* **2011**, *91*, 825–835.
22. Roy, F.; Boye, J.I.; Simpson, B.K. Bioactive proteins and peptides in pulse crops: Pea, chickpea and lentil. *Food Res. Int.* **2010**, *43*, 432–442. [CrossRef]
23. Hefnawy, T.H. Effect of processing methods on nutritional composition and anti-nutritional factors in lentils (Lens culinaris). *Ann. Agric. Sci.* **2011**, *56*, 57–61. [CrossRef]
24. Johnson, C.R.; Thavarajah, D.; Combs, G.F., Jr.; Thavarajah, P. Lentil (*Lens culinaris* L.): A prebiotic-rich whole food legume. *Food Res. Int.* **2013**, *51*, 107–113. [CrossRef]
25. Gibson, G.R.; Hutkins, R.; Sanders, M.E.; Prescott, S.L.; Reimer, R.A.; Salminen, S.J.; Scott, K.; Stanton, C.; Swanson, K.S.; Cani, P.D.; et al. Expert consensus document: The International Scientific Association for Probiotics and Prebiotic s (ISAPP) consensus statement on the definition and scope of prebiotics. *Nat. Rev. Gastroenterol. Hepatol.* **2017**, *14*, 491–502. [CrossRef]
26. Micioni Di Bonaventura, M.V.; Cecchini, C.; Vila-Donat, P.; Caprioli, G.; Cifani, C.; Coman, M.M.; Cresci, A.; Fiorini, D.; Ricciutelli, M.; Silvi, S.; et al. Evaluation of the hypocholesterolemic effect and prebiotic activity of a lentil (*Lens culinaris* Medik) extract. *Mol. Nutr. Food Res.* **2017**, *61*, 1700403. [CrossRef] [PubMed]
27. Johari, A.; Arora, S.; Potaliya, M.; Kawatra, A. Role of Lentil (*Lens culinaris* L.) in human health and nutrition. *Ann. Agri-Bio Res.* **2015**, *20*, 291–294.
28. Bouchenak, M.; Lamri-Senhadji, M. Nutritional quality of legumes, and their role in cardiometabolic risk prevention: A review. *J. Med. Food* **2013**, *16*, 185–198. [CrossRef]
29. Wang, N.; Hatcher, D.W.; Toews, R.; Gawalko, E.J. Influence of cooking and dehulling on nutritional composition of several varieties of lentils (Lens culinaris). *Food Sci. Technol.* **2009**, *42*, 842–848. [CrossRef]
30. Durazzo, A.; Turfani, V.; Azzini, E.; Maiani, G.; Carcea, M. Phenols, lignans and antioxidant properties of legume and sweet chestnut flours. *Food Chem.* **2013**, *140*, 666–671. [CrossRef]
31. Turfani, V.; Narducci, V.; Mellara, F.; Bartoli, L.; Carcea, M. Technological properties and bread characteristics of soft wheat and red lentil flour blends. *Tec. Molit. Int.* **2017**, *68*, 52–72.
32. Mabbott, N.A.; Kobayashi, A.; Sehgal, A.; Bradford, B.M.; Pattison, M.; Donaldson, D.S. Aging and the mucosal immune system in the intestine. *Biogerontology* **2015**, *16*, 133–145. [CrossRef] [PubMed]
33. International Association for Cereal Science and Technology. *ICC Standard Methods*; Methods No. 104/1, 105/2, 110/1, 115/1, 131, 136; ICC: Vienna, Austria, 2003.
34. Lee, S.C.; Prosky, L.; DeVries, J.W. Determination of total, soluble and insoluble, dietary fibre in foods, enzymatic-gravimetric method, MES-TRIS buffer: Collaborative study. *J. Assoc. Off. Anal. Chem.* **1992**, *75*, 395–416.
35. AACC. *International Approved Methods of Analysis*, 11th ed.; Method 10-05.01 "Guidelines for Measurement of Volume by Rapeseed Displacement" and Method 32-40.01 "Resistant Starch in Starch Samples and Plant Materials"; AACC International: St. Paul, MN, USA, 2009.
36. Spackman, D.K.; Stein, W.H.; Moore, S. Chromatography of amino acids on sulfonated polystyrene resin: An improved system. *Anal. Chem.* **1958**, *30*, 1190–1196. [CrossRef]
37. Singleton, V.L.; Orthofer, R.; Lamuela-Raventós, R.M. Analysis of total phenols and other oxidation substrates and antioxidants by means of Folin-Ciocalteu reagent. *Methods Enzymol.* **1999**, *299*, 152–178.
38. Reeves, P.G. Components of the AIN-93 diets as improvements in the AIN-76A diet. *J. Nutr.* **1997**, *127*, 838S–841S. [CrossRef] [PubMed]
39. Hammer, Ø.; Harper, D.A.T.; Ryan, P.D. PAST: Paleontological Statistics Software Package for Education and Data Analysis. *Palaeontol. Electron.* **2001**, *4*, 1–9.
40. Boye, J.; Zare, F.; Pletch, A. Pulse proteins: Processing, characterization, functional properties and applications in food and feed. *Food Res. Int.* **2010**, *43*, 414–431. [CrossRef]
41. Joshi, M.; Aldred, P.; Panozzo, J.F.; Kasapis, S.; Adhikari, B. Rheological and microstructural characteristics of lentil starch-lentil protein composite pastes and gels. *Food Hydrocoll.* **2014**, *35*, 226–237. [CrossRef]
42. Earnshaw, S.R.; McDade, C.L.; Chu, Y.; Fleige, L.E.; Sievenpiper, J.L. Cost-effectiveness of maintaining daily intake of oat β-glucan for coronary heart disease primary prevention. *Clin. Ther.* **2017**, *39*, 804–818. [CrossRef]
43. Roudi, R.; Mohammadi, S.R.; Roudbary, M.; Mohsenzadegan, M. Lung cancer and β-glucans: Review of potential therapeutic applications. *Investig. New Drugs* **2017**, *35*, 509–517. [CrossRef]

44. Pérez-Jiménez, J.; Torres, J.L. Analysis of nonextractable phenolic compounds in foods: The current state of the art. *J. Agric. Food Chem.* **2011**, *59*, 12713–12724. [CrossRef] [PubMed]
45. Carcea, M.; Narducci, V.; Turfani, V.; Giannini, V. Polyphenols in raw and cooked cereals/pseudocereals/legume pasta and couscous. *Foods* **2017**, *6*, 80. [CrossRef] [PubMed]
46. Vitaglione, P.; Napolitano, A.; Fogliano, V. Cereal dietary fibre: A natural functional ingredient to deliver phenolic compounds into the gut. *Trends Food Sci. Technol.* **2008**, *19*, 451–463. [CrossRef]
47. Milder, I.E.; Arts, I.C.; van de Putte, B.; Venema, D.P.; Hollman, P.C.H. Lignan contents of Dutch plants foods: A database inscluding lariciresinol, pinoresinol, secoisolariciresinol and matairesinol. *Br. J. Nutr.* **2005**, *93*, 393–402. [CrossRef]
48. Adlercreutz, H. Lignans and human health. *Crit. Rev. Clin. Lab. Sci.* **2007**, *44*, 483–525. [CrossRef]
49. During, A.; Debouche, C.; Raas, T.; Larondelle, Y. Among plant lignans, pinoresinol has the strongest anti-inflammatory properties in human intestinal Caco-2 cells. *J. Nutr.* **2012**, *142*, 1798–1805. [CrossRef]
50. Dong, S.F.; Chen, J.M.; Zhang, W.; Sun, S.H.; Wang, J.; Gu, J.X.; Boraschi, D.; Qu, D. Specific immune response to HBsAg is enhanced by beta-glucan oligosaccharide containing an alpha-(1–>3)-linked bond and biased towards M2/Th2. *Int. Immunopharmacol.* **2007**, *7*, 725–733. [CrossRef]
51. Bobadilla, F.; Rodriguez-Tirado, C.; Imarai, M.; Galotto, M.J.; Andersson, R. Soluble β-1,3/1,6-glucan in seaweed from the southern hemisphere and its immunomodulatory effect. *Carbohydr. Polym.* **2013**, *92*, 241–248. [CrossRef]
52. Min, H.; Montecino-Rodriguez, E.; Dorshkind, K. Effects of aging on early B-and T-cell development. *Immunol. Rev.* **2005**, *205*, 7–17. [CrossRef]
53. Riley, R.L.; Blomberg, B.B.; Frasca, D. B cells, E2A, and aging. *Immunol. Rev.* **2005**, *205*, 30–47. [CrossRef]
54. Gollapudi, S.; Gupta, S. Reversal of oxidative stress-induced apoptosis in T and B lymphocytes by Coenzyme Q10 (CoQ10). *Am. J. Clin. Exp. Immunol.* **2016**, *5*, 41–47. [PubMed]
55. Xiao, P.; Huang, H.; Chen, J.; Li, X. In vitro antioxidant and anti-inflammatory activities of Radix Isatidis extract and bioaccessibility of six bioactive compounds after simulated gastro-intestinal digestion. *J. Ethnopharmacol.* **2014**, *157*, 55–61. [CrossRef] [PubMed]
56. Gao, S.; Shu, S.; Wang, L.; Zhou, J.; Yuan, Z. Pro-inflammatory and anti-inflammatory cytokine responses of peripheral blood mononuclear cells in apparently healthy subjects. *Nan Fang Yi Ke Da Xue Xue Bao* **2014**, *34*, 1589–1593. [PubMed]
57. Măluţan, A.M.; Drugan, T.; Ciortea, R.; Mocan-Hognogi, R.F.; Bucuri, C.; Rada, M.; Mihu, D. Serum anti-inflammatory cytokines for the evaluation of inflammatory status in endometriosis. *J. Res. Med. Sci.* **2015**, *20*, 668–674. [PubMed]
58. Teimourian, M.; Jafaraian, Z.; Hosseini, S.R.; Rahmani, M.; Bagherzadeh, M.; Aghamajidi, A.; Bijani, A.; Nooreddini, H.; Mostafazadeh, A. Both immune hormone IL-10 and parathormone tend to increase in serum of old osteoporotic people independently of 1, 25 dihydroxy vitamin D3. *Casp. J. Intern. Med.* **2016**, *7*, 283–289.
59. Langmann, G.A.; Perera, S.; Ferchak, M.A.; Nace, D.A.; Resnick, N.M.; Greenspan, S.L. Inflammatory Markers and Frailty in Long-Term Care Residents. *J. Am. Geriatr. Soc.* **2017**, *65*, 1777–1783. [CrossRef]

14

Use of Sourdough in Low FODMAP Baking

Jussi Loponen [1] and Michael G. Gänzle [2,*]

[1] Fazer Group, 01230 Vantaa, Finland; jussi.loponen@fazer.com
[2] Department of Agricultural, Food and Nutritional Science, University of Alberta, Edmonton, AB T6G 2P5, Canada
[*] Correspondence: mgaenzle@ualberta.ca

Abstract: A low FODMAP (fermentable oligosaccharides, disaccharides, monosaccharides, and polyols) diet allows most irritable bowel syndrome (IBS) patients to manage their gastrointestinal symptoms by avoiding FODMAP-containing foods, such as onions, pulses, and products made from wheat or rye. The downside of a low FODMAP diet is the reduced intake of dietary fiber. Applying sourdoughs—with specific FODMAP-targeting metabolic properties—to wholegrain bread making can help to remarkably reduce the content of FODMAPs in bread without affecting the content of the slowly fermented and well-tolerated dietary fiber. In this review, we outline the metabolism of FODMAPs in conventional sourdoughs and outline concepts related to fructan and mannitol metabolism that allow development of low FODMAP sourdough bread. We also summarize clinical studies where low FODMAP but high fiber, rye sourdough bread was tested for its effects on gut fermentation and gastrointestinal symptoms with very promising results. The sourdough bread-making process offers a means to develop natural and fiber-rich low FODMAP bakery products for IBS patients and thereby help them to increase their dietary fiber intake.

Keywords: sourdough; FODMAP; fructan; mannitol; lactobacilli; irritable bowel syndrome (IBS); non-celiac wheat intolerance

---

1. Introduction

Fermentable oligosaccharides, disaccharides, monosaccharides, and polyols (FODMAPs) have beneficial and adverse health effects [1]. Oligosaccharides that are not hydrolyzed and absorbed in the small intestine are rapidly fermented by intestinal microbiota in the terminal ileum and the proximal colon [2,3]. Diverse FODMAPs that are fermented by intestinal microbiota consistently cause adverse symptoms when a dose of about 0.3 g/kg body weight, corresponding to about 15 g/day, is exceeded [4,5]. Adverse symptoms include osmotic diarrhea, intestinal distension, and bloating [5,6]. The extent of the adverse symptoms decreases with the degree of polymerization because of the reduced osmotic load of oligosaccharides in the small intestine, and the reduced rate of fermentation [6]. Adverse effects are not described for non-digestible polysaccharides, which are fermented at a much lower rate [7]. Microbiota in the terminal ileum include proteobacteria and lactic acid bacteria as the dominant representatives; ileal microbiota effectively ferment mono- and disaccharides but typically lack extracellular enzymes for hydrolysis of higher oligosaccharides and polysaccharides [6]. The sensitivity of individuals to adverse symptoms caused by FODMAPs is highly variable; adverse symptoms are often linked to irritable bowel syndrome (IBS). The sensitivity to gas pressure and pain varies highly among individuals; moreover, intestinal microbiota adapt toward the fermentation of specific oligosaccharides; this adaptation reduces or eliminates adverse symptoms [8]. Many FODMAPs are conditionally digestible depending on the genetic status of the host. About 35% of humans are lactase-persistent and digest lactose while lactose is a non-digestible FODMAP in the remainder of the population [9]. A substantial proportion of humans are fructose intolerant; the proportion of fructose intolerant individuals among patients with IBS was reported to be over 60% [10,11]. Fructose absorption is highly dependent on the presence of equimolar amounts of glucose as uptake from the small intestine uses the same transport channels [10]. A rare variation in the sucrose-isomaltase gene reduces the digestibility of sucrose, including sucrose in the FODMAPs; this genetic variant also predisposes for IBS [12].

Health beneficial or prebiotic effects of oligosaccharides relate to the bacterial conversion of oligosaccharides to short chain fatty acids [1,13]. These short chain fatty acids increase the energy harvest from carbohydrates that escape small intestinal hydrolysis and absorption, improve intestinal barrier properties and resistance to enteric infections, and exert systemic effects related to inflammation, cognitive functions, and behavior through specific recognition with G-protein coupled receptors (for reviews, see [1,7,13]). Of note, oligomeric fructans, for which health beneficial prebiotic effects were most consistently demonstrated [13], appear also of particular concern for adverse effects in IBS [6]. Adverse and beneficial effects of FODMAPs are thus interconnected and partially related to the same mechanisms, bacterial fermentation. Consequently, a reduction of adverse symptoms in IBS by a low FODMAP diet also increased the luminal pH and reduced the abundance of bifidobacteria and butyrate-producing colonic bacteria [14,15]. While the term FODMAPs indiscriminately includes all oligosaccharides, different compounds were reported to have divergent effects. Supplementation of a low FODMAP diet with β-galacto-oligosaccharides was reported to improve IBS symptoms relative to a low FODMAP diet [16]. In other words, replacement of FODMAPs with different categories of FODMAPs may improve symptoms of IBS without the adverse consequences of a low fiber diet [1].

Wheat and rye are major contributors to the dietary intake of low molecular weight fructans [17] but whole grain products also are major contributors to the intake of dietary fiber [7]. Fermentation processes during baking may allow conversion or degradation of FODMAPs without reducing the overall dietary fiber content of bread [18]. This review aims to summarize current knowledge on the use of conventional and sourdough baking in the production of low FODMAP bread.

2. FODMAPs as Contributors to Non-Celiac Wheat Sensitivity?

Non-celiac wheat sensitivity refers to syndromes where components of wheat cause intestinal symptoms. Triggers and mechanisms of the syndrome are poorly described; non-celiac wheat sensitivity is often self-diagnosed or assessed after exclusion of celiac disease and wheat allergy [19,20]. Non-celiac wheat sensitivity overlaps significantly with IBS [20]. Non-celiac wheat sensitivity has also been described as non-gluten wheat sensitivity since gluten apparently is not a major trigger in these symptoms [21]. While a contribution of FODMAPs to symptoms in IBS is increasingly supported by clinical trials, their role in non-celiac wheat sensitivity is not as well documented. FODMAPs and amylase trypsin inhibitors (ATIs) were suggested as likely non-gluten triggers of these symptoms [19,20]. It is likely that *Triticeae* cereals other than wheat, such as rye and barley, are also potential triggers of wheat sensitivity because they also contain fructans and ATIs.

3. FODMAPs in Cereals and FODMAP Metabolism in Conventional Sourdoughs

Resting grains of wheat and rye contain only low levels of monosaccharides; the major oligosaccharides are sucrose, raffinose, and fructans (Table 1). During sourdough fermentation, amylase and glucoamylase activities of wheat and rye flour release maltose and glucose, respectively, from damaged starch [18]. The fructans of cereal grains are graminan-type fructans, which are oligosaccharides built of mixed-linkage fructose units [22]. Fructans in wheat and rye are concentrated in the outer layers of the grain and have an average degree of polymerization (DP) of 5–6; 1-kestose and nystose account for only a minor proportion of the overall fructans (Table 1) [23]. Additional non-starch polysaccharides include arabinoxylans and β-glucans as the major components, polysaccharides composed of mannose, galactose, and galacturonic acid, and trace amounts of pectin (Table 1). In addition to polysaccharides and FODMAPs that are present in the grain, polysaccharides, oligosaccharides, and polyols can be produced by bacterial activity during sourdough fermentation.

An overview of the conversion and production of FODMAPs in sourdough fermentation is provided in Figure 1.

During bread making, the fructans undergo partial degradation due to invertase activity present in yeast. The remaining fructan has a lower DP than the native fructan of flour. Low molecular weight fructans may be under-estimated when analyzing fructan in dough; in addition, they are fermented more rapidly than fructans with a higher molecular weight. The fate of fructans is valid for sourdough fermentation, i.e., grain fructans degrade to some extent but in the case of sourdough, the released fructose is also partially converted to mannitol by sourdough lactobacilli. Mannitol is a polyol that is rapidly fermented by gut microbiota. Thus, for accurate FODMAP quantification, mannitol levels in sourdough breads should also be determined. In the following sections, we outline the carbohydrate metabolism in sourdoughs. This is relevant to understand when the focus is in changes of FODMAPs in sourdough bread making.

Table 1. Content of oligosaccharides and non-starch polysaccharides (%) in wheat and rye grains.

Saccharide	Wheat	Rye
Arabinoxylans	6–7	7–12
β-Glucans including lignified cellulose	0.3–3	2–3
Pectin	trace	trace
Mannans, galactans, and galacturonans	1–1.5	n.d.
Fructans	1–2	4.3–5
1-Kestose	0.1	0.3
Nystose	0.03	0.1
Sucrose	0.6–1.0	1.2–1.8
Maltose	trace	trace
Raffinose	0.2–0.7	0.1–0.7
Stachyose	trace	trace

Compiled with information from [17,23–31]; n.d., not determined.

In straight dough processes, the dough is fermented with baker's yeast as the sole fermentation organism; the addition of high cell counts of *S. cerevisiae*, 1–2% biomass corresponding to about 10^8 cfu/g, achieves leavening after a fermentation time of 2 h or less. In sourdough baking, lactic acid bacteria are used as the second group of organisms; moreover, part of the flour is fermented for an extended period of time. The inclusion of lactic acid bacteria extends the metabolic capacity of the fermentation microbiota; the extended fermentation time strongly enhances the contribution of flour enzymes to the conversion and degradation of dough components [18]. Type I sourdoughs are typically fermented between 15 and 30 °C and they have traditionally been used as the sole leavening agent in bread making. To ensure a sufficient metabolic activity and leavening capacity, type I sourdoughs are propagated through one to three fermentation steps prior to mixing the bread dough [27,32]. Fermentation procedures that use sourdough as the sole leavening agent typically result in ~10% of the flour being fermented for >12 h, 20–30% fermented for >6 h, and all of the flour fermented for 2–3 h, i.e., the time required for dough rest and proofing [33,34]. Fermentation organisms in type I sourdoughs generally include *Lactobacillus sanfranciscensis* and *Kazachstania humilis* (syn. *Candida milleri*) and *S. cerevisiae* or *S. exiguus*. Lactobacilli of the *L. brevis*, *L. plantarum*, and *L. reuteri* groups are also represented in type I sourdoughs [32,35]. Industrial bread production generally includes baker's yeast as the leavening agent; sourdough fermentations in industrial baking (type I or II sourdoughs) aim at dough acidification to improve the baking quality of rye flour, at supporting the leavening capacity of baker's yeast, and as baking improver [32–34]. Fermentation conditions depend on the technological aim of the fermentation and are often specific for a specific production site; typically, 5–20% of the flour is fermented for >12 h while the remainder of the flour is fermented for ~2 h, corresponding to dough rest, shaping, and proofing [33,34]. Type II sourdough fermentation takes place at around 40 °C and the microbiota typically comprise organisms of the *L. delbrueckii* group (e.g., *L. amylovorans* and *L. johnsonii*) and organisms of the *L. reuteri* group (e.g., *L. reuteri, L. pontis,* and *L. panis*) [32,36]. Sourdough microbiota are metabolically active if the sourdough is fermented at the bakery but inactivated if the sourdough is stabilized by drying or pasteurization prior to use in baking [34].

Sucrose is metabolized rapidly by invertase activity of *S. cerevisiae*. Yeast invertase is an extracellular or cell wall-bound enzyme and is secreted in excess of the yeast's capacity to ferment the hydrolysis products [37]. Sucrose metabolism in lactic acid bacteria is mediated by sucrose phosphorylase or sucrose-1-phosphate hydrolase [38]. Sucrose metabolism and the metabolism of other oligosaccharides in homofermentative lactic acid bacteria is repressed by glucose [39]; in contrast, sucrose conversion in heterofermentative lactic acid bacteria is induced by the substrate but not repressed by glucose [40,41]. Fructose is utilized as a carbon source by homofermentative lactic acid bacteria but used as an electron acceptor for the regeneration of reduced cofactors by most heterofermentative lactobacilli [41,42]. Sourdough lactic acid bacteria also harbor extracellular glucansucrases or fructansucrases, which convert sucrose to indigestible poly- and oligosaccharides. These enzymes are frequently present in *Leuconostoc* spp., *Weissella* spp., and species of the *L. reuteri* and *L. delbrueckii* groups but are also present in other lactobacilli including *L. sanfranciscensis* [43,44]. Glucansucrases convert sucrose to polymeric glucans, isomalto-oligosaccharides, and fructose; fructansucrases catalyze the conversion to levan or inulin, fructo-oligosaccharides, and glucose [44]. Sucrose conversion by glucansucrases and fructansucrases accumulated isomalto-oligosaccharides and fructo-oligosaccharides, respectively, in wheat and sorghum sourdoughs; however, accumulation of oligosaccharides to relevant concentrations is observed only when sucrose is added to the sourdough [45,46]. Glucansucrases and the hydrolase activity of fructansucrases generally also release fructose, which is converted to the polyol mannitol by heterofermentative lactic acid bacteria [41,43]. In traditional sourdough fermentations, mannitol accumulates to 10–20 mmol/kg in wheat and 50 mmol/kg in rye, corresponding to 0.2–0.4% and 0.9%, respectively; the mannitol concentration is increased in direct proportion to the sucrose addition to sourdoughs [47]. *Weissella* spp. are exceptional because the majority of strains do not produce mannitol from fructose [45].

Lactic acid bacteria metabolize raffinose by sequential activity of extracellular levansucrase to convert raffinose to melibiose and fructose or fructan, followed by melibiose transport and intracellular hydrolysis by α-galactosidase. An alternative pathway involves raffinose transport and sequential hydrolysis by intracellular α-galactosidase to convert raffinose to sucrose and galactose and sucrose phosphorylase [48]. Metabolism by extracellular levansucrase with intracellular α-galactosidase is faster than the alternate pathway using two intracellular enzymes, presumably because the disaccharide melibiose is transported faster than raffinose [48]. Raffinose metabolism in heterofermentative lactobacilli is not subject to carbon catabolite repression [49] and the relatively high concentrations of raffinose and raffinose level oligosaccharides in pulse flours are rapidly degraded during fermentation [48]. Type I sourdough microbiota and most strains of *S. cerevisiae* are raffinose negative. Nevertheless, levansucrase from *L. sanfranciscensis* and/or yeast invertase converts raffinose to fructose and melibiose [43,50].

The content of fructans is reduced in straight dough processing to 1–1.5% fructans in wheat bread and about 3% in rye bread [51]. Fructans are not degraded in simulated sourdoughs without microbial activity but invertase activity of *S. cerevisiae* and *Kazachstania humilis* results in partial hydrolysis of flour fructans [52,53]. In a straight dough process, the rate of fructan hydrolysis decreases in the order trisaccharides > tetrasaccharides > pentasaccharides and only a small proportion of higher fructans are degraded [54]. Hydrolysis of fructans is mediated by yeast. However, dimerization of the enzyme reduces the activity towards kestose and nystose and sterically prevents access of oligosaccharides with a DP of more than four to the catalytic site [55]. Metabolism of fructans in lactobacilli is mediated by oligosaccharide transport through the ATP-Bbinding-Cassette transporter MsmEFGK or the phosphotransferase (PTS) system PTS1Bca, followed by hydrolysis through intracellular fructosidases or phospho-fructosidases, respectively [38]. Oligosaccharide transport by MsmEFGK and PTS1BCA is limited to fructans with a DP of four or less [56,57]. Metabolic enzymes for fructo-oligosaccharide (FOS) catabolism are frequent in homofermentative lactobacilli where FOS degradation is repressed by glucose [58] but are very infrequently found in heterofermentative lactobacilli [38,43,49]. Intracellular metabolism of FOS by lactobacilli thus does not contribute to the degradation of fructans in wheat or rye sourdoughs.

In summary, conventional dough fermentations, including sourdough fermentations, result in decreased levels of FODMAPs but may generate FODMAPs from the digestible carbohydrates sucrose and fructose (Figure 1). Low FODMAP baking thus necessitates dedicated approaches, particularly involving fructan- and mannitol-degrading organisms.

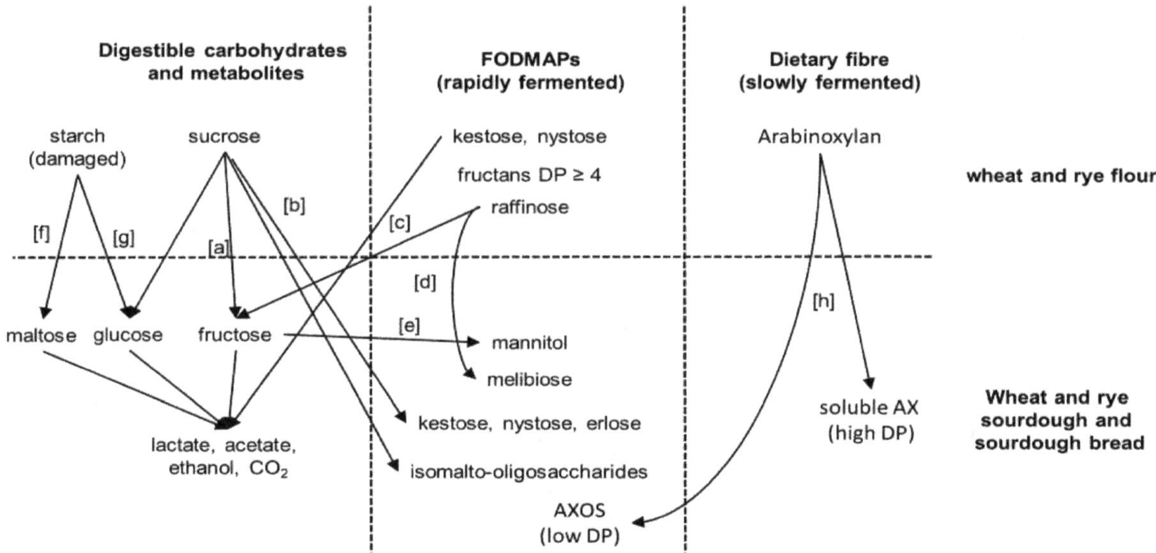

Figure 1. Conversion and generation of fermentable oligosaccharides, disaccharides, monosaccharides, and polyols (FODMAPs) in wheat and rye sourdoughs. Sucrose hydrolysis by yeast invertase or fructosidases of lactic acid bacteria [a]. Oligosaccharide formation by glucansucrases to form isomalto-oligosaccharides, or by fructansucrases to form kestose, nystose, and erlose from sucrose [b]. Kestose and nystose degradation by yeast invertase or by intracellular (phospho)-fructosidases of lactic acid bacteria [c]. Raffinose conversion by yeast invertase and levansucrase from lactic acid bacteria [d]. Fructose conversion by mannitol-dehydrogenase from heterofermentative lactic acid bacteria [e]. Starch conversion to maltose and glucose by flour amylases and gluco-amylase [f,g]. Exogenous xylanases are used in baking to increase the amount of soluble pentosane (arabinoxylan, AX) to improve bread properties, which can produce low DP arabinoxylan oligosaccharides (AXOS) along soluble high-DP arabinoxylan fragments [h].

4. Concepts for Low FODMAP Sourdough Baking

Degradation of fructans with a DP of more than four requires extracellular fructanases. Baker's yeast *S. cerevisiae* does not express extracellular fructanase. However, *Kluyveromyces marxianus* was suggested as an alternative leavening agent with extracellular fructanase activity [53,59]. *K. marxianus* is maltose negative and most strains do not provide sufficient CO_2 production for dough leavening; the use of *K. marxianus* in low FODMAP baking thus requires co-culture with *S. cerevisiae* [53] or selection of *K. marxianus* strains with sufficient leavening power and addition of amyloglucosidase to provide glucose for *K. marxianus* metabolism [53,59]. Dough fermentation with *K. marxianus* alone or in co-culture with *S. cerevisiae* allowed production of experimental breads with a low fructan content and a volume and sensory properties matching those of experimental breads produced with baker's yeast [53,59].

Extracellular glycosyl hydrolases are exceptional in lactobacilli [38]; accordingly, only a few strains with extracellular fructanase activity have been characterized (Figure 2). The extracellular

GH32 β-fructanase FosE was characterized in *L. paracasei* [60]. FosE is an extracellular enzyme that is induced by fructose, sucrose, or inulin but repressed by glucose [60]. BLAST analysis frequently identified homologues of this enzyme in other strains of the *L. casei* group and in few strains of the *L. salivarius* group (Figure 2 and data not shown). The β-fructanase FruA of *Streptococcus mutans* is extracellular with an LPXTG cell wall anchor; the enzyme has less than 40% amino acid identity to FosE ([61] Figure 2). FruA of *S. mutans* plays a critical role in fructan degradation and the virulence of oral streptococci; BLAST analysis frequently identified homologues of FruA in other streptococci (Figure 2). Only five of the more than 1500 genome sequences assigned to the genus *Lactobacillus* harbors FruA homologues; this low frequency suggests that this β-fructanase is not necessary for the lifestyle of lactobacilli but only infrequently acquired by lateral gene transfer. Two of the species with FruA activity, *L. amylovorus* and *L. crispatus*, match species that are typically found in type II sourdoughs.

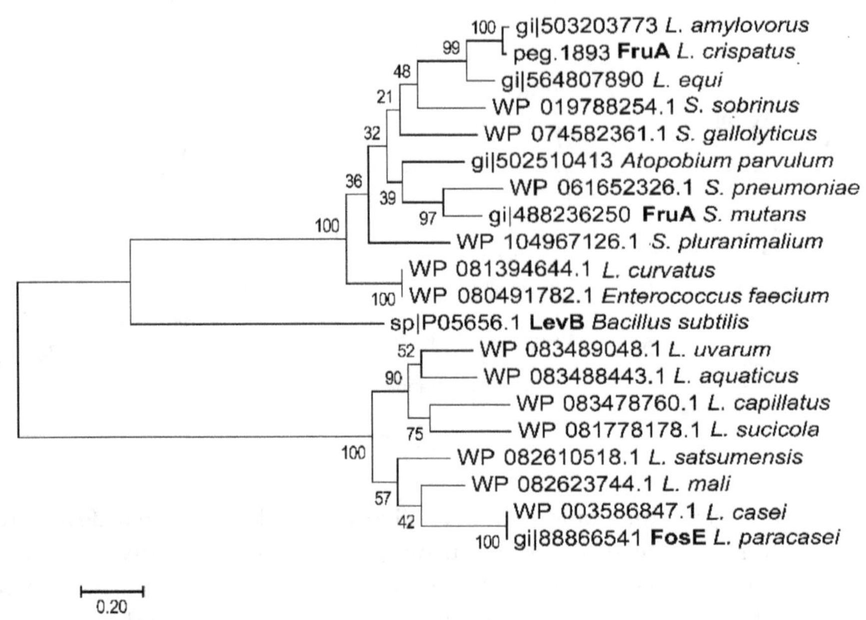

Figure 2. Molecular phylogenetic analysis of extracellular fructanases in lactic acid bacteria by the Maximum Likelihood method. The evolutionary history was inferred by using the Maximum Likelihood method; the tree is drawn to scale with branch lengths measured in the number of substitutions per site. Evolutionary analyses were conducted in MEGA7. Sequences were retrieved by NCBI Blast using the fructanase of *L. crispatus* [62] and the inulinase of *L. paracasei* [60] as query sequence. Sequences from lactic acid bacteria (*Lactobacillales*) with a more than 80% coverage and more than 50% amino acid identity were retrieved and aligned by ClustalW in MEGA 7.0. A levanase of *Bacillus subtilis* was included for comparison. Only one representative sequence for each bacterial species was chosen; sequences of 15 *Streptococcus* spp. which were all similar to sequences of other streptococci were omitted from the tree. The two *Lactobacillus* enzymes that were characterized biochemically are printed in bold.

Type I and type II sourdough microbiota generally include heterofermentative lactobacilli that convert fructose to mannitol. Degradation of mannitol in low FODMAP baking therefore requires mannitol-fermenting lactobacilli. Mannitol metabolism in lactobacilli is mediated by a mannitol-specific PTS system, followed by conversion by mannitol-1-phosphate-dehydrogenase to fructose-1-phospyate [63]. Enzymes for mannitol conversion are present in homofermentative lactobacilli of the *L. delbrueckii*, *L. casei*, *L. plantarum* and *L. salivarius* groups, likely representing trophic relationships with heterofermentative lactobacilli. In analogy to other PTS systems in lactobacilli, mannitol metabolism in homofermentative lactobacilli is repressed by glucose [39,41,58].

Glucose and maltose levels in wheat and rye sourdoughs and consequently carbon catabolite repression in homofermentative lactobacilli and yeasts [38,41] are determined by the level of damaged starch and the β-amylase and amyloglucosidase activity in flour (Figure 1; [18,64]). If enzyme activity and the level of damaged starch in flour are low, sucrose, raffinose, and fructans become the most readily available carbohydrates [64]. The composition of the microbiota in rye sourdoughs that are low in damaged starch match the composition in other type II sourdoughs with organisms of the *L. delbrueckii* group including *L. crispatus*, *L. amylovorus*, and *L. ultuensis*, and organisms of the *L. reuteri* group including *L. frumentii* and *L. pontis* as the dominant members [32,35,65]. The restricted availability of maltose and glucose, however, selects for strains expressing an exceptional fructanase (Figure 2, [62,65]). The prevailing enzyme activity is an extracellular exofructanase (Figure 2), which exhibits more than 80% of the maximum activity in the pH range of 4–6 and the temperature range of 30–60 °C [62]. Fructan hydrolysis in sourdough releases fructose that is partially converted to mannitol by *L. reuteri* group organisms (Figure 3). However, the restriction of carbohydrate sources also allows for mannitol conversion after fructans are completely consumed (Figure 3) and results in a virtually zero FODMAP sourdough. The use of this zero FODMAP sourdough in low FODMAP rye bread making involves the addition of unfermented rye flour, which is fermented for only a short time [65]. Nevertheless, the choice of appropriate raw materials and the use of FruA-positive and mannitol-fermenting lactobacilli allows fructan degradation in rye and rye sourdoughs for the production of bread with a low content of fructans and mannitol but a comparable fiber content when compared to regular bread [66–68].

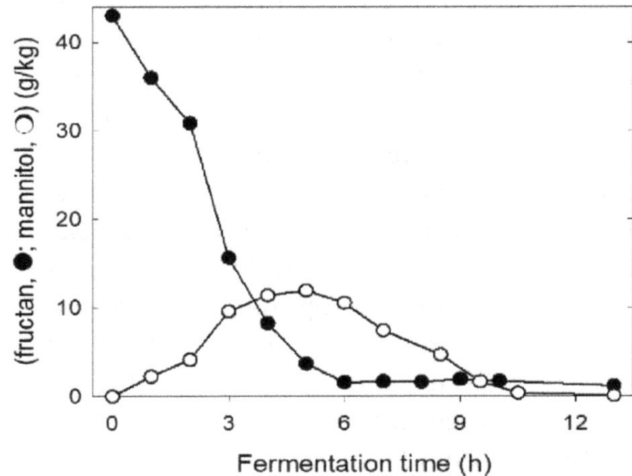

Figure 3. Degradation of fructans (black) and the formation and degradation of mannitol (white) in a type II rye sourdough. Sourdough microbiota consist of fructan-degrading strains of the *L. delbrueckii* group and heterofermentative strains of the *L. reuteri* group, which convert fructose to mannitol. Drawn with data from [65].

5. Proof of Concept from Clinical Trials with Low FODMAP Rye Bread

Two clinical trials done with IBS patients verified that low FODMAP rye bread made by using the above described zero FODMAP sourdough influences the gastrointestinal symptoms and the extent of gas production generated in intestinal fermentation. In the first study in a randomized double-blind controlled crossover study, it was shown that low FODMAP rye bread caused less flatulence, less abdominal pain, fewer cramps, and less stomach rumbling than regular rye bread [66]. Of note, the low FODMAP bread retained a high dietary fiber content (10 g/100 g) although the FODMAP levels were lowered to one third [66]. Including the low FODMAP rye bread thus also increased the dietary fiber intake to the recommended level in IBS patients, avoiding drawbacks of the other low FODMAP diets [15]. A second randomized double-blind controlled crossover study evaluated the amount of breath hydrogen levels after consuming low FODMAP rye bread or regular rye bread [68]. Low FODMAP rye bread reduced the generation of hydrogen by colonic fermentation [68]. This study showed that significant differences between bread types may occur in their postprandial effects.

6. Conclusions and Future Directions

Conventional sourdough baking reduces and converts FODMAPs in rye and wheat flour; however, the extent of FODMAP reduction is dependent on the fermentation organisms, the fermentation process, the grain raw material, and the sourdough dosage to the final bread dough. The production of low FODMAP bread requires extracellular fructanase activity; sourdough fermentation with lactobacilli expressing fructanases or the use of fructanase-positive yeasts provide wheat or rye breads with a low FODMAP content. Low FODMAP bread can help to restrict the intake of FODMAPs but at the same time increase the intake of slowly fermentable dietary fiber in IBS patients. High fiber/low FODMAP bread likely prevents the depletion of intestinal bifidobacteria that has been observed on other low FODMAP diets [14,15] and shows promise in reducing symptoms of IBS.

Anecdotal evidence links sourdough bread to improved tolerance of wheat in individuals with non-celiac wheat sensitivities [69]. In addition to the degradation of FODMAPs during sourdough fermentation, reduction and degradation of wheat amylase trypsin inhibitors may improve wheat tolerance in some individuals [67]. Amylase trypsin inhibitors are suggested to play a role in intestinal and extra-intestinal symptoms as they induce inflammatory reactions [70]. Amylase trypsin inhibitors are highly disulfide-bonded proteins; reduction of disulfide bonds reduces bioactivity and accelerates proteolytic digestion. Sourdough fermentation generates reducing conditions and supports reduction and hydrolysis of highly disulfide-bonded proteins that resist digestion in unfermented dough [71]. A pilot trial recruiting IBS patients with non-celiac wheat sensitivity, however, showed no improvement of intestinal symptoms after consuming sourdough wheat bread compared with industrial wheat bread [67]. Difficulties in identifying the protective effects of sourdough fermentation in non-celiac wheat intolerance relate to the poorly identified and likely multifactorial triggers of (self-diagnosed) non-celiac wheat sensitivity, and the inherent difficulties in blinding consumption of wheat or wheat sourdough products in clinical trials [67]. Despite the lack of support from clinical trials, sourdough-derived solutions likely play a significant role when developing healthier bakery products for people with non-gluten wheat sensitivities.

Author Contributions: Conceptualization, writing and editing: M.G.G. and J.L.

References

1. Yan, Y.L.; Hu, Y.; Gänzle, M.G. Prebiotics, FODMAPs and dietary fibre–conflicting concepts in development of functional food products? *Curr. Opin. Food Sci.* **2018**, *20*, 30–37. [CrossRef]
2. Booijink, C.C.; El-Aidy, S.; Rajilić-Stojanović, M.; Heilig, H.G.; Troost, F.J.; Smidt, H.; Kleerebezem, M.; De Vos, W.M.; Zoetendal, E.G. High temporal and inter-individual variation detected in the human ileal microbiota. *Environ. Microbiol.* **2010**, *12*, 3213–3227. [CrossRef] [PubMed]
3. Zoetendal, E.G.; Raes, J.; van den Bogert, B.; Arumugam, M.; Booijink, C.C.; Troost, F.J.; Bork, P.; Wels, M.; de Vos, W.M.; Kleerebezem, M. The human small intestinal microbiota is driven by rapid uptake and conversion of simple carbohydrates. *ISME J.* **2012**, *6*, 1415–1426. [CrossRef] [PubMed]
4. Oku, T.; Nakamura, S. Digestion, absorption, fermentation, and metabolism of functional sugar substitutes and their available energy. *Pure Appl. Chem.* **2002**, *7*, 1253–1261. [CrossRef]
5. Oku, T.; Nakamura, S. Threshold for transitory diarrhea induced by ingestion of xylitol and lactitol in young male and female adults. *J. Nutr. Sci. Vitaminol. (Tokyo)* **2007**, *53*, 13–20. [CrossRef] [PubMed]

6. Murray, K.; Wilkinson-Smith, V.; Hoad, C.; Costigan, C.; Cox, E.; Lam, C.; Marciani, L.; Gowland, P.; Spiller, R.C. Differential effects of FODMAPs (fermentable oligo-, di-, mono-saccharides and polyols) on small and large intestinal contents in healthy subjects shown by MRI. *Am. J. Gastroenterol.* **2014**, *109*, 110–119. [CrossRef] [PubMed]
7. Hamaker, B.R.; Tuncil, Y.E. A perspective on the complexity of dietary fiber structures and their potential effect on the gut microbiota. *J. Mol. Biol.* **2014**, *426*, 3838–3850. [CrossRef] [PubMed]
8. Azcarate-Peril, M.A.; Ritter, A.J.; Savaiano, D.; Monteagudo-Mera, A.; Anderson, C.; Magness, S.T.; Klaenhammer, T.R. Impact of short-chain galactooligosaccharides on the gut microbiome of lactose-intolerant individuals. *Proc. Natl. Acad. Sci. USA* **2017**, *114*, E367–E375. [CrossRef] [PubMed]
9. Gerbault, P.; Liebert, A.; Itan, Y.; Powell, A.; Currat, M.; Burger, J.; Swallow, D.M.; Thomas, M.G. Evolution of lactase persistence: An example of human niche construction. *Philos. Trans. R. Soc. Lond. B Biol. Sci.* **2011**, *366*, 863–877. [CrossRef] [PubMed]
10. Latulippe, M.E.; Skoog, S.M. Fructose malabsorption and intolerance: Effects of fructose with and without simultaneous glucose ingestion. *Crit. Rev. Food Sci. Nutr.* **2011**, *51*, 583–592. [CrossRef] [PubMed]
11. Wilder-Smith, C.H.; Materna, A.; Wermelinger, C.; Schuler, J. Fructose and lactose intolerance and malabsorption testing: The relationship with symptoms in functional gastrointestinal disorders. *Aliment. Pharmacol. Ther.* **2013**, *37*, 1074–1183. [CrossRef] [PubMed]
12. Henström, M.; Diekmann, L.; Bonfiglio, F.; Hadizadeh, F.; Kuech, E.M.; von Köckritz-Blickwede, M.; Thingholm, L.B.; Zheng, T.; Assadi, G.; Dierks, C.; et al. Functional variants in the sucrase-isomaltase gene associate with increased risk of irritable bowel syndrome. *Gut* **2018**, *67*, 263–270. [CrossRef] [PubMed]
13. Bindels, L.B.; Delzenne, N.M.; Cani, P.D.; Walter, J. Towards a more comprehensive concept for prebiotics. *Nat. Rev. Gastroenterol. Hepatol.* **2015**, *12*, 303–310. [CrossRef] [PubMed]
14. Halmos, E.P.; Christophersen, C.T.; Bird, A.R.; Shepherd, S.J.; Gibson, P.R.; Muir, J.G. Diets that differ in their FODMAP content alter the colonic luminal microenvironment. *Gut* **2015**, *64*, 93–100. [CrossRef] [PubMed]
15. Staudacher, H.M.; Lomer, M.C.; Anderson, J.L.; Barrett, J.S.; Muir, J.G.; Irving, P.M.; Whelan, K. Fermentable carbohydrate restriction reduces luminal bifidobacteria and gastrointestinal symptoms in patients with irritable bowel syndrome. *J. Nutr.* **2012**, *142*, 1510–1518. [CrossRef] [PubMed]
16. Wilson, B.; Rossi, M.; Parkes, G.; Aziz, Q.; Anderson, W.; Irving, P.; Lomer, M.; Whelan, K. Prebiotic B-galacto-oligosaccharide supplementation of the low FODMAP diet improves symptoms of irritable bowel syndrome but does not prevent diet induced decline in bifidobacteria: A randomised controlled trial. Proceed. *Nutr. Soc.* **2017**, *76*. [CrossRef]
17. Campbell, J.M.; Bauer, L.L.; Fahey, G.C.; Hogarth, A.J.C.L.; Wolf, B.W.; Hunter, D.W. Selected fructooligosaccharide (1-kestose, nystose, and 1F-β-fructofuranosylnystose) composition of foods and feeds. *J. Agric. Food Chem.* **1997**, *45*, 3076–3082. [CrossRef]
18. Gänzle, M.G. Enzymatic and bacterial conversions during sourdough fermentation. *Food Microbiol.* **2014**, *37*, 2–10. [CrossRef] [PubMed]
19. De Giorgio, R.; Volta, U.; Gibson, P.R. Sensitivity to wheat, gluten and FODMAPs in IBS: Facts or fiction? *Gut* **2016**, *65*, 169–178. [CrossRef] [PubMed]
20. Schuppan, D.; Pickert, G.; Ashfaq-Khan, M.; Zevallos, V. Non-celiac wheat sensitivity: Differential diagnosis, triggers and implications. *Best Pract. Res. Clin. Gastroenterol.* **2015**, *29*, 469–476. [CrossRef] [PubMed]
21. Biesiekierski, J.R.; Peters, S.L.; Newnham, E.D.; Rosella, O.; Muir, J.G.; Gibson, P.R. No effects of gluten in patients with self-reported non-celiac gluten sensitivity after dietary reduction of fermentable, poorly absorbed, short-chain carbohydrates. *Gastroenterology* **2013**, *145*, 320–328. [CrossRef] [PubMed]
22. Verspreet, J.; Dorneza, E.; Van den Ende, W.; Delcour, C.; Courtin, C.M. Cereal grain fructans: Structure, variability and potential health effects. *Trends Food Sci. Technol.* **2015**, *43*, 32–42. [CrossRef]
23. Verspreet, J.; Pollet, A.; Cuyvers, S.; Vergauwen, R.; Van den Ende, W.; Delcour, J.A.; Courtin, C.M. A simple and accurate method for determining wheat grain fructan content and average degree of polymerization. *J. Agric. Food Chem.* **2012**, *60*, 2102–2107. [CrossRef] [PubMed]
24. Kuo, T.M.; Van Middlesworth, J.F.; Wolf, W.J. Content of raffinose oligosaccharides and sucrose in various plant seeds. *J. Agric. Food Chem.* **1988**, *36*, 32–36. [CrossRef]
25. Vinkx, C.J.A.; Delcour, J.A. Rye (*Secale cereale* L.) arabinoxylans: A critical review. *J. Cereal Sci.* **1996**, *24*, 1–14. [CrossRef]

26. Grausgruber, H.; Scheiblauer, J.; Schönlechner, R.; Ruckenbauer, P.; Berghofer, E. Variability in chemical composition and biologically active constituents of cereals. In *Genetic Variation for Plant Breeding*; Vollmann, J., Grausgruber, H., Ruckenbauer, P., Eds.; EUCARPIA & BOKU: Wien, Austria, 2004; pp. 23–26. ISBN 3-900962-56-1.
27. Brandt, M.J. Bedeutung von Rohwarenkomponenten. In *Handbuch Sauerteig*; Brandt, M.J., Gänzle, M.G., Eds.; Behr's Verlag: Hamburg, Germany, 2005; pp. 41–56. ISBN 3-89947-166-0.
28. Haskå, L.; Nymana, M.; Andersson, R. Distribution and characterisation of fructan in wheat milling fractions. *J. Cereal Sci.* **2008**, *48*, 768–774. [CrossRef]
29. Andersson, A.A.; Andersson, R.; Piironen, V.; Lampi, A.M.; Nyström, L.; Boros, D.; Fraś, A.; Gebruers, K.; Courtin, C.M.; Delcour, J.A.; et al. Contents of dietary fibre components and their relation to associated bioactive components in whole grain wheat samples from the HEALTHGRAIN diversity screen. *Food Chem.* **2013**, *136*, 1243–1248. [CrossRef] [PubMed]
30. Chateigner-Boutin, A.L.; Bouchet, B.; Alvarado, C.; Bakan, B.; Guillon, F. The wheat grain contains pectic domains exhibiting specific spatial and development-associated distribution. *PLoS ONE* **2014**, *9*, e89620. [CrossRef] [PubMed]
31. Saulnier, L.; Guillon, F.; Chateigner-Boutin, A.-L. Cell wall deposition and metabolism in wheat grain. *J. Cereal Sci.* **2012**, *56*, 91–108. [CrossRef]
32. Gänzle, M.; Ripari, V. Composition and function of sourdough microbiota: From ecological theory to bread quality. *Int. J. Food Microbiol.* **2016**, *239*, 19–25. [CrossRef] [PubMed]
33. Brandt, M.J.; Gänzle, M.G. *Handbuch Sauerteig*; Behr's Verlag: Hamburg, Germany, 2005; ISBN 3-89947-166-0.
34. Brandt, M.J. Sourdough products for convenient use in baking. *Food Microbiol.* **2007**, *24*, 161–164. [CrossRef] [PubMed]
35. De Vuyst, L.; Harth, H.; Van Kerrebroeck, S.; Leroy, F. Yeast diversity of sourdoughs and associated metabolic properties and functionalities. *Int. J. Food Microbiol.* **2016**, *239*, 26–34. [CrossRef] [PubMed]
36. Gobbetti, M.; Minervini, F.; Pontonio, E.; Di Cagno, R.; De Angelis, M. Drivers for the establishment and composition of the sourdough lactic acid bacteria biota. *Int. J. Food Microbiol.* **2016**, *239*, 3–18. [CrossRef] [PubMed]
37. Perlman, D.; Halvorson, H.O. Distinct repressible mRNAs for cytoplasmic and secreted yeast invertase are encoded by a single gene. *Cell* **1981**, *25*, 525–536. [CrossRef]
38. Gänzle, M.G.; Follador, R. Metabolism of oligosaccharides and starch in lactobacilli: A review. *Front. Microbiol.* **2012**, *3*, 340. [CrossRef] [PubMed]
39. Andersson, U.; Molenaar, D.; Radström, P.; de Vos, W.M. Unity in organization and regulation of catabolic operons in *Lactobacillus plantarum*, *Lactococcus lactis*, and *Listeria monocytogenes*. *Syst. Appl. Microbiol.* **2005**, *28*, 187–195. [CrossRef] [PubMed]
40. Teixeira, J.S.; Abdi, R.; Su, M.S.; Schwab, C.; Gänzle, M.G. Functional characterization of sucrose phosphorylase and scrR, a regulator of sucrose metabolism in *Lactobacillus reuteri*. *Food Microbiol.* **2013**, *36*, 432–439. [CrossRef] [PubMed]
41. Gänzle, M.G. Lactic metabolism revisited: Metabolism of lactic acid bacteria in food fermentations and food biotechnology. *Curr. Opin. Food Sci.* **2015**, *2*, 106–117. [CrossRef]
42. Gänzle, M.G.; Vermeulen, N.; Vogel, R.F. Carbohydrate, peptide and lipid metabolism of lactic acid bacteria in sourdough. *Food Microbiol.* **2007**, *24*, 128–138. [CrossRef] [PubMed]
43. Zheng, J.; Ruan, L.; Sun, M.; Gänzle, M. A genomic view of lactobacilli and pediococci demonstrates that phylogeny matches ecology and physiology. *Appl. Environ. Microbiol.* **2015**, *81*, 7233–7243. [CrossRef] [PubMed]
44. Galle, S.; Arendt, E.K. Exopolysaccharides from sourdough lactic acid bacteria. *Crit. Rev. Food Sci. Nutr.* **2014**, *54*, 891–901. [CrossRef] [PubMed]
45. Galle, S.; Schwab, C.; Arendt, E.; Gänzle, M. Exopolysaccharide-forming *Weissella* strains as starter cultures for sorghum and wheat sourdoughs. *J. Agric. Food Chem.* **2010**, *58*, 5834–5841. [CrossRef] [PubMed]
46. Schwab, C.; Mastrangelo, M.; Corsetti, A.; Gänzle, M.G. Formation of oligosaccharides and polysaccharides by *Lactobacillus reuteri* LTH5448 and *Weissella cibaria* 10M in sorghum sourdoughs. *Cereal Chem.* **2008**, *85*, 679–684. [CrossRef]

47. Korakli, M.; Rossmann, A.; Gänzle, M.G.; Vogel, R.F. Sucrose metabolism and exopolysaccharide production in wheat and rye sourdoughs by *Lactobacillus sanfranciscensis*. *J. Agric. Food Chem.* **2001**, *49*, 5194–5200. [CrossRef] [PubMed]
48. Teixeira, J.S.; McNeill, V.; Gänzle, M.G. Levansucrase and sucrose phoshorylase contribute to raffinose, stachyose, and verbascose metabolism by lactobacilli. *Food Microbiol.* **2012**, *31*, 278–284. [CrossRef] [PubMed]
49. Zhao, X.; Gänzle, M.G. Genetic and phenotypic analysis of carbohydrate metabolism and transport in *Lactobacillus reuteri*. *Int. J. Food Microbiol.* **2018**, *272*, 12–21. [CrossRef] [PubMed]
50. Ostergaard, S.; Olsson, L.; Nielsen, J. Metabolic Engineering of *Saccharomyces cerevisiae*. *Microbiol. Mol. Biol. Rev.* **2000**, *64*, 34–50. [CrossRef] [PubMed]
51. Whelan, K.; Abrahmsohn, O.; David, G.J.; Staudacher, H.; Irving, P.; Lomer, M.C.; Ellis, P.R. Fructan content of commonly consumed wheat, rye and gluten-free breads. *Int. J. Food Sci. Nutr.* **2011**, *62*, 498–503. [CrossRef] [PubMed]
52. Brandt, J.J.; Hammes, W.P. Einfluss von Fructosanen auf die Sauerteigfermentation. *Getreide Mehl Brot* **2001**, *55*, 341–345.
53. Struyf, N.; Laurent, J.; Verspreet, J.; Verstrepen, K.J.; Courtin, C.M. *Saccharomyces cerevisiae* and *Kluyveromyces marxianus* co-cultures allow reduction of fermentable oligo-, di-, and monosaccharides and polyols levels in whole wheat bread. *J. Agric. Food Chem.* **2017**, *65*, 8704–8713. [CrossRef] [PubMed]
54. Nilsson, U.; Öste, R.; Jägerstad, M. Cereal fructans: Hydrolysis by yeast invertase, in vitro and during fermentation. *J. Cereal Sci.* **1987**, *6*, 53–60. [CrossRef]
55. Sainz-Polo, M.A.; Ramírez-Escudero, M.; Lafraya, A.; González, B.; Marín-Navarro, J.; Polaina, J.; Sanz-Aparicio, J. Three-dimensional structure of *Saccharomyces* invertase: Role of a non-catalytic domain in oligomerization and substrate specificity. *J. Biol. Chem.* **2013**, *288*, 9755–9766. [CrossRef] [PubMed]
56. Kaplan, H.; Hutkins, R.W. Metabolism of fructooligosaccharides by *Lactobacillus paracasei* 1195. *Appl. Environ. Microbiol.* **2003**, *69*, 2217–2222. [CrossRef] [PubMed]
57. Saulnier, D.M.; Molenaar, D.; de Vos, W.M.; Gibson, G.R.; Kolida, S. Identification of prebiotic fructooligosaccharide metabolism in *Lactobacillus plantarum* WCFS1 through microarrays. *Appl. Environ. Microbiol.* **2007**, *73*, 1753–1765. [CrossRef] [PubMed]
58. Barrangou, R.; Azcarate-Peril, M.A.; Duong, T.; Conners, S.B.; Kelly, R.M.; Klaenhammer, T.R. Global analysis of carbohydrate utilization by *Lactobacillus acidophilus* using cDNA microarrays. *Proc. Natl. Acad. Sci. USA* **2006**, *103*, 3816–3821. [CrossRef] [PubMed]
59. Stuyf, N.; Vancdewiele, H.; Herrera-Malaver, B.; Verspreet, J.; Verstrepen, K.J.; Courtin, C.M. *Kluyveromyces marxianus* yeast enables the production of low FODMAP whole wheat breads. *Food Microbiol.* **2018**, *76*, 135–145. [CrossRef]
60. Goh, Y.J.; Lee, J.H.; Hutkins, R.W. Functional analysis of the fructooligosaccharide utilization operon in *Lactobacillus paracasei* 1195. *Appl. Environ. Microbiol.* **2007**, *73*, 5716–5724. [CrossRef] [PubMed]
61. Burne, R.A.; Penders, J.E. Differential localization of the *Streptococcus mutans* GS-5 fructan hydrolase enzyme, FruA. *FEMS Microbiol. Lett.* **1994**, *121*, 243–249. [CrossRef] [PubMed]
62. Loponen, J.; Mikola, M.; Sibakov, J. An Enzyme Exhibiting Fructan Hydrolase Activity. Patent No. WO2017220864A1, 28 December 2017.
63. Wisselink, H.W.; Moers, A.P.; Mars, A.E.; Hoefnagel, M.H.; de Vos, W.M.; Hugenholtz, J. Overproduction of heterologous mannitol 1-phosphatase: A key factor for engineering mannitol production by *Lactococcus lactis*. *Appl. Environ. Microbiol.* **2005**, *71*, 1507–1514. [CrossRef] [PubMed]
64. Struyf, N.; Laurent, J.; Lefevere, B.; Verspreet, J.; Verstrepen, K.J.; Courtin, C.M. Establishing the relative importance of damaged starch and fructan as sources of fermentable sugars in wheat flour and whole meal bread dough fermentations. *Food Chem.* **2017**, *218*, 89–98. [CrossRef] [PubMed]
65. Loponen, J. Low-Fructan Grain Material and a Method for Producing the Same. Patent No. WO2016113465A1, 21 July 2016.
66. Laatikainen, R.; Koskenpato, J.; Hongisto, S.M.; Loponen, J.; Poussa, T.; Hillilä, M.; Korpela, R. Randomised clinical trial: Low-FODMAP rye bread vs. regular rye bread to relieve the symptoms of irritable bowel syndrome. *Aliment. Pharmacol. Ther.* **2016**, *44*, 460–470. [CrossRef] [PubMed]

67. Laatikainen, R.; Koskenpato, J.; Hongisto, S.M.; Loponen, J.; Poussa, T.; Huang, X.; Sontag-Strohm, T.; Salmenkari, H.; Korpela, R. Pilot study: Comparison of sourdough wheat bread and yeast-fermented wheat bread in individuals with wheat sensitivity and irritable bowel syndrome. *Nutrients* **2017**, *9*, E1215. [CrossRef] [PubMed]
68. Pirkola, L.; Laatikainen, R.; Loponen, J.; Hongisto, S.M.; Hillilä, M.; Nuora, A.; Yang, B.; Linderborg, K.M.; Freese, R. Low-FODMAP vs regular rye bread in irritable bowel syndrome: Randomized SmartPill® study. *World J. Gastroenterol.* **2018**, *24*, 1259–1268. [CrossRef] [PubMed]
69. CBC. 2013. Available online: http://www.cbc.ca/news/health/sourdough-breadmaking-cuts-gluten-content-in-baked-goods-1.2420209 (accessed on 26 May 2018).
70. Junker, Y.; Zeissig, S.; Kim, S.J.; Barisani, D.; Wieser, H.; Leffler, D.A.; Zevallos, V.; Libermann, T.A.; Dillon, S.; Freitag, T.L.; et al. Wheat amylase trypsin inhibitors drive intestinal inflammation via activation of toll-like receptor 4. *J. Exp. Med.* **2012**, *209*, 2395–2408. [CrossRef] [PubMed]
71. Loponen, J.; König, K.; Wu, J.; Gänzle, M.G. Influence of thiol metabolism of lactobacilli on egg white proteins in wheat sourdoughs. *J. Agric. Food Chem.* **2008**, *56*, 3357–3362. [CrossRef] [PubMed]

15

Comprehensive Nutrition Review of Grain-Based Muesli Bars in Australia: An Audit of Supermarket Products

Felicity Curtain [1,*] and Sara Grafenauer [1,2]

1 Grains & Legumes Nutrition Council, Mount Street, North Sydney 2060, Australia
2 School of Medicine, University of Wollongong, Northfields Avenue, Wollongong 2522, Australia
* Correspondence: f.curtain@glnc.org.au

Abstract: Muesli bars are consumed by 16% of children, and 7.5% of adults, and are classified as discretionary in Australian Dietary Guidelines, containing "higher fat and added sugars" compared with core food choices. This study aimed to provide a nutritional overview of grain-based muesli bars, comparing data from 2019 with 2015. An audit of muesli bars, grain-based bars, and oat slices was undertaken in January 2019 (excluding fruit, nut, nutritional supplement, and breakfast bars) from the four major supermarkets in metropolitan Sydney. Mean and standard deviation was calculated for all nutrients on-pack, including whole grain per serve and per 100g. Health Star Rating (HSR) was calculated if not included on-pack. Of all bars (n = 165), 63% were ≤ 600 kJ (268–1958 kJ), 12% were low in saturated fat, 56% were a source of dietary fibre, and none were low in sugar. Two-thirds (66%) were whole grain (≥8 g/serve), with an average of 10 g/serve, 16% of the 48 g Daily Target Intake. HSR featured on 63% of bars (average 3.2), with an overall HSR of 2.7. Compared to 2015, mean sugars declined (26.6 g to 23.7 g/100 g; $p < 0.001$), and 31% more bars were whole grain (109 up from 60 bars). Although categorised as discretionary, there were significant nutrient differences across grain-based muesli bars. Clearer classification within policy initiatives, including HSR, may assist consumers in choosing products high in whole grain and fibre at the supermarket shelf.

Keywords: muesli bars; grains; whole grain; dietary fibre; snack foods; nutrition

---

1. Introduction

'Muesli bar' is a generic term that refers to baked or cold-formed cereal-based snack bars, and may contain other ingredients such as fruit, nuts, seeds, chocolate, yoghurt, and a variety of other fillings and/or toppings [1]. They are a popular food in Australia, with consumption per capita considered the third highest worldwide, behind Canada and the USA [2]. An estimated 7.5% of Australian adults ate muesli bars the day prior to the 2011–12 Australian Health Survey, with consumption more common in younger age groups (16% of 4–13 year olds, compared to 12.8% of 14–18 year olds, and less than 8% of those aged 19–50 years) [3]. Their popularity with children was noted in a 2005 paper reviewing the lunchbox content of Australian school children, which found an estimated 41.8% of lunchboxes included a muesli/fruit bar, though this also included non-grain-based bars, excluded from this research [4].

Data from the 2011–12 Australian Health Survey found muesli bars contributed overall less than 1% of total energy, protein, fats, sugars, and dietary fibre to Australians aged 2 years and older [5]. However for females aged between 2–18 years, these figures were slightly higher; 1.1% energy, 1.2% total sugars, and 1.5% dietary fibre, and for males 2–18 years; 1.2% energy, 1% saturated fat, 1.4% total sugars, and 1.6% dietary fibre [5]. There is a lack of consensus on what constitutes a 'snack food', with definitions ranging from foods consumed between main meals or at specific times of day, food-type, or participant-described. Based on 'time of day' consumption, bars can be considered a snack food, generally eaten between main meals, and snacking of this kind has been linked with concern around increased risk of obesity and related chronic disease [6], though importantly, these health outcomes are multifactorial, with food choice and energy balance key in determining whether snacking is a healthful or harmful food behaviour [7,8].

Between 1995 and 2012, the prevalence and frequency of children snacking (defined as a single eating occasion between main meals) rose in Australia, with more than double the number of children snacking four or more times per day in 2012 [9]. Subsequently, the contribution of snacks to total energy intake significantly increased, from 24–30.5%. Foods consumed as snacks were a mix of traditional 'snack' foods such as sweet biscuits, cakes, fresh fruit, and 'meal' foods, such as bread and milk. Fruit and vegetable juice was the top contributor to energy from snacks in 1995, but did not appear in 2012, with pome fruit moving up as the top contributor. Muesli bars did not feature in the top snacks in 1995, but were number seven in 2007, and number nine in 2012, where they contributed an estimated 12.5% of total energy to snacks [9]. In Australian adults, cakes, muffins, scones, breads, and dairy milk were the three greatest contributors to energy from snacks, with 22% of total energy derived from snacking occasions [10]. While no data has reviewed changes in snacking habits among Australian adults, steady increases from 1977–2006 amongst adults in the USA mirror Australian children's results, contributing more kilojoules, mainly from discretionary foods like desserts, sugar sweetened beverages, and salty snacks [11].

The popularity of muesli bars, and increasing levels of consumption [9] have attracted attention from public health groups, government, and the media, not least since they are considered a 'discretionary' food in the Australian Dietary Guidelines, where their consumption is discouraged based on having "higher fat and added sugars" [12]. Importantly, they are not depicted in the accompanying Australian Guide to Healthy eating, which visually represents core and discretionary foods. Instead, muesli bars are listed in the longer form supplementary text, and are therefore hidden from view, so it is unclear how well understood their classification as discretionary is among consumers. Similarly, the New Zealand Eating and Activity Guidelines present muesli bars as an example of a 'highly processed' food that may be refined and contain added saturated fat, sugar, and salt [13], and the United Kingdom's Eat Well Guide cautions that cereal bars may have high levels of added sugars [14].

In 2018, proposed sugar reformulation targets for muesli bars were developed by The Healthy Food Partnership, an initiative established by the Australian Government in 2015, which aims to improve public health nutrition through several policy areas, including food reformulation [1]. Their inclusion was noteworthy, as they did not comply with the initial criteria (contributing significantly (≥1%) to sodium, sugars, and/or saturated fat in the Australian population's intake), instead being included based on their high level of consumption among children [1]. The proposed targets call for a "10% reduction in sugar across defined products containing over 28 g sugar/100 g, and a reduction in sugar to 25 g/100 g for products between 25–28 g sugar/100 g by the end of 2022". It is important to recognise that many companies have their own nutrition policies and commitments, as outlined in a 2018 Australian report, which found 16 of the 19 food companies surveyed included nutrition in their corporate strategy and had a commitment to product reformulation, while 11 out of 19 had committed to implementing the voluntary Health Star Rating (HSR) system [15].

The HSR is an interpretive Front of Pack Labelling system, first introduced in Australia and New Zealand in 2014, as a joint initiative between Government, public health, industry, and consumer groups. The system uses an algorithm to assign a star rating between 0.5–5 stars, and is intended to aid consumers in making healthier choices within categories [16,17]. The HSR algorithm rates foods on a per 100 g basis, considering both 'negative nutrients' (kilojoules, saturated fat, total sugars, and sodium), and 'positive' elements (fruit, vegetables, nuts and legumes, as well as protein and dietary fibre in some cases), which is then converted to a star rating [18]. Muesli bars were a key category of consideration in the ongoing HSR 5-year review, which noted they had received negative media attention based on products scoring "inappropriately high scores", despite their categorisation as discretionary foods [19].

However, grain-based muesli bars may also be a potential source of positive ingredients and nutrients within the diet pattern, particularly considering whole grain and dietary fibre content, which are promoted within Australian Dietary Guidelines [12]. Widespread evidence supports whole grains and whole grain foods for their protective health benefits, including lower total and cause-specific mortality, type 2 diabetes [20–24], weight gain [25], and colorectal cancer [26]. Globally, low whole grain intake has been recognised as the second greatest dietary risk factor for mortality (behind sodium), and the greatest dietary risk factor for morbidity, responsible for more than 80 million Disability-Adjusted-Life-Years [27]. Irrespective of its well-documented health benefits, whole grain intake in Australia is low, with follow up data from the Australian Health Survey recording median intake for children at 16.5 g per day, and adults at 21.2 g/day—both less than half of the established Daily Target Intake (DTI) of 48 g per day for adults, and between 32 and 40 g per day for children [28–30]. Equally, a large body of evidence points to the benefits of dietary fibre and its role in reducing chronic disease risk, yet most Australians fall short, with more than half of children, and more than 70% of adults not meeting their respective targets [31].

Due to their popularity and increasing consumption in Australia, muesli bars are often criticised and met with confusion regarding their nutritional value, with a particular focus on sugar content. This study aimed to provide an overview of the nutritional status of grain-based muesli bars on shelf including muesli bars, grain-based bars, and oat slices in Australian supermarkets, and provide a comparison of 2019 with 2015 data.

2. Materials and Methods

An audit of grain-based muesli bars was conducted January 2019, in four major supermarkets in metropolitan Sydney (Aldi, Coles, IGA, and Woolworths). Collectively, these supermarket chains make up more than 80% of total Australian market share, and were chosen in preference to smaller, independent grocery stores in an attempt to reflect food choices that the majority of Australians are faced with during food shopping [32]. This recognised process has been outlined in previously published research [33] and the same process was utilised in the data collection from 2015. Smartphones were used to capture all information on food packaging, including ingredient lists, Nutrition Information Panels (NIP), health and nutrition claims, HSR, and any additional logos and endorsements. Outlined in Table 1 below, products accounted for in the audit included muesli bars, grain-based bars, (including fruit-filled bars and twists, and those made from wheat, puffed rice, or other grains), and oat slices. Products were further categorised to determine whether they were specifically marketed towards children, by the presence of cartoons, promotions, or sporting figures, as described in previous research [34,35]. Products excluded were fruit-based bars, fruit leather/straps, nutritional supplement bars (e.g. protein/'low-carb' bars), nut/seed based bars, and breakfast bars/biscuits (e.g. those designed as a meal replacement, indicated in the product name), in line with exclusions within the Healthy Food Partnership proposed reformulation targets [1]. A supplementary internet search was conducted through supermarket websites and identified manufacturer websites using key words such as "snack bars", "muesli bars", "grain-based bars", "oat slices", and "snack bars", to ensure all products were captured.

Data from photographs taken at both timeframes (2015 and 2019) were transcribed into a Microsoft® Excel® spreadsheet (Version 2013, Redmond, Washington, DC, USA) for analysis. Information for the data entry included the NIP per serve and per 100 g, ingredients, percentage of whole grains, nutrition and health related claims, including whole grain, protein, dietary fibre, saturated fat, sugars, and sodium. Eligibility for products to make nutrition content claims was also assessed, in line with Food Standards Australia New Zealand and GLNCs Code of Practice for Whole Grain Ingredient Content Claims (The Code) [30], as well as proportion of products meeting the Healthy Food Partnership proposed reformulation targets for sugar reduction. HSR was not collected in 2015 as this was not on pack at this time. Where HSR was not featured on packaging, it was calculated for all products using the HSR website calculator [36]. A second, independent reviewer checked data for any inconsistencies and errors, and results were compared with 2015 data that followed the same process, to assess changes.

Table 1. Classification of categories.

Category	Description
Muesli bar	Baked or cold-formed bars where oats made up ≥5% of the product OR were one of the first five ingredients listed on the Nutrition Information Panel (NIP)
Grain-based bar	Baked or cold-formed bars where grain ingredient (s) (excluding oats) made up ≥5% of the product OR grains (excluding oats) were one of the first five ingredients listed on the NIP
Oat slice	Soft-baked bars with the word 'slice' in the product name, where oats made up ≥5% of the product OR were one of the first five ingredients listed on the NIP

Statistics

All data were checked for normality using Shapiro–Wilk test (IBM SPSS®, version 25.0, IBM Corp., Chicago, IL, USA) and mean and standard deviation were presented. As expected, there were missing values for dietary fibre and whole grain as these are often not presented unless a claim is being made on-pack, therefore dietary fibre and whole grain were analysed separately.

One-way ANOVA with post hoc Tukey analysis (IBM SPSS®, version 25.0, IBM Corp., Chicago, IL, USA) was used to compare differences per serve and per 100 g between (1) muesli bars, (2) grain-based bars, (including fruit-filled bars and twists, and those made from wheat, puffed rice, or other grains), and (3) oat slices for all available nutrients reported on-pack, including where relevant, dietary fibre, whole grain (g and %) and HSR (per 100 g). Independent samples t-test (IBM SPSS®, version 25.0, IBM Corp., Chicago, IL, USA) was used to compare whole grain and refined grain bars, which was defined according to each product's eligibility for registration with The Code (≥8 g whole grain per manufacturer serve), a method that has been described in previously published research [37]. T-tests were also used to determine difference in HSR for all products /100 g, between whole grain and refined grain categories and for data per 100 g from 2015 compared with 2019.

3. Results

Data from 165 bars were collected, including 96 muesli bars, 46 grain-based bars, and 23 oat slices from 18 manufacturers where the top three (Nestle Ltd., Kellogg (Aust) Pty. Ltd. and Carman's Fine Foods Pty. Ltd.), hold more than 60% market share (Retail World, December 2018) and have national distribution. Of these, 28 bars (17%) were identified as being specifically marketed towards children; these were predominantly grain-based bars (71%), with the remaining 8% muesli bars. Overall, mean serve size varied substantially between categories, with grain-based bars the smallest (27 g), followed by 35 g for muesli bars, and 55 g for oat slices.

There was a significant difference in nutrients including whole grain across all categories per serve and per 100 g (Tables 2 and 3). Post hoc Tukey analysis (per serve) comparing muesli bars and grain-based bars revealed no significant differences in saturated fat ($p = 0.181$), carbohydrate ($p = 0.365$), sugars ($p = 0.274$), and sodium ($p = 0.869$). Grain-based bars and oat slices were significantly different across all nutrients and whole grain content. Conversely, muesli bars and oat slices were the closest in composition for dietary fibre and whole grain ($p = 0.273$ and $p = 0.238$ respectively) with grain-based bars significantly lower ($p < 0.001$). Almost all (95%) grain-based bars met the Australian Dietary Guidelines recommendations of 600 kJ or less as a 'serve' of discretionary food, as well as 61% of muesli bars, but only 8% of oat slices.

Table 2. Nutrients per serve (mean & SD): muesli bars, grain-based bars, and oat slices including whole grain.

Nutrient Criteria	Muesli Bars (n = 96)	Grain-Based Bars (n = 46)	Oat Slices (n = 23)	p-Value	Total Bars (n = 165)
Serve Size (g)	35 ± 7.5	27 ± 7.0	55 ± 29.9	<0.001	35 ± 15.7
Energy (kJ)	614.4 ± 155.6	428.4 ± 91.6	1007.7 ± 565.6	<0.001	617.4 ± 301.0
Protein (g)	3.1 ± 1.7	1.5 ± 0.6	4.1 ± 2.5	<0.001	2.8 ± 1.9
Fat (g)	5.6 ± 2.9	2.3 ± 1.4	11.2 ± 7.0	<0.001	5.4 ± 4.4
Saturated Fat (g)	1.7 ± 1.2	1.1 ± 0.7	7.1 ± 4.3	<0.001	2.3 ± 2.7
Carbohydrate (g)	19.7 ± 3.9	18.0 ± 5.0	29.6 ± 15.8	<0.001	20.6 ± 7.9
Sugars (g)	7.3 ± 2.5	8.2 ± 3.4	12.0 ± 5.3	<0.001	8.2 ± 3.6
Dietary Fibre (g)	3.2 ± 1.6	1.6 ± 1.5	3.8 ± 2.4	<0.001	2.8 ± 1.9
Sodium (mg)	39.7 ± 44.1	43.5 ± 19.9	99.0 ± 61.4	<0.001	49.0 ± 46.4
Whole Grain (g)	14.2 ± 4.8	1.0 ± 2.8	16.1 ± 8.2	<0.001	10.7 ± 7.9

One Way ANOVA 95% CI.

Table 3. Nutrients, whole grain, and HSR/100 g (mean & SD) in muesli bars, grain-based bars, and oat slices.

Nutrient Criteria	Muesli Bars (n = 96)	Grain-Based Bars (n = 46)	Oat Slices (n = 23)	p-Value
Energy (kJ)	1770.9 ± 180.3	1633.4 ± 188.2	1817.9 ± 112.7	<0.001
Protein (g)	8.6 ± 3.2	5.4 ± 1.9	7.3 ± 1.0	<0.001
Fat (g)	15.4 ± 5.1	9.1 ± 5.8	20.0 ± 4.4	<0.001
Saturated fat (g)	5.0 ± 3.3	4.3 ± 3.7	12.9 ± 3.3	<0.001
Carbohydrate (g)	56.7 ± 8.3	67.6 ± 7.4	53.9 ± 3.9	<0.001
Sugars (g)	20.9 ± 5.6	29.8 ± 6.4	23.1 ± 4.3	<0.001
Dietary Fibre (g)	9.4 ± 5.1	5.8 ± 6.1	6.6 ± 0.8	<0.001
Sodium (mg)	112.2 ± 121.0	166.7 ± 69.9	174.5 ± 46.7	0.002
HSR	3.1 ± 1.1	2.4 ± 1.0	1.8 ± 0.4	<0.001
% Whole Grain	40.7 ± 11.8	4.8 ± 13.4	29.7 ± 4.6	<0.001

One Way ANOVA 95% CI.

Comparing per 100 g, post hoc Tukey analysis revealed no difference in saturated fat (p = 0.558) between muesli bars and grain-based bars although all other nutrients and HSR were significantly different (p < 0.001). Similarly, all nutrients were significantly different between grain-based bars and oat slices except sodium (p = 0.952) and although muesli bars are most similar to oat slices in terms of dietary fibre and whole grain content as noted earlier, there were significant differences in fat (p = 0.001), saturated fat (p < 0.001), sodium (p = 0.009), and HSR (p = 0.001). Muesli bars were highest in dietary fibre, contributing an average of 9.4 g/100 g, the lowest in sodium (112.2 mg/100 g), and had a significantly higher HSR (3.0). They also contained the highest percentage of whole grain ingredients (40.7%) compared with grain-based bars and oat slices. The average HSR for all products was 2.7, but was higher for the 63% of products that displayed it on-pack (3.2 stars) compared to those that did not (1.8 stars).

The overall results for bars specifically targeted towards children were similar to the averages for grain-based bars, with an average of 1659 kJ ± 120 per 100 g, 6.1 ± 3.3g protein, 9.8 ± 3.5 g total fat, 4.3 ± 2.8 g saturated fat, 67 ± 7.9 g carbohydrate, 26 ±8.1 g sugars, 6.1 ± 4 g dietary fibre, and 161 ± 78.1 mg sodium. Children's bars contained 19 ± 23.8% whole grain ingredients (contributing an average of 4.6 g to the 32–40 g Daily Intake Target for the 4–13 year old age group), and had an average HSR of 2.7 ± 1.1 stars, in line with the mean for the total snack bar category.

The percentage of products meeting nutrition claim criteria are presented in Table 4. More than half of muesli bars and oat slices were eligible for a 'contains whole grain' claim (compared to only 4% of grain-based bars), and 17% of oat slices were considered very high in whole grain. Six products did not report their percentage of whole grain ingredients, required to determine claim eligibility, so these were assumed as ineligible. Similar results were obtained for fibre claim eligibility, with 56% of the total category at least a source of fibre, mostly represented by muesli bars (69%), and oat slices (61%). The greatest proportion of grain-based bars were low in saturated fat (30%), compared to only 5% of muesli bars, and no oat slices. While none of the investigated bars were considered low in sugar, 48% overall met the most stringent proposed sugar reformulation target for muesli bars, (<25 g/100 g), and an additional 13% met the lower level proposed target of between 25–28 g sugar/100 g, with 29% falling outside the criteria.

Table 4. Percentage of products meeting claim criteria and proposed reformulation targets *.

	Muesli Bars (n = 96)	Grain-Based Bars (n = 46)	Oat Slices (n = 23)	Total Snack Bars (n = 165)
Eligible for WG claim (≥8 g/manufacturer serve)	90	4	91	66
Contains WG (≥8 g/manufacturer serve)	58	4	65	43
High in WG (16–24 g/manufacturer serve)	41	0	4	16
Very High in WG (≥24 g/manufacturer serve)	4	0	17	6
Source of Fibre (≥2–<4 g/serve)	69	26	61	56
Good Source of Fibre (≥4–<7 g/serve)	5	2	4	4
Excellent Source of Fibre (≥7 g/serve)	5	2	22	7
Low in Saturated Fat (≤1.5 g/100 g)	5	30	0	12
Low in Sugar (≤5 g/100 g)	0	0	0	0
Meets Proposed Sugar Reformulation Target 25–28 g/100 g *	9	11	4	9
Meets Proposed Sugar Reformulation Target <25 g/100 g *	78	24	65	61

* Healthy Food Partnership proposed reformulation targets (September 2018).

As outlined in Table 5, bars categorised as whole grain (≥8 g per manufacturer serve) were significantly higher in energy, total fat, and dietary fibre, and lower in sugars and sodium than refined grain bars. Interestingly, there was no significant difference noted in HSR between whole grain and refined grain bars, with 0.7 star between those categorised as whole grain and the remaining 'non-whole grain bars' which were categorised as refined grain bars.

Table 5. Whole grain versus refined grain nutrients (per 100 g) (mean and SD).

NIP	Whole Grain * (n = 109)	Refined Grain ** (n = 56)	p-Value
Energy (kJ)	1772.6 ± 171.1	1673.8 ± 199.6	0.044
Protein (g)	8.4 ± 2.9	5.9 ± 2.3	0.384
Fat (g)	16.1 ± 5.2	10.9 ± 7.0	0.034
Saturated Fat (g)	6.2 ± 4.4	5.3 ± 4.3	0.389
Carbohydrate (g)	56.2 ± 7.4	65.4 ± 9.3	0.059
Sugars (g)	20.9 ± 5.1	29.1 ± 6.6	0.043
Dietary Fibre (g)	8.6 ± 4.2	6.6 ± 6.7	0.008
Sodium (mg)	119.5 ± 111.0	168.4 ± 82.2	0.005
HSR	3.1 ± 1.1	2.4 ± 1.0	0.075

Independent samples t-test 95% CI. * Based on eligibility for registration with GLNCs Code of Practice for Whole Grain Ingredient Content Claims (≥8 g per manufacturer serve). ** Includes six bars that did not report percentage of whole grain ingredients.

In regards to other on-pack claims, 'No artificial colours/flavours/preservatives' was the most common claim made on packaging, featuring on almost three-quarters (73%) of the total category, and on 91% of oat slices, 80% of grain-based bars, and 66% of muesli bars. More than half made a dietary fibre claim (56%), including 60% of both oat slices and muesli bars, and 30% of grain-based bars. Similarly, 49% made a whole grain claim on-pack, mainly seen on oat slices (70%), and muesli bars (68%), with only 9% of grain-based bars making this claim. An additional 28 products were eligible, but did not make a whole grain claim.

Compared with 2015 (Table 6), 3.5% fewer bars were captured (171 versus 165), with apparent growth in the number of muesli bars (82 to 96 products), and oat slices (18 to 23 products), but a decline in grain-based bars (71 to 46 products), these being the most nutritionally poor products within the category. Over time, there was a significant decrease in total sugars from 26.6 g/100 g to 23.7 g/100 g ($p < 0.001$) across the total category in the four years since 2015, largely attributed to muesli bars, containing 4.2 g/100 g less sugars, while grain-based bars remained stable, and oat slices decreased by 1.1 g/100 g. The proportion of whole grain bars within the category increased, from 35 to 66% in four years (60/171 up to 109/165 bars). HSR data was not captured in 2015 due to the system being newly introduced, so no comparison of this metric over time was possible.

Table 6. Comparison of nutrients and whole grain in total bars between 2015 and 2019 per 100g (mean and SD).

Nutrient Criteria	Total Bars 2015 (n = 171)	Total Bars 2019 (n = 165)	p-Value
Energy (kJ)	1700 ± 179.9	1739.1 ± 186.7	0.049
Protein (g)	6.6 ± 2.1	7.5 ± 3.0	0.001
Fat (g)	13.1 ± 6.2	14.1 ± 6.2	0.089
Saturated Fat (g)	5.7 ± 4.4	5.9 ± 4.4	0.610
Carbohydrate (g)	62.3 ± 8.4	59.3 ± 9.2	0.002
Sugars (g)	26.6 ± 7.2	23.7 ± 6.8	<0.001
Dietary Fibre (g)	6.6 ± 4.1	7.9 ± 5.2	0.203
Sodium (mg)	143.1 ± 104.5	136.1 ± 104.5	0.540
% Whole Grain	30.0 ± 15.0	38.8 ± 11.2	0.009

Independent samples t-test 95% CI.

4. Discussion

Despite their widespread popularity, consumption of grain-based muesli bars are discouraged by the Australian Dietary Guidelines based on their classification as a discretionary food. This study aimed to provide a comprehensive overview of the nutritional status of grain-based muesli bars on shelf in Australian supermarkets, compared to data collected in 2015.

Overall, wide nutrient ranges were demonstrated between and within the categories examined although muesli bars are treated as a homogenous category in food policy and in advice to consumers. A major factor influencing these differences was the range in average serve sizes, with oat slices more than double that of grain-based bars. Serve size discrepancy may be a point of confusion for shoppers, as nutrient content of the smaller sized grain-based bars may appear more favourable, yet these were the highest in some nutrients of concern on a per 100 g basis. Conversely, oat slices are larger and appear the highest in some positive nutrients per serve, but not when compared per 100 g. This may suggest that the nutrition features of bars may be difficult to compare using the per serve nutrition information at the supermarket shelf. This has been previously described as 'health framing', whereby the impression of a healthier product may lead to overconsumption, however as all bars examined were individually wrapped and therefore portion controlled, this may be less of a concern than in other snack food categories such as cakes and biscuits. These findings are consistent with prior research in Australia which found significant variability in manufacturer serve size within both discretionary [38,39], and core food groups [40,41], and are partly explained by the lack of regulation around standard serving sizes in Australia, which is determined by food manufacturers [40].

Differing ingredients were also a major factor influencing variations in nutrition profile and serve size. Many grain-based bars consisted of puffed or flaked grains (such as corn or rice), which were likely lighter in weight than whole grains, more commonly found in muesli bars and oat slices. Oat slices often contained butter and coconut, both known for their high levels of saturated fat. Additionally, muesli bars and oat slices were all based on oats, which are unique among grains for their higher fat content (6–8%, compared to 2–3% in other grains [42]). The difference in ingredients provides basis for considering further differentiation within this category and at the same time, questions the broad categorisation of 'muesli bars' within the discretionary food group.

Almost one in five bars (17%) in 2019 were specifically marketed towards children, and these were mainly within the grain-based bars category (which are smaller and often made with puffed grains). Generally, these were less nutritious options, being lower in protein, dietary fibre, and whole grain, and higher in sugar than the category on average. Previous research has echoed this finding, with the products designed to appeal to children generally higher in some negative nutrients [34]. Encouragingly, their nutritional value was reflected in the average HSR of less than 3 stars, which has been determined as a cut off point for consumers identifying a food as unhealthy [43].

'Snackification', or the demand for convenience foods to suit modern lifestyles may drive continued innovation and reformulation. New Nutrition Business identified snacking as a key driver of food choice in 2018 and 2019, pointing to examples of manufacturers reinventing foods that were once impossible to eat on-the-go, such as peanut butter in portioned sachets and microwave porridge in individual pots, possibly increasing market competition for muesli bars as traditional snack foods [44]. When considering the top three contributors to adults (19–70+ years) discretionary food intake, the Australian Institute of Health & Welfare's 2018 Nutrition Across the Life Stages report listed alcohol, cakes/muffins/pastries, and soft drinks [45]. Similarly, a 2017 review analysing Australian children's discretionary food intake identified cakes/muffins/slices (4.2%), sweet biscuits (2.9%), and potato crisps/similar snacks (2.7%) as the top contributors to total energy, and the greatest contributors to added sugar were sugar-sweetened soft drinks (18.6%), cakes, muffins, and slices (10.6%), and cordials (6.7%). Conversely, 'sweet snack bars' (which included muesli/cereal bars, and fruit/nut/seed bars) contributed only 1.2% to total energy, and 1.6% added sugars [46]. When this is considered in the context of a typical Australian school lunchbox, including "about one sandwich, two biscuits, a piece of fruit, a snack of either a muesli/fruit bar or some other packaged snack, and a drink of fruit juice/cordial or water" [4], the particular focus on muesli bars as a food of concern may need to be reassessed against the full range of options that could be included in this meal occasion. Discretionary foods such as biscuits, cakes, potato chips, and cordial offer minimal nutritional benefits, so encouraging healthier options within the muesli bar category, alongside core foods in preference to these may be more beneficial advice to consumers and parents who are already under pressure to provide convenient, nutritious snacks.

Comparisons with 2015 data (in Table 6) are suggestive of improvements in terms of added sugars and whole grain content made by food industry. Reformulation aims to improve the nutritional content of manufactured foods, either by increasing beneficial nutrients, or reducing risk-associated nutrients. Often, manufacturers make modest nutritional changes over a period of time to allow consumers' tastes to adjust accordingly, referred to as "health by stealth" [47], but in recent years Australian muesli bar manufacturers have openly shared efforts to reduce salt, fat, sugar, and increase dietary fibre [48]. There is evidence to show reduction targets are effective, with a 2018 review of voluntary sodium reduction targets in soup demonstrating a 6% reduction in sodium levels in soup products between 2011 and 2014, with 67–74% of products compliant with targets [49]. Similarly, Australia's National Heart Foundation has reported significant reductions in line with targets set by the Food and Health Dialogue, such as 10% less sodium in bread and processed meats, and 32% less sodium in breakfast cereals [50], indicating that proposed targets set by the Healthy Food Partnership may encourage further improvements in the added sugars content of muesli bars.

Authors of the 2017 Global Burden of Disease study speculated that dietary policies focused on promoting consumption of whole grains, fruits. and vegetables, and other core food groups may have a greater effect than policies targeting excess consumption of sugar and fat [27]. Within the current study, whole grain bars were clearly identified as a healthier option overall, providing more protective nutrients, and fewer negative nutrients than refined grain bars. Across categories, the majority of oat slices and muesli bars were whole grain (≥8 g per manufacturer serve), and provided the equivalent of at least 30% of an adult's 48 g Daily Target Intake for whole grain, and up to half of a child's daily whole grain requirement (32–40 g/day) [30]. In light of this, whole grain bars may present a convenient, portion controlled, and accepted vehicle for whole grain, and their consumption over refined grain bars could aid in bridging the significant gap in consumption. Unlike other nutrients, whole grain claims are not regulated by Food Standards Australia New Zealand, but are instead encouraged through

GLNCs voluntary Code of Practice for Whole Grain Ingredient Content Claims (The Code), introduced in Australia and New Zealand in 2013 to encourage evidence-based promotion of whole grain foods. GLNC utilises audits of grain-based foods to monitor the operation of The Code and provide feedback to industry as necessary. While 60% of eligible bars were registered with The Code, its voluntary nature, and the fact that the percentage of whole grain ingredients is not mandatory in the ingredients list means deciphering which are whole grain options is not always clear to consumers. This was highlighted by the six bars identified that contained whole grain ingredients (such as rolled oats, and whole grain wheat), but did not report their percentages, so it was unclear whether they met The Code's whole grain criteria. Encouragingly, the number of whole grain bars have increased by 31% since 2015, suggesting positive changes have been made by manufacturers to existing products, new whole grain products have been added to the market due to consumer demand, or that labelling has been updated to more clearly communicate whole grain content.

The variability in nutrients supplied within the grain-based muesli bar category, combined with their popularity, may point towards education as the more powerful tool in supporting consumers to choose healthier products, in preference to discouraging consumption. The concept of 'knowledge-is-power' has been explored in previous research, with a review from the USA determining consumers with greater nutrition knowledge were more likely to consult nutrition labels, which may lead to healthier food choices [51]. The HSR attempts to clarify complex nutrition information and arm consumers with the knowledge to make healthier choices within food categories, and has been shown to perform well in directing consumers towards healthier, higher-scoring foods [43,52,53]. HSR scores for the bars category ranged from 1–5 stars, yet there was no significant difference between refined and whole grain varieties, with only 0.7 of a star between products. This finding highlights a shortcoming of the algorithm used to assign products a star rating, and builds on previous research that demonstrated an inability to differentiate whole grain and refined grain breads, breakfast cereals, rice, and flour products, as it does not directly account for, or reward foods for whole grain content [37]. There is a clear opportunity to refine the HSR by recognising whole grain as a positive food component, which could play a role in discerning healthier food choices across numerous categories, including muesli bars. However, to meet its objective of simple nutrition comparisons within categories, widespread uptake of a voluntary front-of-pack labelling system such as the HSR is required. Almost two-thirds (63%) of bars examined displayed a HSR, comparatively higher than overall uptake, which is estimated at 28% [16]. Consistent with existing literature, bars displaying a HSR tended to have higher scores, suggesting the system may be used strategically within and across brands [16,54]. Conversely, industry appear to be using the HSR as an incentive to improve a product's nutritional value, with recent studies in Australia and New Zealand identifying upwards of 83% of products displaying a HSR had been reformulated to increase their score [54,55].

Strengths of this study include its comprehensive nature, and to our knowledge, it is the first study that has reviewed muesli bars on shelf in Australia, with a comparison made to previously collected data. Also, where HSR was not provided, we calculated this for a more accurate representation of HSR across the category. However, there were some limitations. The research was focused only on grain-based bars, excluding others—such as nut bars and protein and low-carb bars—which may also be consumed as snacks though to a lesser extent than muesli bars [56]. While all efforts were made to capture the category in its entirety, differences may exist between geographic areas. As previously stated, reporting of dietary fibre and whole grain within the ingredients and Nutrition Information Panel is not mandatory in the absence of an on-pack claim, so was not always declared, and thus there was some missing data. Finally, we did not conduct an independent nutrition analysis, and were reliant on manufacturer information.

5. Conclusions

Although categorised as discretionary, there are significant nutrient differences across grain-based muesli bars, with well-chosen bars providing valuable amounts of whole grain and dietary fibre.

Muesli bars are a widely consumed snack food, particularly among younger age groups in Australia, yet their contribution and role in the diet is controversial, based on their classification at discretionary by Australian Dietary Guidelines. This study demonstrated significant variation between and within the category, with the whole grain options emerging as more nutritious compared to refined grain bars, and an indication of sugar reduction since 2015. Within a balanced diet, it is clear that some muesli bars can offer a convenient and nutritious snack, with many bars providing around 30% of an adult's, and up to half of a child's daily requirement for whole grain, and more than half of all products are at least a source of fibre. Both whole grains and dietary fibre are encouraged within Dietary Guidelines yet intakes across age groups tend to fall short of dietary targets. The current HSR algorithm does not appear to be overly favouring muesli bars (with an overall score of 2.7), and instead, could be improved to capture and differentiate whole grain options. Ongoing promotion of the higher HSR scoring bars, alongside proposed voluntary sugar reformulation targets and trends such as snackification, may be suggestive of opportunities and incentives for manufacturers to further improve the current range of products. Clearer classification within policy initiatives utilising evidence-based assessment of available products may help refine advice from healthcare professionals, and may be key in providing better direction for consumers to make healthier and acceptable snack food and lunchbox choices.

Author Contributions: Conceptualization, F.C. and S.G.; Methodology, F.C.; Formal analysis, S.G.; Original draft preparation, F.C.; Review and editing, S.G.

Acknowledgments: Thanks to James Sze, Student Dietitian from the University of Wollongong, NSW, who was involved in data collection as part of his university studies, and to Joanna Russell for statistical advice.

References

1. Department of Health; Australian Government. Healthy Food Partnership Voluntary Food Reformulation Targets-Public Consultation. Available online: https://consultations.health.gov.au/population-health-and-sport-division-1/hfp-reformulation/ (accessed on 10 July 2019).
2. Mintel. A Year of Innovation in Snack Bars. 2019. Available online: https://clients.mintel.com/report/a-year-of-innovation-in-snack-bars-2019 (accessed on 10 July 2019).
3. Australian Bureau of Statistics. 4364.0.55.007-Australian Health Survey: Nutrition First Results-Foods and Nutrients, 2011–2012. Available online: http://www.abs.gov.au/ausstats/abs@.nsf/lookup/4364.0.55.007main+features12011-12 (accessed on 9 July 2019).
4. Sanigorski, A.M.; Bell, A.C.; Kremer, P.J.; Swinburn, B.A. Lunchbox contents of Australian school children: Room for improvement. *Eur. J. Clin. Nutr.* **2005**, *59*, 1310–1316. [CrossRef] [PubMed]
5. Australian Bureau of Statistics. 4364.0.55.012-Australian Health Survey: Consumption of Food Groups from the Australian Dietary Guidelines, 2011–2012. Available online: http://www.abs.gov.au/ausstats/abs@.nsf/Lookup/by%20Subject/4364.0.55.007~{}2011-12~{}Main%20Features~{}Cereals%20and%20cereal%20products~{}720 (accessed on 10 July 2019).
6. Wang, D.; van der Horst, K.; Jacquier, E.F.; Afeiche, M.C.; Eldridge, A.L. Snacking Patterns in Children: A Comparison between Australia, China, Mexico, and the US. *Nutrients* **2018**, *10*, 198. [CrossRef]
7. Mattes, R. Snacking: A cause for concern. *Physiol. Behav.* **2018**, *193*, 279–283. [CrossRef] [PubMed]
8. Mielmann, A.; Brunner, T.A. Consumers' snack choices: Current factors contributing to obesity. *Br. Food J.* **2019**, *121*, 347–358. [CrossRef]
9. Fayet-Moore, F.; Peters, V.; McConnell, A.; Petocz, P.; Eldridge, A.L. Weekday snacking prevalence, frequency, and energy contribution have increased while foods consumed during snacking have shifted among Australian children and adolescents: 1995, 2007 and 2011–12 National Nutrition Surveys. *Nutr. J.* **2017**, *16*, 65. [CrossRef] [PubMed]
10. Fayet-Moore, F.F.; McConnell, A.A.; Keighley, T.T. Adult snacking in Australia: Understanding who, what, when, and how much. *J. Nutr. Intermed. Metab.* **2016**, *4*, 15. [CrossRef]
11. Piernasm, C.; Popkin, B.M. Snacking Increased among U.S. Adults between 1977 and 2006. *J. Nutr.* **2009**. [CrossRef]

12. NHMRC. Australian Dietary Guidelines. Available online: https://www.nhmrc.gov.au/_files_nhmrc/file/publications/n55_australian_dietary_guidelines1.pdf (accessed on 9 July 2019).
13. New Zealand Ministry of Health. *Eating and Activity Guidelines for New Zealand Adults*; The Ministry of Health: Wellington, New Zealand, 2015.
14. England, P.H. The Eatwell Guide. Available online: https://assets.publishing.service.gov.uk/government/uploads/system/uploads/attachment_data/file/742750/Eatwell_Guide_booklet_2018v4.pdf (accessed on 10 July 2019).
15. Sacks, G.; Robinson, E. *For Informas. Inside Our Food and Beverage Manufacturers: Assessment of Company Policies and Commitments Related to Obesity Prevention and Nutrition, Australia*; Deakin University: Melbourne, Australia, 2018.
16. Jones, A.; Shahid, M.; Neal, B. Uptake of Australia's Health Star Rating System. *Nutrients* **2018**, *10*, 997. [CrossRef]
17. Commonwealth of Australia. About Health Star Ratings. Available online: http://healthstarrating.gov.au/internet/healthstarrating/publishing.nsf/Content/About-health-stars (accessed on 12 July 2019).
18. Jones, A.; Rådholm, K.; Neal, B. Defining 'Unhealthy': A Systematic Analysis of Alignment between the Australian Dietary Guidelines and the Health Star Rating System. *Nutrients* **2018**, *10*, 501. [CrossRef]
19. Mpconsulting. Five Year Review of the Health Star Rating System—Consultation Paper: Options for System Enhancement. Available online: http://www.healthstarrating.gov.au/internet/healthstarrating/publishing.nsf/Content/news-20181510/$File/HSR%20System%20Consultation%20Paper%20-%20October%202018.pdf (accessed on 10 July 2019).
20. Wu, H.; Flint, A.J.; Qi, Q.; van Dam, R.M.; Sampson, L.A.; Rimm, E.B.; Holmes, M.D.; Willett, W.C.; Hu, F.B.; Sun, Q. Association Between Dietary Whole Grain Intake and Risk of Mortality: Two Large Prospective Studies in US Men and Women. *JAMA Intern. Med.* **2015**. [CrossRef]
21. Aune, D.; Keum, N.; Giovannucci, E.; Fadnes, L.T.; Boffetta, P.; Greenwood, D.C.; Tonstad, S.; Vatten, L.J.; Riboli, E.; Norat, T. Whole grain consumption and risk of cardiovascular disease, cancer, and all cause and cause specific mortality: Systematic review and dose-response meta-analysis of prospective studies. *Br. Med. J.* **2016**, *353*, 2716. [CrossRef] [PubMed]
22. Zhang, B.; Zhao, Q.; Guo, W.; Bao, W.; Wang, X. Association of whole grain intake with all-cause, cardiovascular, and cancer mortality: A systematic review and dose-response meta-analysis from prospective cohort studies. *Eur. J. Clin. Nutr.* **2018**, *72*, 57–65. [CrossRef] [PubMed]
23. Zong, G.; Gao, A.; Hu, F.B.; Sun, Q. Whole Grain Intake and Mortality From All Causes, Cardiovascular Disease, and Cancer: A Meta-Analysis of Prospective Cohort Studies. *Circulation* **2016**, *133*, 2370–2380. [CrossRef] [PubMed]
24. Li, B.; Zhang, G.; Tan, M.; Zhao, L.; Jin, L.; Tang, X.; Jiang, G.; Zhong, K. Consumption of whole grains in relation to mortality from all causes, cardiovascular disease, and diabetes: Dose-response meta-analysis of prospective cohort studies. *Medicine (Baltim.)* **2016**, *95*, 4229. [CrossRef] [PubMed]
25. Maki, K.C.; Palacios, O.M.; Koeche, K.; Sawicki, C.M.; Livingston, K.A.; Bell, M.; Cortes, H.M.; McKeown, N.M. The Relationship between Whole Grain Intake and Body Weight: Results of Meta-Analyses of Observational Studies and Randomized Controlled Trials. *Nutrients* **2019**, *11*, 1245. [CrossRef] [PubMed]
26. Aune, D.; Chan, D.S.; Lau, R.; Vieira, R.; Greenwood, D.C.; Kampman, E.; Norat, T. Dietary fibre, whole grains, and risk of colorectal cancer: Systematic review and dose-response meta-analysis of prospective studies. *BMJ* **2011**, *343*, 6617. [CrossRef] [PubMed]
27. GBD 2017 Diet Collaborators. Health effects of dietary risks in 195 countries, 1990–2017: A systematic analysis for the Global Burden of Disease Study 2017. *Lancet* **2019**, *393*, 1958–1972. [CrossRef]
28. Griffiths, T. Towards an Australian 'daily target intake' for wholegrains. *Food Aust.* **2007**, *59*, 600–601.
29. Galea, L.; Beck, E.; Probst, Y.; Cashman, C. Whole grain intake of Australians estimated from a cross-sectional analysis of dietary intake data from the 2011-13 Australian Health Survey. *Public Health Nutr.* **2017**, *20*, 2166–2172. [CrossRef]
30. GLNC. Code of Practice for Whole Grain Ingredient Content Claims. Available online: http://www.glnc.org.au/codeofpractice/ (accessed on 25 July 2019).
31. Fayet Moore, F.; Cassettari, T.; Tuck, K.; McConnell, A.; Petocz, P. Dietary Fibre Intake in Australia. Paper I: Associations with Demographic, Socio-Economic, and Anthropometric Factors. *Nutrients* **2018**, *10*, 599. [CrossRef]

32. Roy Morgan. Woolworths and Aldi Grow Grocery Market Share in 2018. Available online: http://www.roymorgan.com/findings/7936-australian-grocery-market-december-2018-201904050426 (accessed on 8 August 2019).
33. Grafenauer, S.; Curtain, F. An Audit of Australian Bread with a Focus on Loaf Breads and Whole Grain. *Nutrients* **2018**, *10*, 1106. [CrossRef]
34. Mehta, K.; Phillips, C.; Ward, P.; Coveney, J.; Handsley, E.; Carter, P. Marketing foods to children through product packaging: Prolific, unhealthy and misleading. *Public Health Nutr.* **2012**, *15*, 1763–1770. [CrossRef] [PubMed]
35. Chapman, K.; Nicholas, P.; Banovic, D.; Supamaniam, R. The extent and nature of food promotion directed to children in Australian supermarkets. *Health Promot. Int.* **2006**, *21*. [CrossRef] [PubMed]
36. Commonwealth of Australia. Health Star Rating Calculator. Available online: http://www.healthstarrating.gov.au/internet/healthstarrating/publishing.nsf/Content/online-calculator#/step/1 (accessed on 1 July 2019).
37. Curtain, F.; Grafenauer, S.J. Health Star Rating in Grain Foods—Does It Adequately Differentiate Refined and Whole Grain Foods? *Nutrients* **2019**, *11*, 415. [CrossRef] [PubMed]
38. Haskelberg, H.; Neal, B.; Dunford, E.; Flood, V.; Rangan, A.; Thomas, B.; Cleanthous, X.; Trevena, H.; Zheng, J.M.; Louie, J.C.Y.; et al. High variation in manufacturer-declared serving size of packaged discretionary foods in Australia. *Br. J. Nutr.* **2016**, *115*, 1810–1818. [CrossRef] [PubMed]
39. Watson, W.L.; Kury, A.; Wellard, L.; Hughes, C.; Dunford, E.; Chapman, K. Variations in serving sizes of Australian snack foods and confectionery. *Appetite* **2016**, *96*, 32–37. [CrossRef] [PubMed]
40. Cleanthous, X.; Mackintosh, A.M.; Anderson, S. Comparison of reported nutrients and serve size between private label products and branded products in Australian supermarkets. *Nutr. Diet.* **2011**, *68*, 120–126. [CrossRef]
41. Yang, S.; Gemming, L.; Rangan, A. Large Variations in Declared Serving Sizes of Packaged Foods in Australia: A Need for Serving Size Standardisation? *Nutrients* **2018**, *10*, 139. [CrossRef]
42. Decker, E.A.; Rose, D.J.; Stewart, D. Processing of oats and the impact of processing operations on nutrition and health benefits. *Br. J. Nutr.* **2014**, *112*, S58–S64. [CrossRef] [PubMed]
43. Talati, Z.; Pettigrew, S.; Kelly, B.; Ball, K.; Dixon, H.; Shilton, T. Consumers' responses to front-of-pack labels that vary by interpretive content. *Appetite* **2016**, *101*, 205–213. [CrossRef]
44. Mellentin, J. *10 Key Trends in Food, Nutrition & Health 2019*; New Nutrition Business: London, UK, 2018.
45. Australian Institute of Health and Welfare. *Nutrition Across the Life Stages*; Australian Institue of Health and Weldare: Canberra, Australia, 2018.
46. Johnson, B.J.; Bell, L.K.; Zarnowiecki, D.; Rangan, A.M.; Golley, R.K. Contribution of Discretionary Foods and Drinks to Australian Children's Intake of Energy, Saturated Fat, Added Sugars and Salt. *Children* **2017**, *4*, 104. [CrossRef] [PubMed]
47. Regan, A.; Potvin Kent, M.; Raats, M.M.; McConnon, A.; Wall, P.; Dubois, L. Applying a Consumer Behavior Lens to Salt Reduction Initiatives. *Nutrients* **2017**, *9*, 901. [CrossRef] [PubMed]
48. Han, E. Uncle Tobys Cuts Fat, Salt and Sugar from Muesli Bars to Boost Health Star Rating. Available online: https://www.smh.com.au/business/companies/uncle-tobys-cuts-fat-salt-and-sugar-from-museli-bars-to-boost-health-star-rating-20151013-gk7n4j.html (accessed on 15 July 2019).
49. Levi, R.; Probst, Y.; Crino, M.; Dunford, E. Evaluation of Australian soup manufacturer compliance with national sodium reduction targets. *Nutr. Diet.* **2018**, *75*, 200–205. [CrossRef] [PubMed]
50. National Heart Foundation of Australia. *Report on the Evaluation of the Nine Food Categories for Which Reformulation Targets Were Set under the Food and Health Dialogue*; National Heart Foundation: Victoria, Australia, 2016.
51. Soederberg Miller, L.M.; Cassady, D.L. The effects of nutrition knowledge on food label use. A review of the literature. *Appetite* **2015**, *92*, 207–216. [CrossRef] [PubMed]
52. Actona, R.; Vanderleeb, L.; Hammond, D. Influence of front-of-package nutrition labels on beverage healthiness perceptions: Results from a randomized experiment. *Prev. Med.* **2018**, *115*, 83–89. [CrossRef] [PubMed]
53. Neal, B.; Crino, M.; Dunford, E.; Gao, A.; Greenland, R.; Li, N.; Ngai, J.; Ni Mhurchu, C.; Pettigrew, S.; Sacks, G.; et al. Effects of Different Types of Front-of-Pack Labelling Information on the Healthiness of Food Purchases—A Randomised Controlled Trial. *Nutrients* **2017**, *9*, 1284. [CrossRef] [PubMed]

54. Morrison, H.; Meloncelli, N.; Pelly, F.E. Nutritional quality and reformulation of a selection of children's packaged foods available in Australian supermarkets: Has the Health Star Rating had an impact? *Nutr. Diet.* **2019**, *76*, 296–304. [CrossRef] [PubMed]
55. Ni Mhurchu, C.; Eyles, H.; Choi, Y.-H. Effects of a Voluntary Front-of-Pack Nutrition Labelling System on Packaged Food Reformulation: The Health Star Rating System in New Zealand. *Nutrients* **2017**, *9*, 918. [CrossRef]
56. Mpconsulting. Five Year Review of the Health Star Rating (HSR) System: Snack Bar. Available online: http://www.mpconsulting.com.au/wp-content/uploads/2018/10/Snack-bars.pdf (accessed on 22 July 2019).

16

Lutein Esterification in Wheat Flour Increases the Carotenoid Retention and is Induced by Storage Temperatures

Elena Mellado-Ortega and Dámaso Hornero-Méndez *

Chemistry and Biochemistry of Pigments Group, Food Phytochemistry Department, Instituto de la Grasa (CSIC), Campus Universidad Pablo de Olavide, Ctra. de Utrera km. 1, 41013 Seville, Spain; melladoortegae@gmail.com
* Correspondence: hornero@ig.csic.es

Abstract: The present study aimed to evaluate the effects of long-term storage on the carotenoid pigments present in whole-grain flours prepared from durum wheat and tritordeum. As expected, higher storage temperatures showed a catabolic effect, which was very marked for free carotenoid pigments. Surprisingly, for both cereal genotypes, the thermal conditions favoured the synthesis of lutein esters, leading to an enhanced stability, slower degradation, and, subsequently, a greater carotenoid retention. The putative involvement of lipase enzymes in lutein esterification in flours is discussed, particularly regarding the preferential esterification of the hydroxyl group with linoleic acid at the 3′ in the ε-ring of the lutein molecule. The negative effects of processing on carotenoid retention were less pronounced in durum wheat flours, which could be due to an increased esterifying activity (the de novo formation of diesterified xanthophylls was observed). Moreover, clear differences were observed for tritordeum depending on whether the lutein was in a free or esterified state. For instance, lutein-3′-*O*-monolinoleate showed a three-fold lower degradation rate than free lutein at 37 °C. In view of our results, we advise that the biofortification research aimed at increasing the carotenoid contents in cereals should be based on the selection of varieties with an enhanced content of esterified xanthophylls.

Keywords: carotenoids; lutein esters; tritordeum; *Triticum turgidum* conv. *durum*; carotenoid retention; whole-grain flour

---

1. Introduction

Carotenoids, the most widespread pigments in nature, are liposoluble antioxidants produced by plants, algae, fungi, and some bacteria. In plants, carotenoids contribute to the photosynthetic process by acting as light collectors and photoprotectors [1]. Moreover, carotenoids are found in high concentrations in most fruits and flowers where they contribute to the bright colours that attract animals for seed and pollen dispersion. These ubiquitous pigments can also be found in some roots, tubers, and grains, mostly due to the selection of coloured varieties as desired traits for plant domestication by man [2]. Animals are not able to synthetize carotenoids de novo; consequently carotenoids must be acquired through dietary consumption.

Different carotenoids are associated with different health benefits. The provitamin A activity of carotenoids with at least one unsubstituted β-ring end-group in their structure is well-known and of nutritional significance [3]. Moreover, epidemiological studies have correlated carotenoid intake with protection against a range of chronic diseases, such as cardiovascular diseases and cancer [4,5]. In particular, lutein and zeaxanthin play important roles in the prevention of eye diseases such as age related macular degeneration (AMD), cataracts, and retinitis pigmentosa [6].

Wheat (*Triticum* spp.), one of the most important crops for human consumption worldwide, contains low carotenoid contents compared to most vegetables and fruits. However, the widespread and daily-based consumption of cereals and derived products makes these staple foods an important source of these antioxidants in the diet, particularly in disadvantaged populations. The main objective of biofortification programs is the breeding of crops for better nutrition. The major carotenoid present in wheat is lutein [7]. Among the different *Triticum* species, durum wheat (*Triticum turgidum* ssp. *durum*) grains are characterized for presenting a yellowish colour due to carotenoids. In fact the yellow colour of pasta is a major quality trait [8]. Manipulating the carotenoid content of several cereals, or other crops, by means of biofortification strategies has the potential to provide significant health benefits without altering normal dietetic habits [9]. Remarkable progress has been made in this area; a good example is HarvestPlus, part of the Consultative Group on International Agriculture Research (CGIAR) Program on Agriculture for Nutrition and Health (A4NH). HarvestPlus collaborators have developed staple crops with increased densities of micronutrients through plant breeding techniques, such as pro-vitamin A cassava, which provides up to 40% of the daily vitamin A requirement, iron pearl millet, which provides up to 80% of daily iron needs, and zinc rice, which provides up to 60% of the daily zinc requirement (http://www.harvestplus.org/).

The *Triticeae* tribe, which includes wheat, barley (*Hordeum vulgare*), and rye (*Secale cereale*) species, is a series of closely related polyploids. Fertile amphiploid hybrids can be generated among the different cultivated members of this tribe and some wild cereal species. Tritordeum (*Tritordeum*; $2n = 6x = 42$, $AABBH^{ch}H^{ch}$) is a cereal obtained from the cross between a wild barley (*Hordeum chilense* Roem. & Schult.) with diploid genome ($H^{ch}H^{ch}$) and durum wheat (*Triticum turgidum* conv. *durum*; [10]). The lutein content in tritordeum is about 5–8 times higher than durum wheat and is characterized by a specific esterification profile involving two major fatty acids (linoleic and palmitic acids) [11,12]. The latter characteristic is derived from the genetic background of *H. chilense* [13]. The detailed composition of the lutein esters present in tritordeum has been determined and consists of four monoesters (lutein 3′-*O*-linoleate, lutein 3-*O*-linoleate, lutein 3′-*O*-palmitate, and lutein 3-*O*-palmitate) and four diesters (lutein dilinoleate, lutein 3′-*O*-linoleate-3-*O*-palmitate, lutein 3′-*O*-palmitate-3-*O*-linoleate, and lutein dipalmitate) [12]. Tritordeum is currently the subject of an intense breeding program at the Institute of Sustainable Agriculture (IAS; http://www.ias.csic.es/en/) in Cordoba, Spain, to optimize its use as a cereal for incorporation into the formulation of both functional and novel foods.

Cereal grains are traditionally processed for human consumption. The influence of processing techniques on the composition of phytonutrients and bioactive compounds of many staple foods, including cereal grains, has been extensively studied. For example, in cassava, maize, and sweet potato, the conditions and duration of storage have a more significant negative impact on the retention of provitamin A carotenoids than drying or cooking [14]. Similarly, Mugode et al. [15] concluded that the degradation of provitamin A carotenoids in maize mostly occurred during storage and this effect varied among genotypes. Whole-grain wheat flour contains substantially more vitamins, minerals, antioxidants, and other nutrients, including carotenoids, than refined wheat flour [16]. In addition to milling, the subsequent storage of grains and flours can have a significant impact on the composition of phytochemicals. In fact, cereal flour is usually stored during prolonged periods as part of their industrial and technological treatments, and, therefore, an important impact on the carotenoid content is expected as a result of storage. In the case of wheat flour, the main cause of carotenoid degradation is oxidation (including both enzymatic and non-enzymatic processes) during the storage period. Oxygen present in the medium is considered to be the major factor affecting the stability of carotenoids [17]. Therefore, in addition to considering the "high pigment content" trait of *Triticeae* genotypes, the "carotenoid retention ability" should also be considered when screening and selecting strains for their inclusion in breeding programs [18]. Moreover, new technological treatments are emerging for the processing of cereals and their derived products in order to preserve and enhance the content of carotenoids and other phytonutrients of nutritional relevance (reviewed by Hemery et al. [19]).

The natural process by which xanthophylls are esterified with fatty acids is an important part of post-carotenogenic metabolism and mediates their accumulation in plants. To assist in the development of carotenoid-enhanced cereals, the biochemical characterization of the xanthophyll esterification process and studies of the capacity of the cereal endosperm tissue to store these pigments are necessary. Some studies have highlighted the importance of the carotenoid retention capacity, and its influence on the stability during the postharvest storage of crops [20,21]. However, only a few studies investigated the involvement of xanthophyll esterification in the retention of carotenoids during the storage of cereals and derived products [22,23].

We recently assessed the effect of long-term storage on the biosynthesis of lutein esters in durum wheat and tritordeum grains and found that xanthophyll esterification was induced by environmental conditions (especially the temperature) [24]. We also found the xanthophyll esterification process to be highly specific (with the preferential esterification of lutein at position 3 of the β-end ring) and that the fatty acids involved in the esterification and their position in the lutein molecule had a significant effect on the carotenoid stability. Although the results from our previous study increased our understanding of the effects of long-term storage on carotenoid metabolism, characterization of the xanthophyll esterification process was lacking. Therefore, the main goal of the present study was to fully categorize the stability of carotenoid pigments in cereal flours and the influence of pigment esterification during the long-term storage of whole-grain flours in different temperature-controlled conditions.

2. Materials and Methods

2.1. Plant Material, Sample Preparation and Storage Conditions

A commercial durum wheat variety (Don Pedro) and a high-carotenoid tritordeum line (HT621, germplasm line developed in the framework of the Cereal Breeding Program carried out at the Institute for Sustainable Agriculture, Córdoba, Spain) [25] were used in the present study. Both samples are considered representatives of these two cereal genotypes and have been previously characterized regarding their carotenoid profile [11,12,23,26]. Plants were grown in 1-L pots, until maturity, under greenhouse conditions with supplementary lights providing a day/night regime of 12/12 h at 22/16 °C. Immediately after harvesting, seeds were preserved for 2 months at 4 °C in a desiccator before the beginning of experiment. After this storage period, and for each cereal genotype, whole-grain flour was obtained from 500 g of grains by using an oscillating ball mill Retsch Model MM400 (Retsch, Haan, Germany) at 25 Hz for 1 min. Subsequently, the resulting flour was distributed in lots of approximately 4 g in round-capped polypropylene 15-mL centrifuge tubes. Flour samples were stored under controlled temperature conditions (−32, 6, 20, 37 and 50 °C) for a period of 12 months. A control sample (t = 0 days) consisting of 5 subsamples was taken and analysed for each cereal type. Triplicate samples (three tubes for each temperature and time) were taken at monthly intervals and analysed in duplicate. The dry matter content (%) in the samples at each sampling date was measured in triplicate by using an Ohaus moisture balance model MB35 (Ohaus, Greifensee, Switzerland). During the course of the experience a continuous monitoring of the storage temperature was performed.

2.2. Chemicals and Reagents

Deionised water (HPLC-grade) was produced with a Milli-Q Advantage A10 system (Merck Millipore, Madrid, Spain). HPLC-grade acetone was supplied by BDH Prolabo (VWR International Eurolab, S.L., Barcelona, Spain). The rest of reagents were all of analytical grade.

2.3. Extraction of Carotenoids

Carotenoid pigments were extracted from flours with the following procedure. Briefly, 1 g of flour was placed into 25 mL stainless-steel grinding jar together with two stainless-steel balls (15 mm ø), 6 mL of acetone containing 0.1% (w/v) BHT and a known amount of internal standard (β-apo-8′-carotenal; 1.75 and 3.50 μg for durum wheat and tritordeum samples, respectively). Samples were crushed in an oscillating ball mill Retsch Model MM400 (Retsch, Haan, Germany) at 25 Hz for 1 min. Most of the resulting slurry was transferred into a tube and centrifuged at 4500× *g* for 5 min at 4 °C and the clear supernatant collected in a clean tube. The solvent was gently evaporated under a nitrogen stream, and the pigments were dissolved in 0.5 mL of acetone. Prior to the chromatographic analysis, samples were centrifuged at 13,000× *g* for 5 min at 4 °C. The analyses were carried out in duplicate for each sample. All operations were performed under dimmed light to prevent isomerization and photo-degradation of carotenoids.

2.4. HPLC Analysis of Carotenoids

The procedures for the isolation and identification of carotenoid pigments and its esters have already been described in previous works [11,12]. Quantitative analysis of carotenoids was carried out by HPLC according to Atienza et al. [11]. The HPLC system consisted of a Waters e2695 Alliance chromatograph fitted with a Waters 2998 photodiode array detector, and controlled with Empower2 software (Waters Cromatografía, S.A., Barcelona, Spain). A reversed-phase column (Mediterranea SEA18, 3 μm, 20 × 0.46 cm; Teknokroma, Barcelona, Spain) was used. Separation was achieved by a binary-gradient elution using an initial composition of 75% acetone and 25% deionized water, which was increased linearly to 95% acetone in 10 min, then raised to 100% in 2 min, and maintained constant for 10 min. Initial conditions were reached in 5 min. An injection volume of 10 μL and a flow rate of 1 mL/min were used. Detection was performed at 450 nm, and the UV-visible spectra were acquired online (350–700 nm wavelength range). Quantification was carried out using calibration curves prepared with lutein, zeaxanthin and β-carotene standards isolated and purified from natural sources [27]. Calibration curves including eight-points were prepared in the pigment concentration range of 0.5–45 μg/mL. Lutein ester content were estimated by using the calibration curve for free lutein, since the esterification of xanthophylls with fatty acids does not modify the chromophore properties [28]. Accordingly, the concentration of lutein esters was expressed as free lutein equivalents. The calibration curve of free lutein was also used to determine the concentration of the (Z)-isomers of lutein. Data were expressed as μg/g dry weight (μg/g dw).

2.5. Degradation Kinetics Model

In order to investigate the effects of the esterification on the carotenoid degradation during the storage period, the reaction order and derived kinetic parameters were only investigated in those time ranges where the occurrence of catabolic reactions was dominant for each pigment (that is a decline in the concentration with time was clearly observed). For this purpose zero- and first-order kinetics were hypothesized. The general reaction rate expression was applied, $-dC/dt = kC^n$, where C is the concentration of the compound (μg/g dw), k is the reaction rate constant (months^{-1}), t is the reaction time (months), and n is the order of the reaction [29]. The reaction rate expression and the kinetic parameters for zero- and first-order models are summarized in Table 1. The selected order of the reaction was that showing the best correlation (R^2) and the best correspondence among the experimental values and the half-life of the compound ($t_{1/2}$) and D ($t_{1/10}$) [time needed for the concentration of a reactant to fall to half and one tenth its initial value respectively, where $t_{1/2} = C_0/2k$ and $t_{1/10} = 0.9C_0/k$ for zero-order and $t_{1/2} = (\mathrm{Ln}2)/k$ and $t_{1/10} = (\mathrm{Ln}10)/k$ for first-order]. Kinetic parameters derived from fitted models with $R^2 < 0.8$ were not considered in the discussion.

Table 1. Expression of the reaction rate depending on the reaction order (n) and kinetic parameters derived.

Reaction Order	Reaction Rate Expression	Integrated Expression	Graphical Representation	Half-Life [a] ($t_{1/2}$)	D [b] ($t_{1/10}$)
Zero $n = 0$	$-dC/dt = kC^0 = k$	$C\text{-}C_0 = -kt$	$C\text{-}C_0$ vs. t Slope $= -k$	$t_{1/2} = C_0/2k$	$t_{1/10} = 0.9C_0/k$
First $n = 1$	$-dC/dt = kC^1 = kC$	$\mathrm{Ln}(C/C_0) = -kt$	$\mathrm{Ln}(C/C_0)$ vs. t Slope $= -k$	$t_{1/2} = \mathrm{Ln}(2)/k$	$t_{1/10} = \mathrm{Ln}(10)/k$

[a] Time needed for the concentration of a reactant to fall to half of its initial value. [b] Time needed for the concentration of a reactant to fall one tenth of its initial value.

2.6. Statistical Analysis

Pigment contents are expressed as mean and standard error of the mean (SEM). Significant differences between means was determined by one-way ANOVA, followed by a post-hoc test of mean comparison using the Duncan test for a confidence level of 95% ($p < 0.05$) utilizing the STATISTICA 6.0 software (StatSoft Inc., Tulsa, OK, USA).

3. Results and Discussion

3.1. Carotenoid Content in Whole-Grain Flours: Effect of Long-Term Storage

The initial carotenoid composition for the flours of durum wheat (*Triticum turgidum* conv. *durum*, Don Pedro) and tritordeum (Tritordeum HT621 line) was consistent with previous studies (see Table 2 at t = 0 months) [11,12,23,26]. The initial concentrations of individual pigments were higher in whole-grain tritordeum flour than durum wheat flour, with the exception of (all-*E*)-zeaxanthin, which is not present in tritordeum. On average, the total initial carotenoid content was six times higher in tritordeum (HT621 line) with respect to durum wheat (Don Pedro).

Table 2. Initial carotenoid composition in *Triticum turgidum* cv. *durum* (Don Pedro variety) and *Tritordeum* (HT621 line) whole-grain flours subjected to long-term storage (12 months) under controlled temperature.

HPLC Peak [a]	Pigment	Concentration (μg/g Dry Weight) [b]	
		Durum Wheat (Don Pedro Variety)	**Tritordeum (HT621 Advanced Line)**
1	(all-*E*)-Zeaxanthin	0.08 ± 0.00	-
2	(all-*E*)-Lutein	1.08 ± 0.02	3.95 ± 0.04
3	(9Z)-Lutein	0.06 ± 0.00	0.19 ± 0.01
4	(13Z)-Lutein	0.12 ± 0.00	0.30 ± 0.01
5	Lutein-3′-*O*-linoleate	0.01 ± 0.00	0.15 ± 0.00
6	Lutein-3-*O*-linoleate	0.01 ± 0.00	0.72 ± 0.01
5 + 6	Lutein monolinoleate	0.03 ± 0.00	0.87 ± 0.00
7	Lutein-3′-*O*-palmitate	0.00 ± 0.00	0.49 ± 0.01
8	Lutein-3-*O*-palmitate	0.00 ± 0.00	1.01 ± 0.02
7 + 8	Lutein monopalmitate	0.01 ± 0.00	1.50 ± 0.01
9	(all-*E*)-β-Carotene	0.02 ± 0.00	0.06 ± 0.00
10	Lutein-3,3′-dilinoleate	n.d. [c]	0.12 ± 0.00
11	Lutein-3′-*O*-linoleate-3-*O*-palmitate plus Lutein-3′-*O*-palmitate-3-*O*-linoleate	n.d.	0.42 ± 0.01
12	Lutein-3,3′-dipalmitate	n.d.	0.41 ± 0.01
	Lutein monoesters	0.04 ± 0.00	2.37 ± 0.01
	Lutein diesters	-	0.96 ± 0.01
	Total lutein esters	0.04 ± 0.00	3.33 ± 0.02
	Total free lutein	1.26 ± 0.02	4.44 ± 0.09
	Total lutein	1.29 ± 0.02	7.77 ± 0.07
	Total carotenoids	1.39 ± 0.03	7.83 ± 0.07
	Regioisomers ratios		
	Lutein-3-*O*-linoleate/Lutein-3′-*O*-linoleate	1	5
	Lutein-3-*O*-palmitate/Lutein-3′-*O*-palmitate	1	2

[a] Peak numbers according to Figure S1 (Supplementary Materials). [b] Data represent the mean ± standard error (n = 5). [c] n.d. not detected.

The evolution of total carotenoids revealed significant losses for both cereals at the higher examined temperatures of 37 and 50 °C (Figure 1; see also Figure S1, and Tables S1 and S2). The total degradation of pigments was observed by the end of the 12-month storage period in the durum wheat and tritordeum samples kept at the higher temperature (50 °C). In accordance with Gayen et al. [30], the experimental conditions tested in the present study may facilitate the action of degradative enzymes, such as lipoxygenase (LOX), leading to the co-oxidation of carotenoid pigments. LOX is mostly located in the germ and bran of the grain kernel and its main substrate is linoleic acid [31]. In addition to LOX degradation, the susceptibility of carotenoids to oxygen and high temperatures should be responsible for the decrease in the pigment levels observed during our experiments. The pigment content reduction at the end of the 12-month storage period at −32, 6, and 20 °C were similar in all cases for both cereal genotypes. In contrast, significant differences were observed between the two cereals at 37 °C, with a greater retention of pigments observed in tritordeum (pigment losses of 84% for durum wheat compared to 72% for tritordeum) (Figure 1).

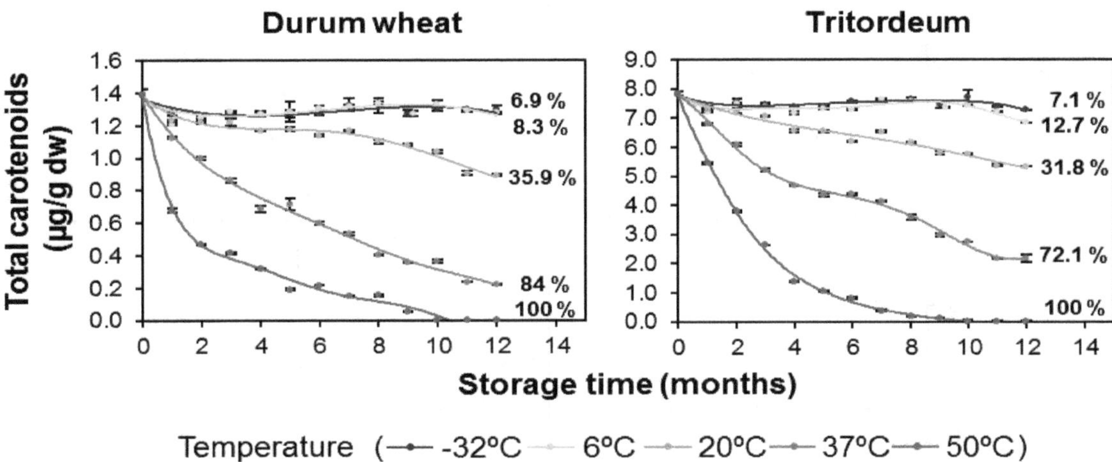

Figure 1. Evolution of the total carotenoid content (µg/g dry weight) in durum wheat (Don Pedro variety) and tritordeum (HT621 advanced line) whole-grain flours during long-term storage under temperature controlled conditions (−32, 6, 20, 37 and 50 °C). The values shown are the mean and standard error (n = 5 for the starting sample, n = 3 for the rest of the samples). Pigment losses (%) are indicated at the end of storage.

The changes observed for the individual free pigments in durum wheat (Figure 2) were similar to the trend described for total carotenoid content: The carotenoid content remained fairly constant at the lowest storage temperatures of −32 and 6 °C while higher carotenoid losses were observed with increased storage temperature. Thus, the carotenoid losses after 12 months of storage at 20 °C were 51% and 63% for (all-*E*)-lutein and (all-*E*)-zeaxanthin, respectively (Table S1). The declines were lower at 20 and 37 °C for the (Z)-isomers of lutein (39% and 89%, respectively), which is consistent with a *trans* to *cis* isomerization process, as reported in other similar studies [32]. At the end of the storage period at 37 °C, (all-*E*)-lutein, (all-*E*)-zeaxanthin, and (all-*E*)-β-carotene had been degraded to trace levels. For the durum wheat flour maintained at 50 °C, (all-*E*)-zeaxanthin and (all-*E*)-β-carotene were already undetectable at the seventh month. These results suggest that both zeaxanthin and β-carotene are less thermostable than lutein at higher temperatures. Some authors have suggested that (all-*E*)-β-carotene is the most thermolabile carotenoid, especially in low-water environments as in the case of cereal flour [33].

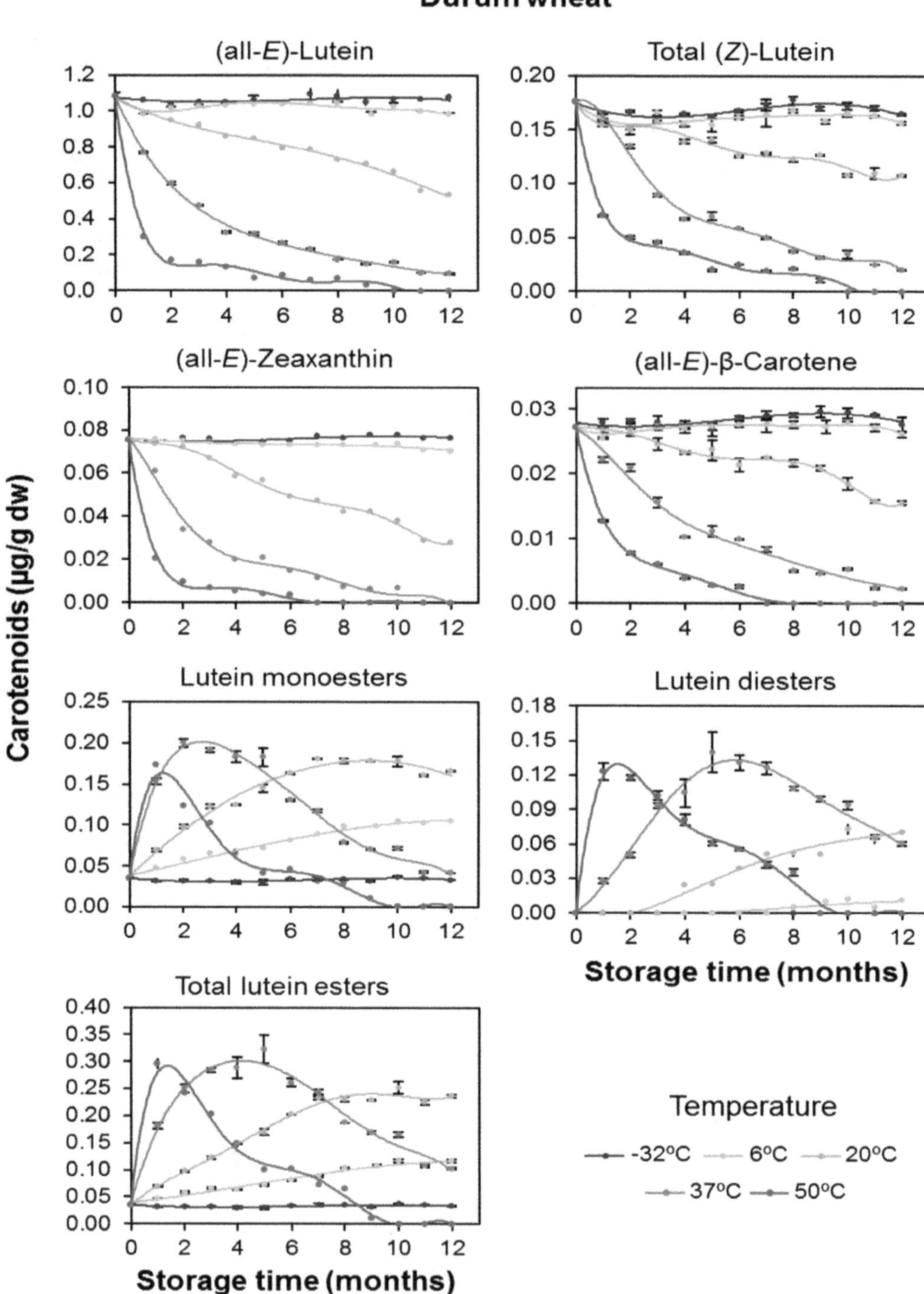

Figure 2. Evolution of the individual carotenoid content and esterified fractions (μg/g dry weight) in durum wheat (Don Pedro variety) whole-grain flours during long-term storage under temperature controlled conditions (−32, 6, 20, 37 and 50 °C). The values shown are the mean and standard error (n = 5 for the starting sample, n = 3 for the rest of the samples).

For whole-grain tritordeum flour, greater losses of the individual free pigments were also observed at the higher storage temperatures (Figure 3). For tritordeum flour stored at 37 °C, (all-*E*)-lutein, (*Z*)-lutein, and (all-*E*)-β-carotene had decreased by 83–98% by the end of the 12-month storage period (Table S2). Similar to durum wheat, the total pigments in tritordeum were completely destroyed after 10 months of storage at 50 °C, and (all-*E*)-β-carotene was already undetectable after 4 months.

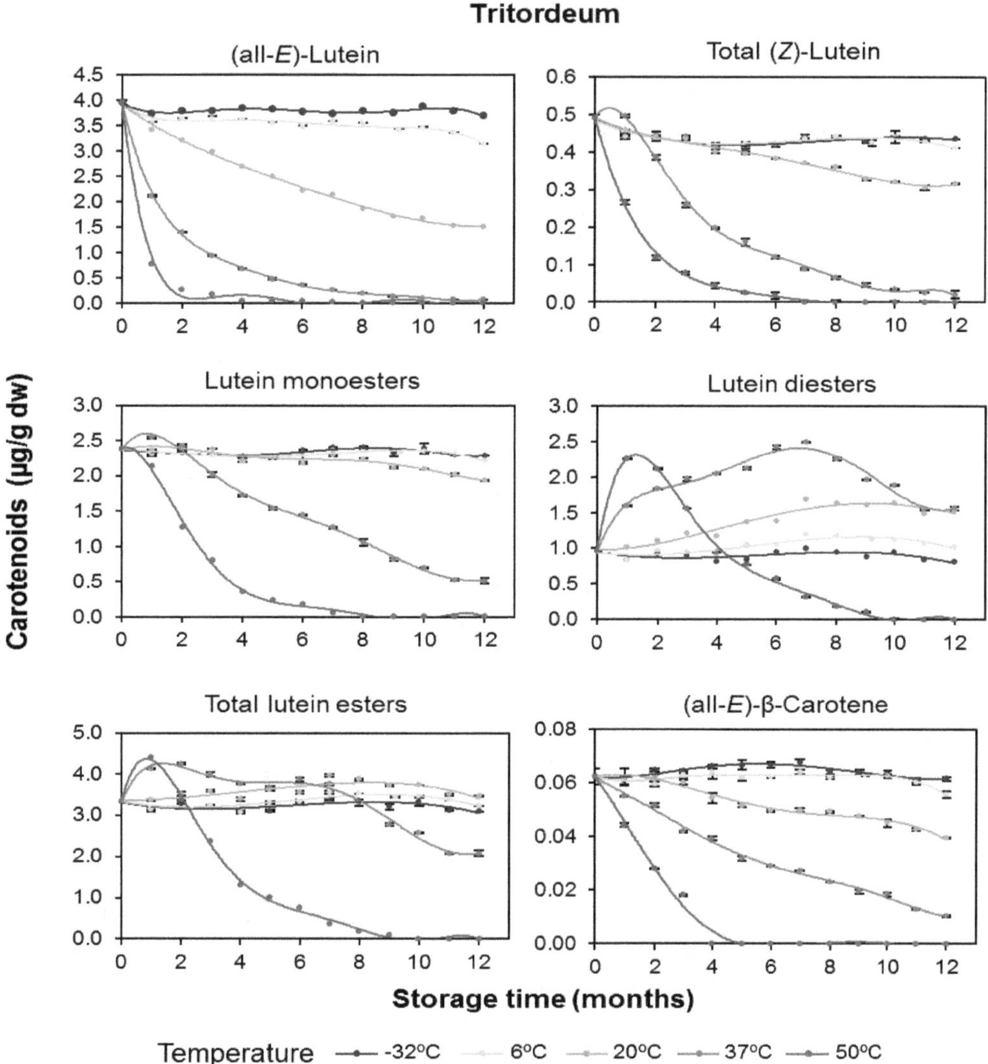

Figure 3. Evolution of the individual carotenoid content and esterified fractions (µg/g dry weight) in tritordeum (HT621 advanced line) whole-grain flours during long-term storage under temperature controlled conditions (−32, 6, 20, 37 and 50 °C). The values shown are the mean and standard error ($n = 5$ for the starting sample, $n = 3$ for the rest of the samples).

In contrast to the free carotenoids, the lutein esters showed increased levels with increasing temperature. This distinction was particularly striking for durum wheat, and especially the monoester fraction, stored at the milder conditions of 6 and 20 °C (Figure 2). For example, the concentration of lutein monoesters increased by 3.7 and 5.7 times the initial values after 12 months at 6 and 20 °C, respectively. At the higher temperatures (37 and 50 °C), competition and/or compensation was observed between the increases promoted by the temperature (de novo esterification) and decreases caused by oxidative degradation. After the storage of durum wheat for 12 months, concentration increases of 2–3 fold were recorded at 37 °C for the lutein ester fraction (sum of monoesters and diesters), revealing an intense esterifying activity under these conditions. The concomitant formation of lutein diesters associated with the rise in storage temperature and time was prompted by the increase in the pool of monoesters.

The free pigments in tritordeum showed a general pattern of degradation with increasing temperature; in contrast, analysis of the esterified fractions in tritordeum revealed clear differences in the evolution profile of lutein monoesters and diesters (Figure 3). Similar to the free pigments, the monoesters fraction decreased by 18.4% and 78.3% with respect to initial levels after 12-months storage at 20 and 37 °C, respectively. However, the diester fraction showed a similar behaviour to that found in durum wheat, with increases of 7%, 60%, and 63% with respect to initial levels after 12-months storage at 6, 20, and 37 °C, respectively. These results might indicate either the occurrence of different isoforms of the esterifying enzymes in the two cereals, or a more intensive esterifying activity of the enzymes in durum wheat. The *H. chilense* genetic background of tritordeum could be responsible for these differences.

The synthesis of lutein esters in cereal flours could possibly take place through a different metabolic pathway from the one operating in intact grains. In fact, in a preliminary study carried out with durum wheat flour [23], the formation of lutein esters was observed, especially at high temperatures; however, the trace levels of the pigments impaired their quantification. The present results underline the importance of controlling the storage conditions of cereals and derived products in order to prevent or promote changes in the profile of carotenoids and other phytochemicals. One possibility is that the esterification of xanthophylls in flours is mediated by the activity of lipases, which are concentrated in the bran in the case of cereals [34]. Lipases catalyse the hydrolysis of carboxyl-ester linkages leading to the release of fatty acids and organic alcohols. However, under low-water conditions, lipases may catalyse the reverse reaction (esterification) or various transesterification reactions involving acids, alcohols, and esters [35]. The acyl transferase activity of lipases has already been suggested to be involved in the formation of sterol esters during the long-term storage of wheat flour [36]. These authors also observed the esterification of lutein, although the data obtained were inconclusive. More recently, Ahmad et al. [37] have provided sound data concluding that lutein esterification in bread wheat was genetically controlled and likely due to a GDSL-lipase located on the 7D chromosome and co-located with a QTL (Quality Trait Loci) associated with ester formation. Moreover, Mattera et al. [38,39] demonstrated that lutein esterification in wheat endosperm is controlled by chromosomes of the homoeologous group 7 (7D and $7H^{ch}$), and suggested differential fatty acid enzyme specificity depending on the cereal species (for instance, common wheat and *H. chilense*).

3.2. Effect of Long-Term Storage on the Esterified Lutein Fractions

The evolution of individual lutein monoesters (lutein monolinoleate and monopalmitate) was similar and consistent with the corresponding changes observed for the total esters fraction during the entire storage of both cereal flours. The profiles at 37 and 50 °C presented two distinctive areas of net synthesis (peaks) and degradation (troughs). This was particularly evident in durum wheat (Figure 4). At 37 °C, lutein monolinoleate showed a synthesis period over the first 2 months of storage, with a 4-fold concentration increase, followed by a degradation period during the remaining storage time, reaching up to 78% total degradation. Similarly, at 50 °C, the maximum synthesis was observed after the first month, accounting for concentrations of up to 3 times the initial content. Lutein monopalmitate showed a more pronounced synthesis, with a 10-fold increase observed after two months at 37 °C and an 8-fold increase after the first month at 50 °C (Figure 4). These data indicate differences in relation to the preferential formation of lutein monoesters with both fatty acids, with the palmitic acid esters being more abundant. On the other hand, the degradation rate was similar for lutein monopalmitate and lutein monolinoleate during the storage of durum wheat flour at 37 and 50 °C. Thus, the ratio between lutein monopalmitate and lutein monolinoleate remained constant across the whole storage period (Table S1). However, in a previous study with durum wheat grains submitted to long-term storage, a higher thermostability for lutein monolinoleate was reported [24].

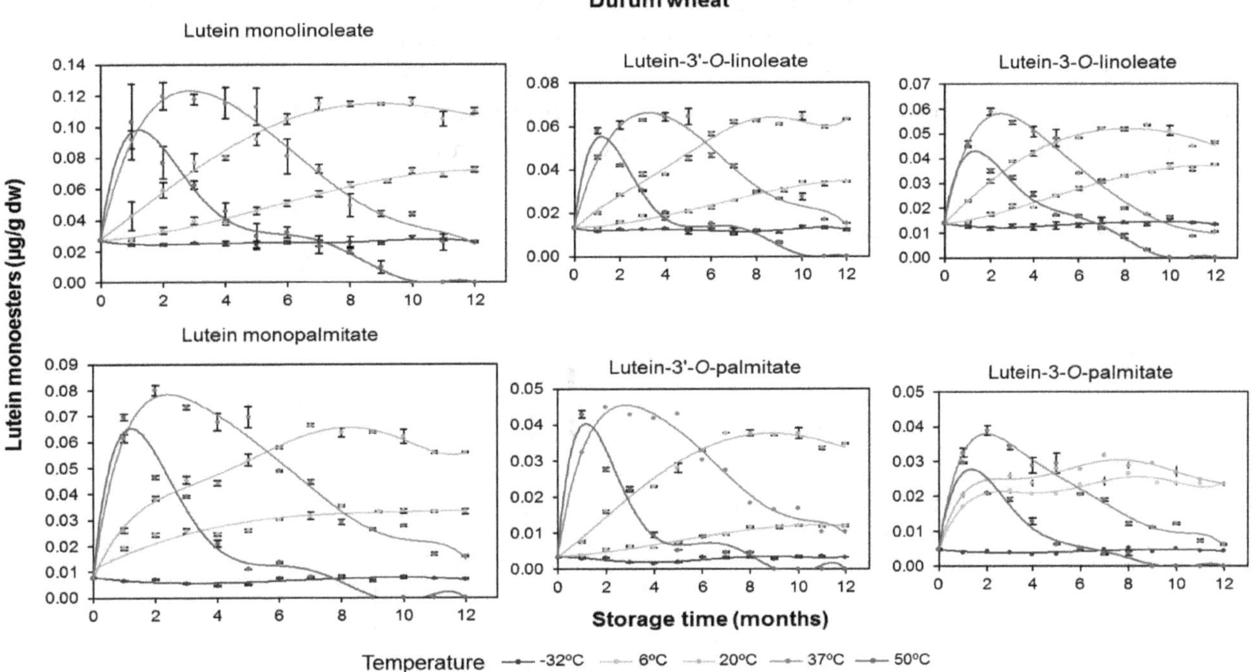

Figure 4. Quantitative changes in the xanthophyll ester fractions (µg/g dry weight) in durum wheat (Don Pedro variety) whole-grain flours during long-term storage under temperature controlled conditions (−32, 6, 20, 37 and 50 °C). The values shown are the mean and standard error (n = 5 for the starting sample, n = 3 for the rest of the samples).

In tritordeum, the maximum concentration increase for lutein monolinoleate was registered after two months at 37 °C and one month at 50 °C (Figure 5). In contrast to durum wheat, stability differences between both monoesters were observed in tritordeum. Lutein monolinoleate remained mostly constant at −32, 6, and 20 °C, whereas lutein monopalmitate showed a progressive decrease with increasing temperature and storage time. Nevertheless, the degradation rates for lutein monoesters were consistently lower than the rates recorded for free lutein (Figure 3). The degradation after 12 months at 37 °C was greater for lutein monopalmitate (85.9%) than for lutein monolinoleate (65.1%).

With respect to the increases in the lutein ester contents observed in durum wheat (Figures 2 and 4), the putative lipase enzyme could exhibit greater activity for palmitic acid than for linoleic acid due to a higher specificity for palmitic acid as a substrate or a better availability of this saturated fatty acid. These results are in line with those obtained by O'Connor et al. [40] who reported the lipase activity in different cereals. However, the evolution of the esterified fraction in tritordeum flour suggested a different scenario compared to durum wheat. In order to interpret this data, it should be taken into consideration that tritordeum is a novel hybrid cereal in which the *H. chilense* genome contributes and interacts with that of durum wheat. Therefore, it is likely that these genetic differences are the cause for the lower esterification activity in tritordeum flour.

Regarding the two regioisomers for each lutein monoester, the 3′ position of the lutein molecule appears to be the preferred site for esterification mediated by lipases in both cereals (Figures 4 and 5), and gives rise to a more stable compound (i.e., lutein-3′-*O*-linoleate and lutein-3′-*O*-palmitate are more stable than lutein-3-*O*-linoleate and lutein-3-*O*-palmitate, respectively). These observations reinforced the idea that the enzyme systems involved in the esterification of lutein in cereal flours are different from those operating in intact grains [12].

In both cereal flours, lutein diesters presented remarkable net increases during the duration of the storage period, especially for lutein dilinoleate and particularly at the storage temperature of 37 °C (Figures 6 and 7). The evolution of diesterified xanthophylls over the storage period clearly suggests that their formation is due to induction of the esterification process by temperature, with this synthesis being particularly prominent in durum wheat. As the storage temperature increased, the rate and amounts of synthesis were also increased, but, on the other hand, the degradative processes due to oxidative stress were also induced. Interestingly, the higher the degree of esterification (diester > monoester > free), the higher the xanthophyll's stability and, consequently, the more delayed the degradation (Figures 4 and 6 for durum wheat and Figures 5 and 7 for tritordeum).

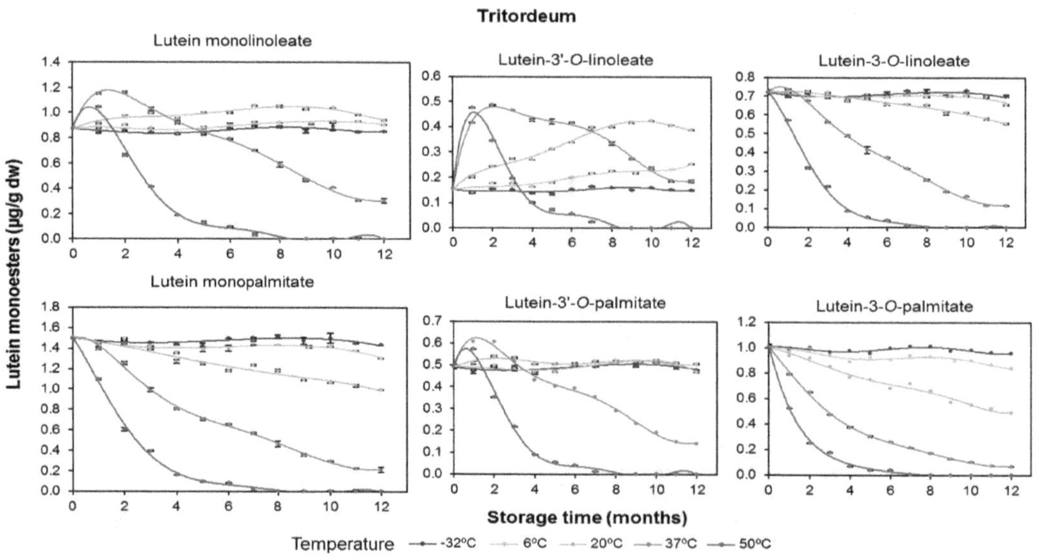

Figure 5. Evolution of the monoesterified lutein (µg/g dry weight), including the regioisomers, in tritordeum (HT621 advanced line) whole-grain flours during long-term storage under temperature controlled conditions (−32, 6, 20, 37 and 50 °C). The values shown are the mean and standard error (n = 5 for the starting sample, n = 3 for the rest of the samples).

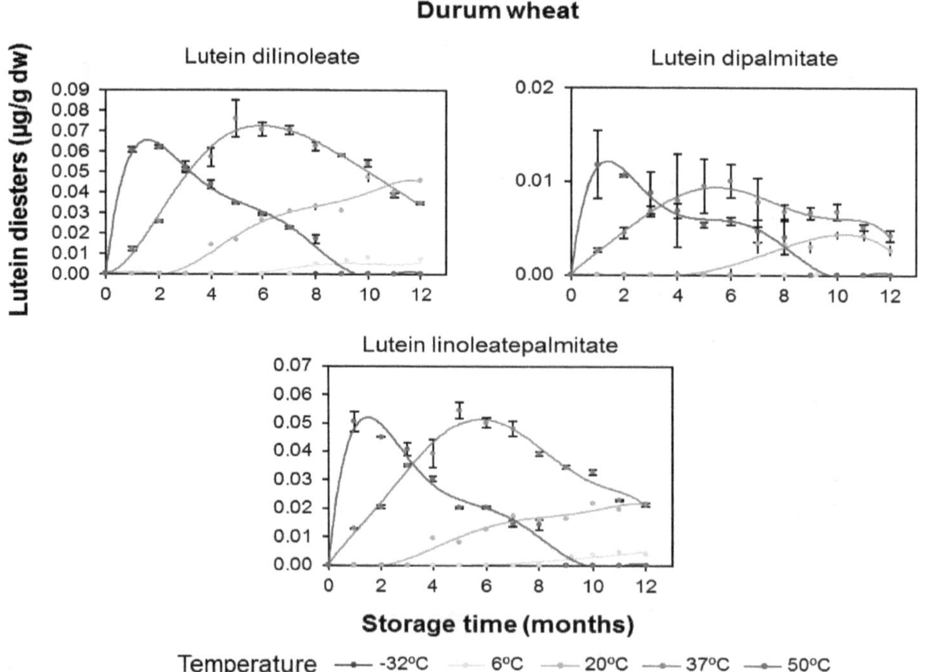

Figure 6. Evolution of the diesterified lutein (µg/g dry weight) in durum wheat (Don Pedro variety) whole-grain flours during long-term storage under temperature controlled conditions (−32, 6, 20, 37 and 50 °C). The values shown are the mean and standard error (n = 5 for the starting sample, n = 3 for the rest of the samples).

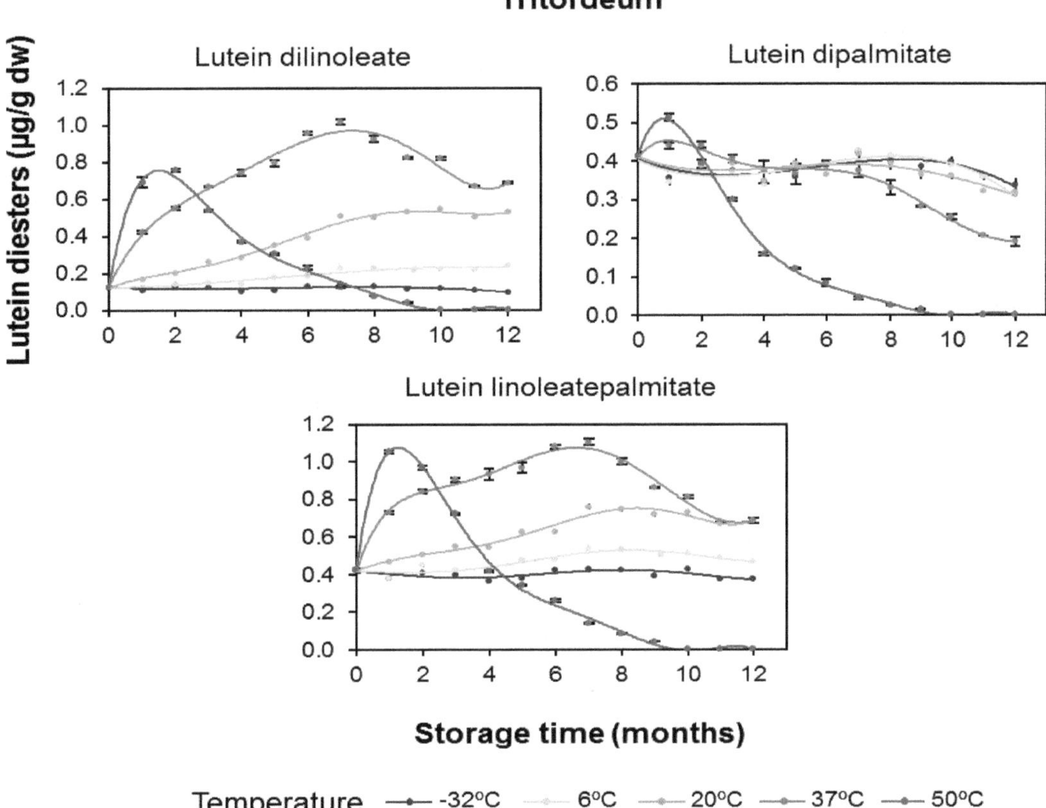

Figure 7. Evolution of the diesterified lutein (µg/g dry weight) in tritordeum (HT621 advanced line) whole-grain flours during long-term storage under temperature controlled conditions (−32, 6, 20, 37 and 50 °C). The values shown are the mean and standard error (n = 5 for the starting sample, n = 3 for the rest of the samples).

3.3. *Kinetics of Retention of Carotenoids during the Long-Term Storage of Wheat Flours*

A kinetic study indicated a progressive increase of the rate constants (k) with the rise of temperature for both cereal genotypes. Tables 3 and 4 summarized the kinetic data characterizing the evolution of both free and total pigments (including esterified pigments) during long-term storage assuming zero- and first-order kinetic models, respectively. As deducted from the correlation coefficient values, the first-order kinetic model showed best adjustment to the data, indicating that the degradation reaction rate is directly proportional to the pigment concentration ($-dC/dt = kC$; see Materials and Methods and Table 1). These results are consistent with those reported by other authors [32,41]. The reaction rates were higher in tritordeum for all pigments at 20, 37, and 50 °C, with β-carotene being an exception. At 50 °C, the k values for all xanthophylls were approximately double in tritordeum compared to durum wheat. Pigment structure (free or esterified with fatty acids), matrix effects (including the presence of oxidative enzymes and other antioxidants), and the oxidative stressing environment are likely to be key factors for this phenomena. The milling process, involving cell and tissue disruption, and the subsequent storage of cereal flours have also previously been found to affect carotenoid stability [42]. The possible presence of other antioxidants might also produce a protective effect on the carotenoids. For example, the changes and/or interactions between tocopherols and carotenoids during cereal processing have been analysed by several authors [43,44]. However, there is no information about such interactions in tritordeum, with further work needed in this area.

Table 3. Reaction rate constant (k; month^{-1}) for the total carotenoid content in durum wheat (Don Pedro variety) and tritordeum (HT621 line) whole-grain flours during a long-term storage period (12 months) at −32, 6, 20, 37, and 50 °C following the zero-order kinetic model (C-C_0 = $-kt$).

Pigment	T (°C)	Durum Wheat (Don Pedro Variety)		Tritordeum (HT621 Advanced Line)	
		k (×10^{-3} Month^{-1})	R^2	k (×10^{-3} Month^{-1})	R^2
(all-E)-Zeaxanthin	−32	0.2	0.33	-	-
	6	0.4	0.80	-	-
	20	4	0.98	-	-
	37	5	0.80	-	-
	50	3	0.43	-	-
(all-E)-Lutein	−32	1	0.06	7	0.15
	6	3	0.18	41	0.72
	20	42	0.98	198	0.96
	37	68	0.80	232	0.65
	50	51	0.47	160	0.33
Total free (Z)-Lutein	−32	0.3	0.04	2	0.14
	6	0.2	0.01	3	0.31
	20	5	0.92	15	0.97
	37	12	0.86	42	0.87
	50	10	0.63	28	0.57
(all-E)-β-Carotene	−32	0.1	0.35	0.1	0.02
	6	0.5	0.06	0.2	0.12
	20	8	0.93	2	0.95
	37	2	0.90	4	0.97
	50	1	0.62	4	0.62
Total free lutein	−32	1	0.06	9	0.19
	6	3	0.15	42	0.70
	20	47	0.98	213	0.95
	37	80	0.82	273	0.70
	50	60	0.50	188	0.36
Total free carotenoids	−32	1	0.01	9	0.19
	6	6	0.20	44	0.70
	20	50	0.96	215	0.96
	37	85	0.80	277	0.70
	50	64	0.48	192	0.36
Total lutein	−32	2	0.08	10	0.07
	6	4	0.15	29	0.21
	20	23	0.88	191	0.95
	37	85	0.95	432	0.95
	50	80	0.73	546	0.75
Total carotenoids	−32	0.8	0.01	10	0.07
	6	1	0.01	29	0.21
	20	33	0.88	192	0.95
	37	90	0.94	436	0.95
	50	83	0.71	550	0.75

Table 4. Reaction rate constant (k; month^{-1}), half-life ($t_{1/2}$; months), and D ($t_{1/10}$; months) for the total carotenoid content in durum wheat (Don Pedro variety) and tritordeum (HT621 line) whole-grain flours during a long-term storage period (12 months) at −32, 6, 20, 37, and 50 °C following the first-order kinetic model ($Ln(C/C_0) = -kt$).

Pigment	T (°C)	Durum Wheat (Don Pedro Variety)				Tritordeum (HT621 Advanced Line)			
		k (×10^{-3} Month^{-1})	R^2	$t_{1/2}$ (Months)	$t_{1/10}$ (D) (Months)	k (×10^{-3} Month^{-1})	R^2	$t_{1/2}$ (Months)	$t_{1/10}$ (D) (Months)
(all-*E*)-Zeaxanthin	−32	3	0.33	277	921	-	-	-	-
	6	5	0.79	141	470	-	-	-	-
	20	85	0.96	8	27	-	-	-	-
	37	252	0.97	3	9	-	-	-	-
	50	473	0.87	1	5	-	-	-	-
(all-*E*)-Lutein	−32	1	0.06	693	2302	2	0.15	385	1279
	6	3	0.18	217	719	12	0.72	60	198
	20	53	0.96	13	43	82	0.99	8	28
	37	191	0.97	4	12	329	0.99	2	7
	50	300	0.84	2	8	596	0.88	1	4
Total free (*Z*)-lutein	−32	2	0.04	385	1279	4	0.13	165	548
	6	0.7	0.00	990	3289	6	0.31	110	365
	20	38	0.93	18	60	39	0.98	18	59
	37	177	0.98	4	13	283	0.99	2	8
	50	249	0.88	3	9	559	0.99	1	4
(all-*E*)-β-Carotene	−32	5	0.35	139	460	1	0.02	576	1918
	6	2	0.06	462	1535	3	0.12	210	698
	20	45	0.90	16	52	38	0.95	19	62
	37	203	0.96	3	11	141	0.98	5	16
	50	387	0.95	2	6	417	0.99	2	6
Total free lutein	−32	1	0.07	693	2302	2	0.19	330	1096
	6	3	0.15	248	822	11	0.71	63	209
	20	51	0.97	14	45	76	0.99	9	30
	37	189	0.98	4	12	321	0.99	2	7
	50	290	0.85	2	8	630	0.94	1	4
Total free carotenoids	−32	0.7	0.01	990	3289	2	0.19	347	1151
	6	5	0.20	151	500	11	0.70	64	211
	20	53	0.96	13	44	75	0.99	9	31
	37	191	0.97	4	12	311	0.99	2	7
	50	296	0.85	2	8	636	0.94	1	4
Total lutein	−32	1	0.08	533	1771	1	0.07	495	1644
	6	3	0.15	248	822	4	0.21	178	590
	20	27	0.86	25	84	30	0.96	23	77
	37	145	0.98	5	16	103	0.98	7	22
	50	285	0.93	2	8	465	0.98	1	5
Total carotenoids	−32	0.5	0.00	1386	4604	1	0.07	495	1644
	6	0.9	0.01	770	2558	4	0.21	178	590
	20	30	0.87	23	78	30	0.96	23	77
	37	148	0.98	5	16	103	0.98	7	22
	50	290	0.93	2	8	466	0.98	1	5

The k values obtained for durum wheat were similar for xanthophylls and carotenes (β-carotene) with some exceptions (Table 4). (all-*E*)-Zeaxanthin was the pigment that was degraded most rapidly at all temperatures. As expected, the k value for zeaxanthin was maximum at 50 °C (473 × 10^{-3} month^{-1}), which is consistent with its complete disappearance at the seventh month in these conditions (Figure 2). Markedly, the differences between the k values for carotenes and xanthophylls were more evident in tritordeum flour. These results are in line with those obtained by Dhuique-Meyer et al. [45], whose study about the thermal degradation kinetics of vitamin C and carotenoids in citrus juices reported lower degradation rates for β-carotene than for xanthophylls.

The kinetic data obtained for the total carotenoids (which included the esterified pigments) confirmed a faster degradation in tritordeum than in durum wheat, especially at the higher storage temperatures, as indicated by the k values at 50 °C (Table 4). In the case of durum wheat flours, the k values at 20, 37, and 50 °C were consistently lower for total lutein and total carotenoids (including the xanthophyll esters) than for the respective free fractions, underlining the contribution of the esters to the greater stability of such fractions. Accordingly, this effect was more pronounced in tritordeum due to the higher content and proportion of esterified lutein.

The rate constants for lutein esters, including the distinction between regioisomers, are summarized in Table 5. In line with the results for total carotenoids (Table 4), the esterified fractions showed a higher degradation rate in tritordeum with compared to durum wheat. Notably, the k value for lutein diesters at 50 °C in tritordeum was double the k value in durum wheat. This result highlights an important turnover of diesters in durum wheat in accordance with a possible esterifying activity in this cereal. The differential content of other pro-oxidant and antioxidant substances in both cereal genotypes should also be considered. In any case, the k values decreased with an increase in the degree of esterification, with k lutein diester < k lutein monoester < k free lutein, resulting in an increased thermostability thereof. Regarding the regioisomers of the lutein monoesters (lutein monolinoleate and lutein monopalmitate), both positions 3 and 3′ had similar degradation rates for each lutein monoester. No relevant differences between free and esterified lutein (Tables 4 and 5) were found in durum wheat, with the exception of the diesters. In tritordeum, lower degradation rates were recorded for lutein monoesters and diesters, even at 50 °C, despite the intense degradative conditions at that temperature. Lutein-3′-*O*-monolinoleate showed a degradation rate approximately 3-fold lower compared to free lutein at 37 °C. Within the monoester fraction, lutein monolinoleate presented a slower degradation than lutein monopalmitate; the same trend was observed for the monoesters at position 3′ compared with the counterpart regioisomer at position 3. These data are consistent with the evolution described for the esterified fractions. In the case of the diesters, the degradation rates were even lower with no differences between the different acylated forms.

Table 5. Reaction rate constants (k; month^{-1}) for the esterified carotenoid content in durum wheat (Don Pedro variety) and tritordeum (HT621 line) whole-grain flours during a long-term storage period (12 months) at 20, 37, and 50 °C following the first-order kinetic model ($Ln(C/C_0) = -kt$).

Pigment	T (°C)	Durum Wheat (Don Pedro Variety)		Tritordeum (HT621 Advanced Line)	
		k ($\times 10^{-3}$ Month^{-1})	R^2	k ($\times 10^{-3}$ Month^{-1})	R^2
Lutein monolinoleate	20	-	-	-	-
	37	210	0.96	113	0.87
	50	262	0.96	388	0.90
Lutein-3′-*O*-linoleate	20	-	-	-	-
	37	184	0.94	103	0.91
	50	230	0.90	487	0.98
Lutein-3-*O*-linoleate	20	-	-	22	0.92
	37	200	0.95	140	0.94
	50	284	0.91	526	0.96
Lutein monopalmitate	20	-	-	34	0.97
	37	204	0.95	158	0.98
	50	332	0.94	544	0.96
Lutein-3′-*O*-palmitate	20	-	-	-	-
	37	201	0.95	147	0.97
	50	329	0.87	606	0.98
Lutein-3-*O*-palmitate	20	-	-	59	0.98
	37	186	0.96	228	1
	50	336	0.96	632	0.96
Total monoesters	20	-	-	13	0.78
	37	208	0.95	114	0.91
	50	310	0.94	471	0.95
Lutein-3,3′-dilinoleate	20	-	-	-	-
	37	111	0.90	85	0.92
	50	188	0.97	370	0.97
Lutein-3′-*O*-linoleate-3-*O*-palmitate plus Lutein-3′-*O*-palmitate-3-*O*-linoleate	20	-	-	-	-
	37	139	0.95	103	0.96
	50	201	0.96	400	0.97

Table 5. *Cont.*

Pigment	T (°C)	Durum Wheat (Don Pedro Variety)		Tritordeum (HT621 Advanced Line)	
		k ($\times10^{-3}$ Month^{-1})	R^2	k ($\times10^{-3}$ Month^{-1})	R^2
Lutein-3,3′-dipalmitate	20	-	-	-	-
	37	90	0.78	66	0.83
	50	156	0.96	451	0.98
Total diesters	20	-	-	-	-
	37	122	0.93	88	0.93
	50	190	0.98	395	0.97
Total esters	20	-	-	-	-
	37	162	0.96	-	-
	50	333	0.81	472	0.98

Half-life values ($t_{1/2}$; months) and D values ($t_{1/10}$; months) (Table 4) are a very useful tool for estimating the pigment concentration that will be retained in flours stored under controlled temperature conditions. Both parameters are inversely related to k values, so that an increase in the storage temperature results in a reduction in the $t_{1/2}$ and $t_{1/10}$ values. The half-life and D values were generally higher for durum wheat for all pigments at all storage temperatures. Thus, total free lutein and free carotenoids showed longer half-life values by 2 and 1 extra month, and D values of 5 and 4 extra months at 37 °C and 50 °C, respectively, for durum wheat compared to tritordeum. As an exception, the observed half-life and D values at 37 °C for total lutein and total carotenoids revealed the opposite situation, with tritordeum flour having higher values. These results are directly related to the higher content and proportion of esterified pigments in tritordeum, and they are in line with the lower carotenoid losses in tritordeum compared to durum wheat at 37 °C (Figure 1).

4. Conclusions

This comparative study evaluated the effects of processing and storage of whole-grain durum wheat and tritordeum flours on the total carotenoid content. The influence of the cereals' different genetic backgrounds was found to be important and the effect of storage was more severe on the carotenoid content of tritordeum. Tritordeum flour showed a lower retention of free and esterified carotenoids than durum wheat flour. This could be mediated by an increased esterifying activity in durum wheat flours and/or greater oxidative enzymatic activity, or a more oxidative environment in tritordeum flour. These results could be influenced by the fact that durum wheat varieties have generally suffered domestication and selective pressure by man for the preservation of the yellow colour trait. Our results suggest the occurrence of an enzymatic process, maybe a lipase, involved in the esterification of xanthophylls during the storage of these flours. The enzyme showed a preferential action for esterification of the hydroxyl group at position 3′ in the ε-ring of the lutein molecule with linoleic acid. We hypothesize that this process could be different to the one described in intact grains in which the responsible enzymes (XAT: xanthophyll acyltransferase) showed a preferential acylation for the β-ring and a higher selectivity for palmitic acid, and therefore further research needs to be carried out to contrast this hypothesis. In any case, the increase in esterified xanthophylls eventually derived in a higher stability and retention capacity for total carotenoids in both cereal flours. This study provides valuable information to inform the optimization of storage conditions for flours of durum wheat and the novel hybrid cereal tritordeum with the aim of preserving their phytochemicals. This information could also be used in crop biofortification programs for the selection of cereal varieties, such as tritordeum, with an enhanced content of esterified xanthophylls.

Acknowledgments: This work was supported by the Ministerio de Ciencia e Innovación (Spanish Government, Project AGL2010-14850/ALI) and the Consejería de Economía, Innovación, Ciencia y Empleo (Junta de Andalucía, Project P08-AGR-03477). E.M.-O. was the recipient of a JAE-Predoctoral grant (CSIC) co-financed by the ESF. D.H.-M. is member of CaRed Network funded by MINECO (BIO2015-71703-REDT) and EUROCAROTEN COST Action (CA15136). We acknowledge support of the publication fee by the CSIC Open Access Publication Support Initiative through its Unit of Information Resources for Research (URICI). We are grateful to Sergio G. Atienza (IAS-CSIC) for providing the plant material, and to Ruth Stuckey for language manuscript editing.

Author Contributions: D.H.-M. conceived and designed the experiments; E.M.-O. performed the experiments; D.H.-M. and E.M.-O. analyzed the data; D.H.-M. contributed reagents/materials/analysis tools; D.H.-M. and E.M.-O. wrote the paper.

References

1. Britton, G.; Liaaen-Jensen, S.; Pfander, H. *Carotenoids. Volume 1A: Isolation and Analysis*; Birkhäuser Verlag: Basel, Switzerland, 1995.
2. Howitt, C.A.; Pogson, B.J. Carotenoid accumulation and function in seeds and non-green tissues. *Plant Cell Environ.* **2006**, *29*, 435–445. [CrossRef] [PubMed]
3. Mayne, S.T. β-Carotene, carotenoids and disease prevention in humans. *FASEB J.* **1996**, *10*, 690–701. [PubMed]
4. Cooper, D.A. Carotenoids in health and disease: Recent scientific evaluations, research recommendations and the consumer. *J. Nutr.* **2004**, *134*, 221S–224S. [PubMed]
5. Britton, G.; Liaaen-Jensen, S.; Pfander, H. *Carotenoids Volume 5: Nutrition and Health*; Birkhäuser Verlag: Basel, Switzerland, 2009.
6. Landrum, J.T.; Bone, R.A. Lutein, zeaxanthin, and the macular pigment. *Arch. Biochem. Biophys.* **2001**, *385*, 28–40. [CrossRef] [PubMed]
7. Hentschel, V.; Kranl, K.; Hollmann, J.; Lindhauer, M.G.; Böhm, V.; Bitsch, R. Spectrophotometric determination of yellow pigment content and evaluation of carotenoids by high-performance liquid chromatography in durum wheat grain. *J. Agric. Food Chem.* **2002**, *50*, 6663–6668. [CrossRef] [PubMed]
8. Ficco, D.B.M.; Mastrangelo, A.M.; Trono, D.; Borrelli, G.M.; De Vita, P.; Fares, C.; Beleggia, R.; Platani, C.; Papa, R. The colours of durum wheat: A review. *Crop Pasture Sci.* **2014**, *65*, 1–15. [CrossRef]
9. Bai, C.; Twyman, R.M.; Farré, G.; Sanahuja, G.; Christou, P.; Capell, T.; Zhu, C.A. Golden era—Provitamin A enhancement in diverse crops. *In Vitro Cell. Dev. Biol. Plant* **2011**, *47*, 205–221. [CrossRef]
10. Martín, A.; Sanchez-Monge, E.L. Citology and morphology of the amphiploid *Hordeum chilense-Triticum turgidum* conv. *Durum*. *Euphytica* **1982**, *31*, 261–267. [CrossRef]
11. Atienza, S.G.; Ballesteros, J.; Martín, A.; Hornero-Méndez, D. Genetic variability of carotenoid concentration and degree of esterification among tritordeum (×*Tritordeum* Ascherson et Graebner) and durum wheat accessions. *J. Agric. Food Chem.* **2007**, *55*, 4244–4251. [CrossRef] [PubMed]
12. Mellado-Ortega, E.; Hornero-Méndez, D. Isolation and identification of lutein esters, including their regioisomers, in tritordeum (×*Tritordeum* Ascherson et Graebner) grains. Evidences for a preferential xanthophyll acyltransferase activity. *Food Chem.* **2012**, *135*, 1344–1352. [CrossRef] [PubMed]
13. Mellado-Ortega, E.; Hornero-Méndez, D. Carotenoid profiling of *Hordeum chilense* grains: The parental proof for the origin of the high carotenoid content and esterification pattern of tritordeum. *J. Cereal Sci.* **2015**, *62*, 15–21. [CrossRef]
14. Chavez, A.L.; Sanchez, T.; Ceballos, H.; Rodriguez-Amaya, D.B.; Nestel, P.; Tohme, J.; Ishitani, M. Retention of carotenoids in cassava roots submitted to different processing methods. *J. Sci. Food Agric.* **2007**, *87*, 388–393. [CrossRef]
15. Mugode, L.; Ha, B.; Kaunda, A.; Sikombe, T.; Phiri, S.; Mutale, R.; Davis, C.; Tanumihardjo, S.; De Moura, F. Carotenoid retention of biofortified provitamin A maize (*Zea mays* L.) after Zambian traditional methods of milling, cooking and storage. *J. Agric. Food Chem.* **2014**, *62*, 6317–6325. [CrossRef] [PubMed]
16. Fardet, A. New hypotheses for the health-protective mechanisms of wholegrain cereals: What is beyond fibre? *Nutr. Res. Rev.* **2010**, *23*, 65–134. [CrossRef] [PubMed]
17. Britton, G.; Khachik, F. Carotenoids in food. In *Carotenoids Volume 5: Nutrition and Health*; Britton, G., Liaaen-Jensen, S., Pfander, H., Eds.; Birkhäuser Verlag: Basel, Switzerland, 2009; pp. 45–66.

18. De Moura, F.F.; Miloff, A.; Boy, E. Retention of provitamin A carotenoids in staple crops targeted or biofortification in Africa: Cassava, maize, and sweet potato. *Crit. Rev. Food Sci. Nutr.* **2015**, *55*, 1246–1269. [CrossRef] [PubMed]
19. Hemery, Y.; Rouau, X.; Lullien-Pellerin, V.; Barron, C.; Abecassis, J. Dry processes to develop wheat fractions and products with enhanced nutritional quality. *J. Cereal Sci.* **2007**, *46*, 327–347. [CrossRef]
20. Li, L.; Yong, Y.; Qiang, X.; Owsiany, K.; Welsch, R.; Chitchumroonchokchai, C.; Lu, S.; Van Eck, J.; Deng, X.; Failla, M.; et al. The *Or* gene enhances carotenoid accumulation and stability during post-harvest storage of potato tubers. *Mol. Plant* **2012**, *5*, 339–352. [CrossRef] [PubMed]
21. Ortiz, D.; Rocheford, T.; Ferruzzi, M.G. Influence of temperature and humidity on the stability of carotenoids in biofortified maize (*Zea mays* L.) genotypes during controlled postharvest storage. *J. Agric. Food Chem.* **2016**, *64*, 2727–2736. [CrossRef] [PubMed]
22. Ahmad, F.T.; Asenstorfer, R.E.; Soriano, I.R.; Mares, D.J. Effect of temperature on lutein esterification and lutein stability in wheat grain. *J. Cereal Sci.* **2013**, *58*, 408–413. [CrossRef]
23. Mellado-Ortega, E.; Hornero-Méndez, D. Carotenoid evolution during short-storage period of durum wheat (*Triticum turgidum* conv. *durum*) and tritordeum (×*Tritordeum* Ascherson et Graebner) whole-grain flours. *Food Chem.* **2016**, *192*, 714–723. [CrossRef] [PubMed]
24. Mellado-Ortega, E.; Hornero-Méndez, D. Effect of long-term storage on free and esterified carotenoids in durum wheat (*Triticum turgidum* conv. *durum*) and tritordeum (×*Tritordeum* Ascherson et Graebner) grains. *Food Res. Int.* **2017**, *99*, 877–890. [CrossRef] [PubMed]
25. Ballesteros, J.B.; Ramírez, M.C.; Martínez, C.; Atienza, S.G.; Martín, A. Registration of HT621, a high carotenoid content tritordeum germplasm line. *Crop Sci.* **2005**, *45*, 2662–2663. [CrossRef]
26. Mellado-Ortega, E.; Atienza, S.G.; Hornero-Méndez, D. Carotenoid evolution during postharvest storage of durum wheat (*Triticum turgidum* conv. *durum*) and tritordeum (×*Tritordeum* Ascherson et Graebner) grains. *J. Cereal Sci.* **2015**, *62*, 134–142. [CrossRef]
27. Mínguez-Mosquera, M.I.; Hornero-Méndez, D. Separation and quantification of the carotenoid pigments in red peppers (*Capsicum annuum* L.), paprika and oleoresin by reversed-phase HPLC. *J. Agric. Food Chem.* **1993**, *43*, 1613–1620. [CrossRef]
28. Britton, G. UV/visible spectroscopy. In *Carotenoids. Volume 1B: Spectroscopy*; Britton, G., Liaaen-Jensen, S., Pfander, H., Eds.; Birkhäuser Verlag: Basel, Switzerland, 1995; pp. 13–62.
29. Upadhyay, S.K. Elementary. In *Chemical Kinetics and Reaction Dynamics*; Anamaya Publishers: New Delhi, India, 1996; pp. 1–45.
30. Gayen, D.; Ali, N.; Sarkar, S.N.; Datta, S.K.; Datta, K. Down-regulation of lipoxygenase gene reduces degradation of carotenoids of golden rice during storage. *Planta* **2015**, *242*, 353–363. [CrossRef] [PubMed]
31. Rani, K.U.; Prasada Rao, U.J.S.; Leelavathi, K.; Haridas Rao, P. Distribution of enzymes in wheat flour mill streams. *J. Cereal Sci.* **2001**, *34*, 233–242. [CrossRef]
32. Li, D.; Song, J.; Liu, C. Kinetic stability of lutein in freeze-dried sweet corn powder stored under different conditions. *Food Sci. Technol. Res.* **2014**, *20*, 65–70. [CrossRef]
33. Choe, E.; Lee, J.; Park, K.; Lee, S. Effects of heat pretreatment on lipid and pigments of freeze-dried spinach. *J. Food Sci.* **2001**, *66*, 1074–1079. [CrossRef]
34. Urquhart, A.A.; Altosaar, I.; Matlashewski, G.J.; Sahasrabudhe, M.R. Localization of lipase activity in oat grains and milled oat fractions. *Cereal Chem.* **1983**, *60*, 181–183.
35. Barros, M.; Fleuri, L.F.; Macedo, G.A. Seed lipases: Sources, applications and properties—A review. *Braz. J. Chem. Eng.* **2010**, *27*, 15–29. [CrossRef]
36. Farrington, F.F.; Warwick, M.J.; Shearer, G. Changes in the carotenoids and sterol fractions during the prolonged storage of wheat flour. *J. Sci. Food Agric.* **1981**, *32*, 948–950. [CrossRef]
37. Ahmad, F.T.; Mather, D.E.; Law, H.; Li, M.; Yousif, S.; Chalmers, K.J.; Asenstorfer, R.E.; Mares, D.J. Genetic control of lutein esterification in wheat (*Triticum aestivum* L.) grain. *J. Cereal Sci.* **2015**, *64*, 109–115. [CrossRef]
38. Mattera, G.; Cabrera, A.; Hornero-Méndez, D.; Atienza, S.G. Lutein esterification in wheat endosperm is controlled by the homoeologous group 7, and is increased by the simultaneous presence of chromosomes 7D and $7H^{ch}$ from *Hordeum chilense*. *Crop Pasture Sci.* **2015**, *66*, 912–921. [CrossRef]
39. Mattera, G.; Hornero-Méndez, D.; Atienza, S.G. Lutein ester profile in wheat and tritordeum can be modulated by temperature: Evidences for regioselectivity and fatty acid preferential of enzymes encoded by genes on chromosomes 7D and $7H^{ch}$. *Food Chem.* **2017**, *219*, 199–206. [CrossRef] [PubMed]

40. O'Connor, J.; Perry, H.J.; Harwood, J.L. A comparison of lipase activity in various cereal grains. *J. Cereal Sci.* **1992**, *16*, 153–163. [CrossRef]
41. Hidalgo, A.; Brandolini, A. Kinetics of carotenoids degradation during the storage of einkorn (*Triticum monococcum* L. ssp. *monococcum*) and bread wheat (*Triticum aestivum* L. ssp. *aestivum*) flours. *J. Agric. Food Chem.* **2008**, *56*, 11300–11305. [CrossRef] [PubMed]
42. Borrelli, G.M.; Troccoli, A.; Di Fonzo, N.; Fares, C. Durum wheat lipoxygenase activity and other quality parameters that affect pasta colour. *Cereal Chem.* **1999**, *76*, 335–340. [CrossRef]
43. Leenhardt, F.; Lyan, B.; Rock, E.; Boussard, A.; Potus, J.; Chanliaud, E.; Remesy, C. Wheat lipoxygenase activity induces greater loss of carotenoids than vitamin E during breadmaking. *J. Agric. Food Chem.* **2006**, *54*, 1710–1715. [CrossRef] [PubMed]
44. Fratianni, A.; Di Criscio, T.; Mignogna, R.; Panfili, G. Carotenoids, tocols and retinols evolution during egg pasta-making processes. *Food Chem.* **2012**, *131*, 590–595. [CrossRef]
45. Dhuique-Mayer, C.; Tbatou, M.; Carail, M.; Caris-Veyrat, C.; Dornier, M.; Amiot, M.J. Thermal degradation of antioxidant micronutrients in citrus juice: Kinetics and newly formed compounds. *J. Agric. Food Chem.* **2007**, *55*, 4209–4216. [CrossRef] [PubMed]

17

A Survey of Sodium Chloride Content in Italian Artisanal and Industrial Bread

Marina Carcea *, Valentina Narducci, Valeria Turfani and Altero Aguzzi

Research Centre for Food and Nutrition, Council for Agricultural Research and Economics (CREA-AN), Via Ardeatina 546, 00178 Roma, Italy; valentina.narducci@crea.gov.it (V.N.); valeria.turfani@crea.gov.it (V.T.); altero.aguzzi@crea.gov.it (A.A.)

* Correspondence: marina.carcea@crea.gov.it

Abstract: A nationwide survey on salt content in both artisanal and industrial bread was undertaken in Italy to establish a baseline for salt reduction initiatives. Excess sodium intake in the diet is associated with high blood pressure and the risk of cardiovascular diseases. Bread has been identified as a major contributor to salt intake in the Italian diet. Most of the bread consumed in Italy comes from artisanal bakeries so 135 artisanal bread were sampled in 56 locations from Northern to Southern Italy together with 19 samples of industrial bread representative of the entire Italian production. Sodium chloride content was analysed according to the Volhardt's method. A salt content between 0.7% and 2.3% g/100 g (as is basis) was found, with a mean value of 1.5% (Standard Deviation, 0.3). However, the majority of samples (58%) had a content below 1.5%, with 12% having a very low salt content (between 0.5% and 1.0%), whereas the remaining 42% had a salt content higher than the mean value with a very high salt content (>2.0%) recorded for 3% of samples. As regards the industrial bread, an average content of 1.6% was found (SD, 0.3). In this group, most of the samples (56%) had a very high content between 2.0% and 2.5%, whereas 5% only had a content between 1.1% and 1.5%. Statistics on salt content are also reported for the different categories of bread.

Keywords: salt; sodium chloride; artisanal bread; industrial bread

---

1. Introduction

One third of global deaths are due to cardiovascular diseases, including heart attacks, strokes and related diseases (World Health Organization, 2007). High blood pressure is the major risk factor and, according to a substantial body of epidemiological and interventional studies, an excess of sodium in the diet is the primary cause of hypertension [1–5]. Salt intake is thus being increasingly monitored and evaluated worldwide. The human physiological need of sodium is rated around 130–230 mg/day by the World Health Organization (WHO), but in many industrialized countries sodium intake is actually 3600–4800 mg/day [6]. This indicates that the mean salt intake of populations is well in excess of dietary needs and far from the WHO recommendation to have a salt intake <5 g/day [6], that is, 2000 mg/day of sodium.

In the last decades, a wide range of initiatives aimed at salt reduction (DASH: Dietary Approaches to Stop Hypertension, WASH: World Action on Salt and Health, National Salt Reduction Weeks, CASH: Consensus Action on Salt and Health) have been started at the international level to sensitize people about salt consumption and salt content in some food categories, to educate the population about the dangers of salt in excess, and to translate scientific evidence into public health policies and plans for reformulation of processed foods [1,3,5,7–11]. In fact, processed foods are the main source of salt in the diet, with cereal products contributing the most of the overall intake [6,10,12,13], especially in those countries where bread is consumed daily at every meal. A recent survey highlighted an average yearly consumption per capita of 64 kg in Europe with Italy ranking third after Germany and France (57 kg) [14].

When in 2008 the European Commission (EC) launched the EU Framework for National Salt Initiatives, an interdisciplinary Working Group for reduction of salt intake (GIRCSI) was established in Italy at the Ministry of Health [3] with the main objective to device strategies to reduce salt consumption in the population. Bread was identified as one of the first processed foods to address and the first steps to be taken were to measure and monitor the sodium content of bread to promote reformulation of foods containing less salt. Other European countries have launched initiatives to reduce salt content in bread and recently news has appeared on the Internet that Portugal will set mandatory maximum salt levels in bread by 2019 [15].

This paper represents the first comprehensive survey on the salt content in bread consumed by the Italian population, and the data reported here represent the baseline for the reformulation of salt reduced bread. Most of the bread consumed in Italy is produced by artisans in artisanal bakeries according to different recipes and procedures and only a small proportion of the market (around 10%) is covered by the industrial production: consequently, a great variability in salt content was expected. Several breads in Italy are also protected by European authenticity labels such as Protected Designation of Origin (PDO) and Protected Geographical Indication (PGI) labels. Both artisanal and industrial bread was considered in the present study. Moreover, a comparison between methods to determine Na content in flour and bread was made on selected bread samples to assess the reliability of the quick method which was used for sodium chloride determination in bread.

2. Materials and Methods

2.1. Samples and Sampling Method

Artisanal bread was purchased at selected bakeries in Northern, Central and Southern Italy particularly in places with a specific identity in terms of bread production. In each bakery, the most consumed types of bread were sampled. For the industrial sector, samples of all the Italian production available on the market were purchased at supermarkets and included sliced pan bread (12 samples) and "traditional-like" bread (6 samples). In total, 154 bread samples (kinds of bread) were collected, between winter 2009 and spring 2010. For each type of sample, a spreadsheet was filled with data concerning origin, ingredients, weight and baking method.

In detail, 19 samples of industrial bread were collected together with 135 samples of artisanal bread from 56 locations (Figure 1). Seven out of 154 samples (1 sample of industrial bread and 6 samples of artisanal bread) were declared, at purchase, without salt and subsequent analysis performed by us, confirmed this feature.

Samples of baking wheat flour (*Triticum aestivum* L. flour, which is the kind of flour mostly used in bread baking in Italy) of two different extraction rates according to the Italian law (0 and 00, ash content maximum 0.65% and 0.55% on dry matter, respectively) were purchased at a local supermarket and analysed for their sodium content.

2.2. Analytical Methods

Soon after purchase, representative portions of each type of bread were cut in small pieces, well homogenised and used for the following analyses. A portion of the sample was used to determine moisture according to ICC Standard No. 110/1 [16], whereas another portion was prepared according to AACC method 62-05 "Preparation of sample: bread" [17] by drying it at 35 °C overnight and grinding it by a MLI 204 laboratory mill (Bühler, Uzwil, Switzerland). The residual moisture in the sample was also determined according to the previous ICC Standard. The determination of chloride ion in bread samples was carried out by titration according to the AACC method 40-33 "Chloride in yeast foods—quantitative method (Volhardt's method)" [17]. Sodium chloride content was finally calculated based on the content of chloride ions in sample. Duplicate analysis was carried out for each sample. Duplicates differing by more than 0.20 were rejected and analysis repeated. Salt content in bread was expressed as percentage, as is basis.

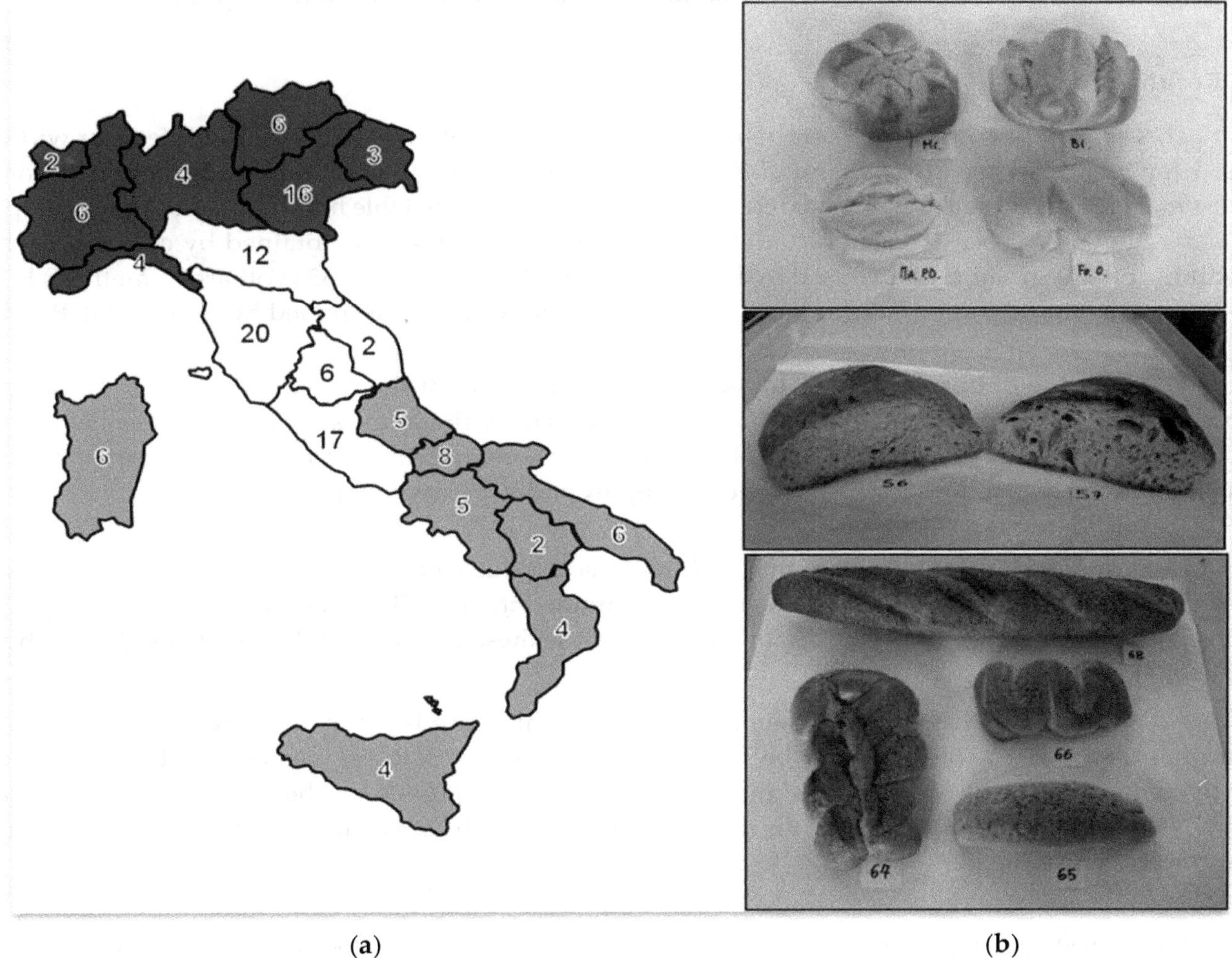

Figure 1. Bread samples collected in the different regions of Northern, Central and Southern Italy. (**a**) Number of samples from each Italian region. Northern regions are coloured in dark grey, Central regions in white and Southern regions in light grey (division according to the Italian Central Institute of Statistics). (**b**) Bread samples of different size, shape and ingredients.

A selection of bread and wheat flour samples were also analysed by Inductively Coupled Plasma Spectroscopy (ICP) on a Perkin-Elmer Plasma Optima 3200XL (Perkin-Elmer, Waltham, MA, USA) in order to determine sodium content in the raw material, and confirm that the results obtained by the AACC method were in good match with those obtained by ICP. Samples were first mineralized in nitric acid (6 mL HNO_3 + 1 mL H_2O_2) in a microwave oven (Milestone 1200 Mega, FKV srl, Torre Boldone, Italy). Standard CRM 189 (whole meal flour) from the Community Bureau of Reference (BCR, Brussels, Belgium) was used as a Reference Material.

2.3. Statistics

The seven samples of bread without salt were excluded from statistical elaboration. Statistical determination of mean, standard deviation and percentage distribution were performed using Microsoft Office Excel 2007. For easiness of results understanding and interpretation, it was decided to establish 4 classes of salt content (as is basis): (i) 0.5–1.0% (low salt content); (ii) 1.1–1.5% (medium salt content); (iii) 1.6–2.0% (high salt content); and (iv) 2.1–2.5% (very high salt content).

The percentage distribution in the above-mentioned salt content classes was calculated for 14 groups that represented all the different commercial categories that could be found in our sample population: all samples together, industrial vs. artisanal samples, 4 categories according to weight, 5 categories according to ingredients, and 2 categories according to leavening method.

3. Results

This section presents the results of analyses of sodium content in soft wheat white flour widely used for bread baking in Italy, and eight samples, selected for their different characteristics and presumably different salt content, are reported in Table 1. The same table briefly describes each sample compositional or processing characteristics. One column reports data obtained by calculating the sodium content in samples analysed by the standard AACC method 40-33 (Volhardt's method) [17], whereas the other column refers to the sodium content in samples determined by means of ICP.

The purpose of this study was to assess the contribution of the raw material flour to the salt content in bread, to verify whether the bread declared to be without any salt actually had a negligible sodium content, and whether the data obtained by the Volhardt's method could be compared with those obtained by a more sensitive but more complex and expensive method.

Data reported in Table 1 show that sodium was not detected in both types of commercial soft wheat white flours, even in the 0 type which is less refined than 00. Based on this result obtained with a very sensitive instrument, it was decided not to analyse these two samples by the Volhardt's method.

No sodium was detected following both analytical procedures in the three different bread samples declared by the bakers to be without salt addition. Sodium was detected by means of both methods in the five remaining samples and values ranged 03–06 for the Volhardt's method and 0.1970–0.4902 g/100 g (as is sample) for the ICP method. In both cases, the highest value was obtained for durum wheat bread.

Table 1. Sodium content in flour and bread samples as measured by two methods of different sensitivity.

Sample	Sodium Content Volhardt * (g/100 g)	Sodium Content ICP * (g/100 g)
Commercial white flour (Italian type 00)	not analysed	not detected
Commercial white flour (Italian type 0)	not analysed	not detected
Sample 1 (bread without salt, 500 g)	not detected	not detected
Sample 4 (bread without salt, 500 g)	not detected	not detected
Sample 14 (bread without salt, 500 g)	not detected	not detected
Sample 32 (common bread, 95 g)	0.3	0.2249
Sample 38 (wholemeal sourdough bread, 1.5 kg)	0.4	0.3283
Sample 25 (durum wheat bread, 170 g)	0.6	0.4902
Sample 57 (sourdough bread, 2 kg)	0.3	0.1970
Sample 67 (special bread, 200 g)	0.6	0.4552

* Average of two determinations on as is sample.

The statistical elaboration of salt content data referring to the 147 samples of salty bread is reported in Figures 2–5. In our survey, a salt content in bread ranging between 0.7% and 2.3% (as is basis) was found, with a mean value of 1.5% and a standard deviation (SD) of 0.3 (Figure 3). If we look at the distribution of salt content in the different classes as specified in the Materials and Methods Section, we can see that the majority of bread samples (58%) had a salt content below the reported mean value (>1.5%) (Figure 2a) with 12% having a very low salt content falling within the range 0.5–1.0%, whereas the remaining 42% had a salt content higher than the mean value with a very high salt content (>2.0%) recorded for 3% of samples.

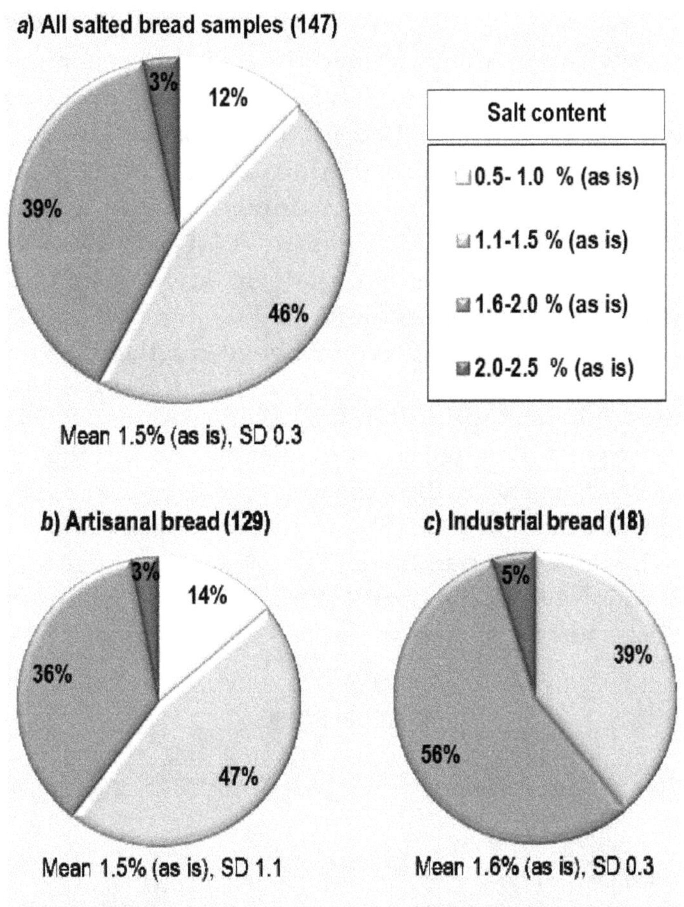

Figure 2. Percent distribution of bread samples according to salt content classes.

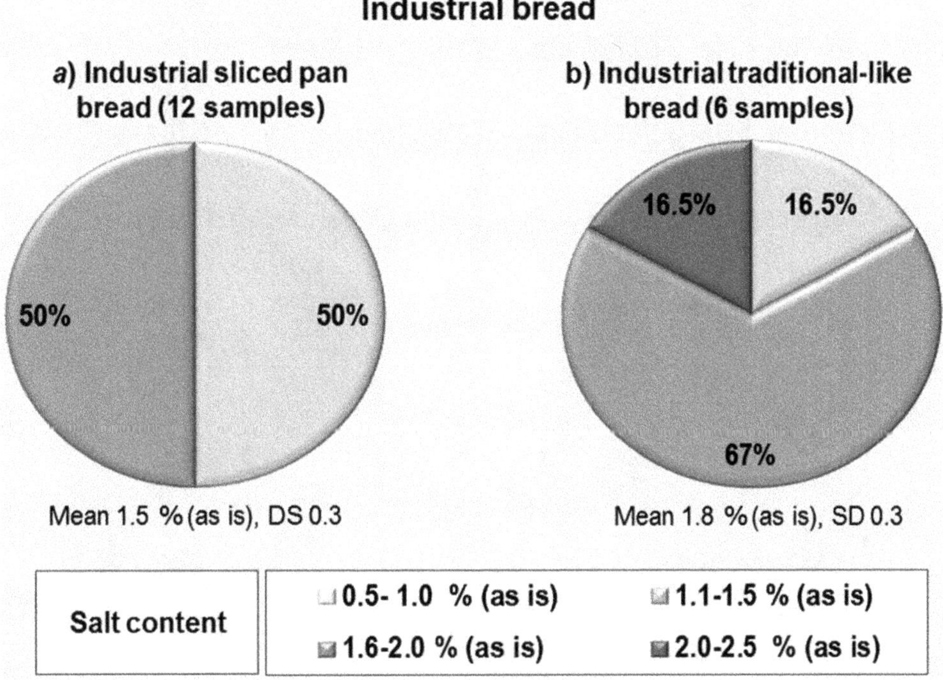

Figure 3. Percent distribution of industrial bread samples according to salt content classes.

If we have a separate look at the artisanal and the industrial production (Figure 2b,c), we can say that, although the average salt content in bread is very similar (1.5 and 1.6 g/100 g as is basis with standard deviations of 1.1 and 0.3, respectively), the distribution of our samples in the different salt content classes is different. In the artisanal bread, the majority of bread samples (61%) had a salt content below the reported mean value (>1.5%) (Figure 2a) with 14% having a very low salt content falling within the range 0.5–1.0%, whereas the remaining 39% had a salt content higher than the mean value with a very high salt content (>2.0%) recorded for only 3% of samples. In the industrial production, only three classes were represented, the very low salt content class (<1.0 g/100 g as is) having disappeared. Most of the samples (56%) had a very high salt content between 2.0 and 2.5 g/100 g (as is) whereas only 5% had a salt content between 1.1 and 1.5 g/100 g (as is).

A further differentiation can be made within the industrial bread by considering separately the sliced pan bread, which represents the most consumed category, and the so-called "traditional-like" bread which resembles more in its shape the artisanal bread (Figure 3). In the pan bread, a mean value of 1.5 g/100 g (as is) was obtained (SD 0.3) and two salt content classes (1.1–2.0%) were found, each having a 50% share, whereas in the traditional-like bread an average value of 1.8% g/100 g (as is) was found (SD 0.3) which derived from the contribution of three salt content classes (1.1–2.5%) with the very high salt content class having a share of 16.5%.

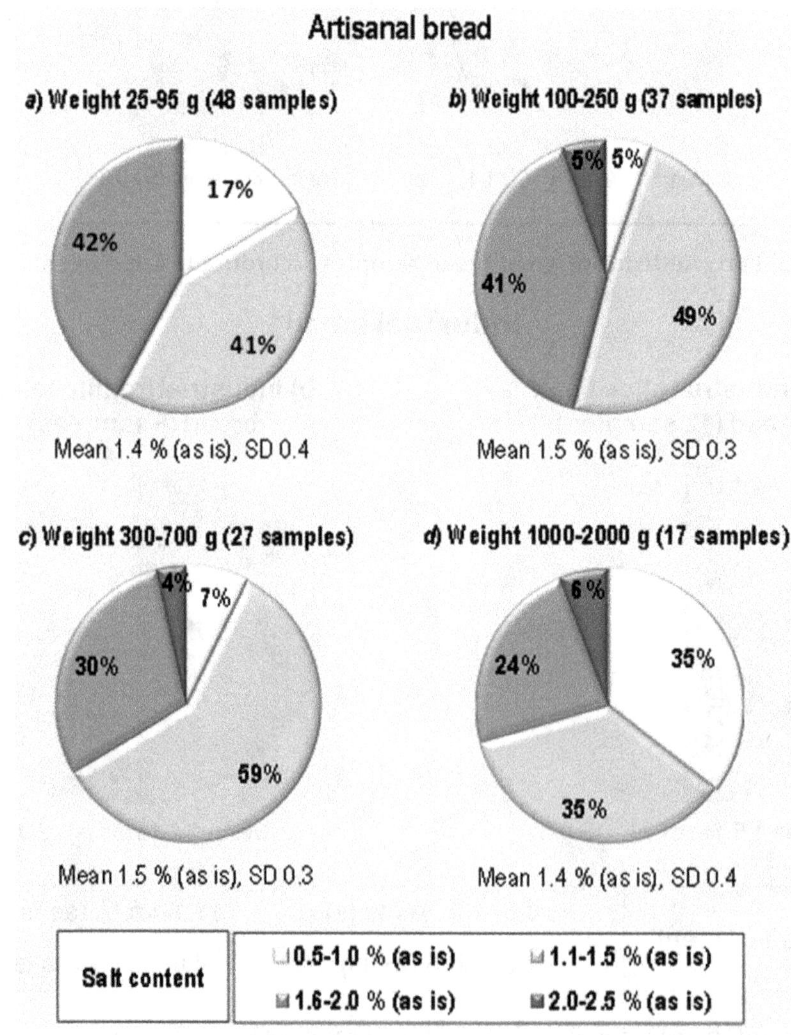

Figure 4. Percent distribution of artisanal bread samples of different weight according to salt content classes.

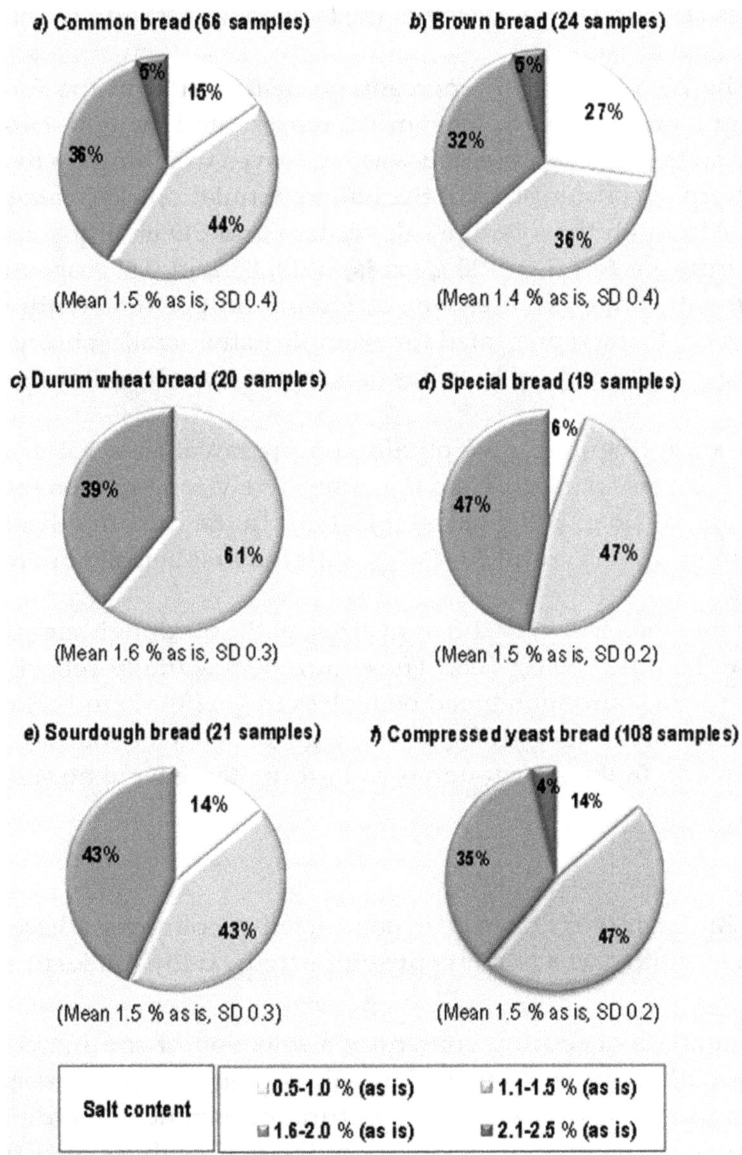

Figure 5. Per cent distribution of artisanal bread samples, differing in dough formulation and leavening method, according to salt content classes.

Given the great variety of artisanal bread, we thought it would be interesting to compare the salt content in different types of bread to determine whether there was any relationship between specific bread characteristics and salt content: weight, ingredients and leavening method were identified as interesting quality traits. The 129 artisanal bread loaves were, therefore, grouped into three different categories according to their weight, ingredients and leavening method. Within the "weight" category, four classes were identified based also on the bread shape: (i) 25–95 g (48 samples); (ii) 100–250 g (37 samples); (iii) 300–700 g (27 samples); and (iv) 1000–2000 g (17 samples), with rolls, typical of the bread production in Northern Italian regions, and big loaves typical of Central and Southern regions. Four classes were also established in the "ingredients" category as follows: common white bread, whose dough is typically formulated with just soft wheat flour, water and salt (66 samples); brown bread, with different amounts of soft wheat whole-meal flour in addition to the common white bread ingredients (24 samples); durum wheat bread (20 samples), typical of Southern Italy but also appreciated and consumed all over Italy made with remilled durum wheat semolina, water and salt; and "special" bread, that is, soft wheat white bread with other ingredients such as oil, milk, and potatoes (19 samples). As regards the leavening method, two classes were established: sourdough and compressed yeast.

Figure 4 reports the pie charts of the percentage distribution in the four salt content classes according to the weight of the bread. The most represented weight class was small breads, i.e., rolls (48 samples), and the least represented was big loaves weighing up to 2 kg. This distribution actually reflects the pattern of consumption of the Italian population. The categories up to 250 g were the most represented. Although the average salt content and SD is very similar or identical in the four groups and goes from 1.4 to 1.5 g/100 g (as is), (SD, 03 and 0.5, respectively), the percentage distribution of the four salt content classes was different and peculiar within each group with the highest salt content class not being represented for example in the smallest bread group and the biggest loaves having the highest percentage of samples (6%) having a salt content between 2.0% and 2.5% (as is).

For dough formulation (Figure 5), we obtained a mean value of 1.4 g/100 g (as is) (SD, 0.4), for brown bread, 1.5 g/100 g (as is) (SD, 0.4 and 0.2, respectively, for common bread and special bread), and for durum wheat bread, 1.6 g/100 g (as is) (SD, 0.3). In the durum wheat group, only two salt classes were found, namely 1.1–1.5% and 1.6–2.0%, with the first being more represented (61%) than the latter (39%).

The two leavening methods had very different sizes, with sourdough samples being only 21 while compressed yeast bread samples being 108. These numbers actually reflect the presence of these categories on the market with sourdough bread being less frequently found. However, the two groups had the same average salt content, 1.5 g/100 g (as is) (with SD = 0.3 for sourdough bread, and SD = 0.2 for compressed yeast bread). In the sourdough bread group, there were no samples with a very high salt content ($\geq$2.1%).

4. Discussion

Recently, several similar surveys have been conducted in countries where bread is a staple food and has therefore been identified as a major contributor to the daily intake of salt and sodium in the population [18–21].

In our study, the analysis of sodium content in a selection of commercial refined wheat flour and bread samples by ICP analysis showed that salt content in white bread, which is the most consumed type of bread in Italy, is not due to a natural occurrence of sodium in the flour, but to the salt added in the recipe. The higher sensitivity of the ICP analysis than the Volhardt's method enabled to confirm, in fact, that sodium naturally occurring in the white flour is negligible (Table 1) and, moreover, it showed that salt content in some of the sampled bread samples, declared at purchase to be "without salt", was, in fact, below 0.1%.

Even if there is no perfect correspondence between the results obtained by the two methods (Table 1), it is nevertheless interesting to notice that the ranking of the samples as regards their sodium content was the same. These results confirmed the practical value of the Volhardt's method for the determination of sodium chloride in bread and for the purpose of our study.

Although the average salt content found in all our bread samples (1.5% g/100 g, as is basis) is similar to that reported in the literature for other European countries [22], the range of values found was very wide with the highest values around 2.3%. This means that there is room for improvement and that salt reduction initiatives and campaigns are advisable also in Italy.

The statistical elaboration of data also showed an interesting variation of salt content in bread at geographical level. It emerged that the mean salt content in bread produced and consumed in Central Italy is slightly lower than in the north and south of the country. In fact, the mean salt content was 1.3% in the 52 bread samples from Central Italy with a SD of 0.4, whereas it was 1.6% with a SD of 0.2 in the 38 bread samples from Northern Italy, and 1.5% with a SD of 0.3 in the 39 bread samples from Southern Italy. In detail, it emerged that in Northern Italy there is no share of bread with a salt content below 1.0%, whereas 21% of analysed samples purchased in Central Italy and 15% of bread types sampled in Southern Italy were in this range. These figures confirm the existence of a well-established tradition in some regions of central Italy, e.g., Umbria, Marche and Tuscany, of producing bread loaves with a very low or null salt content. This evidence also hints at the fact that the main problem in salt reduction might be consumers' acceptance and salt content in bread might be reduced at the artisanal level without encountering too many technological problems.

Considering separately the artisanal production from the industrial production, even though in Italy the latter represents one fourth of the former, it is interesting to notice that the average salt content is higher in industrial bread (1.6% g/100 g, as is basis, with a SD of 0.3) than in the artisanal bread (1.5% g/100 g, as is, and a wider SD 1.1). and no samples were found falling within the class containing a small amount of salt (0.5–1.0%). Most industrial samples (56%) fall in the high salt content class (1.6–2.0%), whereas artisanal bread's most represented category (47%) is that of 1.1–1.5% salt content (medium salt content). The industrial production can easily be subdivided into two categories, namely pan bread (which is always sliced) and traditional-like bread which is more similar in shape and appearance to artisanal bread. They represent the two most common types of industrial bread that are produced by a few manufacturers in a homogeneous and standardized way, and distributed all over the national territory. It is interesting to notice that the pan bread had a more homogeneous salt content, ranging from 1.1% to 2.0% with an average of 1.5%, as is, and a SD of 0.3, whereas the traditional-like bread had 16.5% of samples having a salt content between 2.1% and 2.5% and a higher average content of 1.8% and the same value (0.3) of standard deviation.

The average content in Italian industrial bread is higher than that reported in other European countries such as UK, where in 2011 a National survey, promoted by the Consensus Action on Salt and Health (CASH), reported for industrial pre-packaged bread a salt content ranging between 0.58% and 0.83% [7].

In addition, in the industrial Italian production, it is advisable to reduce the salt content and, considering that most of the production is in the hands of few manufacturers, it should not be too difficult to reach this target. Moreover, being industrial bread generally supplied to canteens, hospitals and caterings, there are high chances that salt reduction initiatives can reach a broad number of consumers in a very short time even if the artisanal market share represents the biggest challenge for any future salt reduction initiative.

The analysis of salt content in bread according to its weight showed two significant pieces of evidence. In big loaves weighing 1000–2000 g (Figure 4d), there is a more consistent percentage of samples (35%) with a very low salt content (0.5–1.0%, as is basis). On the other hand, rolls weighing 25–95 g (Figure 4a) proved to be the only weight class with a salt content always below 2.0% and never reaching the very high content. Comparing the results obtained for the four classes under consideration with the mean salt content obtained for artisanal bread (1.5%, as is basis, with SD of 1.1), it emerged that a very good share of samples for each class has values below this mean: 57% of rolls (class 25–95 g), 54% of small loaves (class 100–250 g), 66% of medium loaves (class 300–700 g) and 70% of big loaves (class 1000–2000 g).

Considering dough formulation, i.e., the different raw materials used in bread making (Figure 5), it emerged that durum wheat bread had a more homogeneous salt content than common, brown or special bread: all samples belonged to only two salt classes, namely 1.1–1.5% and 1.6–2.0%. The main share (61%) is due to the lower salt content class. Considering the mean value of salt content in artisanal bread as a reference point for discussion, it was observed that 59% of common bread (Figure 5a), 63% of brown bread (Figure 5b), 61% of durum wheat bread (Figure 5c) and 53% of special bread (Figure 5d) samples have a salt content lower than this mean.

Bread samples with a salt content exceeding 2% belonged only to the class "common bread" and "brown bread", but at the same time brown bread is the category with the highest percentage (27%) of samples with a very low salt content (0.5–1.0%, as is basis) followed by common bread (15% of samples). The main difference between the sourdough and compressed yeast bread categories can be seen in the presence of 4% samples with a very high salt content (2.1–2.5%). The average content is the same for both categories, i.e., 1.5%, as is, but the SD is higher (0.3 versus 0.2) for sourdough bread. By focusing on the results obtained for the sourdough bread and brown bread categories, which had a significant percentage of the very low salt content, it could be speculated that the use of the sourdough and the formulation with wholemeal flours, can add to bread a natural flavour that prevents an excessive addition of salt to the dough.

5. Conclusions

The present study represents the first extensive survey on the actual salt content in Italian bread and provides the baseline for national salt reduction initiatives, as recommended by the European Commission (EC) to each country within the EU Salt Reduction Framework [8].

As regards artisanal bread, which is the type of bread mostly consumed by the Italian population, the survey highlighted a great variability of values obtained for salt content (from 0.7% to 2.3%, as is basis) that enabled both the identification of a market share offering bread with a high-salt content (2.0–2.5%) that should be immediately addressed by salt reduction policies and education campaigns, as well as the existence of a substantial share of bread with a low salt content that is in line with the EC and WHO recommendations. A good share of the Italian bakery market is represented by the long-established tradition of bread produced with a low salt content (0.5–1.0%) and widely consumed in some regions of Central Italy, e.g., Marche, Toscana and Umbria. This evidence indicates that technological strategies for low-salt bread manufacturing and campaigns for consumer education to gradual salt reduction in bread are possible with high chances of success.

As regards industrial bread, there is less variation in salt content compared to artisanal bread but it is on the high content side. However, future initiatives for salt reduction are more likely to be successful and reach in shorter times a major share of consumers because industrial bread production is controlled by a few manufacturers that distribute their standardized products all over Italy.

Author Contributions: M.C. planned and led the research and wrote the paper. M.C., V.N. and V.T. sampled the bread. V.N. and V.T. performed the experiments helped by A.A. who performed the ICP analysis. V.N. performed the statistical calculations and produced the figures.

Acknowledgments: The authors wish to thank Vittorio Vivanti (INRAN, Italy) and Licia Iacoviello (University of Molise, Italy) for their valuable collaboration in bread sampling, Paolo Fantauzzi for his technical assistance and Francesca Melini for her bibliographical help.

References

1. He, F.J.; MacGregor, G.A. A comprehensive review on salt and health and current experience of worldwide salt reduction programmes. *J. Human Hypertens.* **2009**, *23*, 363–384. [CrossRef] [PubMed]
2. Campbell, N.; Correa-Rotter, R.; Neal, B.; Cappuccio, F.P. New evidence relating to the health impact of reducing salt intake. *Nutr. Metab. Cardiovasc. Dis.* **2011**, *21*, 617–619. [CrossRef] [PubMed]
3. Strazzullo, P.; Cairella, G.; Campanozzi, A.; Carcea, M.; Galeone, D.; Galletti, F.; Giampaoli, S.; Iacoviello, L.; Scalfi, L. Population based strategy for dietary salt intake reduction: Italian initiatives in the European framework. *Nutr. Metab. Cardiovasc. Dis.* **2011**, *22*, 161–166. [CrossRef] [PubMed]
4. Wyness, L.A.; Butriss, J.L.; Stanner, S.A. Reducing the population's sodium intake: The UK Food Standards Agency's salt reduction programme. *Public Health Nutr.* **2011**, *15*, 254–261. [CrossRef] [PubMed]
5. Brindsen, H.C.; Farrand, C.E. Reducing salt; preventing stroke. *Nutr. Bull.* **2012**, *37*, 57–63.
6. World Health Organisation. Reducing Salt Intake in Populations. Report of a WHO Forum and Technical Meeting. Geneva, Switzerland, 2007. Available online: http://www.who.int/dietphysicalactivity/Salt_Report_VC_april07.pdf (accessed on 19 October 2018).
7. CASH Consensus Action on Salt and Health. 1996. Available online: http://www.actiononsalt.org.uk/about (accessed on 19 October 2018).

8. European Union. Implementation of the EU Salt Reduction Framework. Results of Member States Survey. 2012. Available online: http://ec.europa.eu/health/nutrition_physical_activity/high_level_group/nutrition_salt_en.htm (accessed on 19 October 2018).
9. He, F.J.; MacGregor, G.A. Reducing population salt intake worldwide: From evidence to implementation. *Prog. Cardiovasc. Dis.* **2010**, *52*, 363–382. [CrossRef] [PubMed]
10. Quilez, J.; Salas-Salvado, J. Salt in bread in Europe: potential benefits of reduction. *Nutr. Rev.* **2011**, *70*, 666–678. [CrossRef] [PubMed]
11. WASH World Action on Salt and Health. 2012. Available online: http://www.worldactiononsalt.com/ (accessed on 19 October 2018).
12. Lynch, E.J.; Dal Bello, F.; Sheehan, E.M.; Cashman, K.D.; Arendt, E.K. Fundamental studies on the reduction of salt on dough and bread characteristics. *Food Research Int.* **2009**, *42*, 885–891. [CrossRef]
13. Dötsch, M.; Busch, J.; Batenburg, M.; Liem, G.; Tareilus, E.; Mueller, R.; Meijer, G. Strategies to reduce sodium consumption: A food industry perspective. *Crit. Rev. Food Sci. Nutr.* **2010**, *49*, 841–851. [CrossRef] [PubMed]
14. Food. Pane Italia al terzo posto in Europa per i consumi. 2018. Available online: https://www.foodweb.it/2016/06/pane-italia-al-terzo-posto-per-i-consumi/ (accessed on 19 October 2018).
15. Food Navigator. Portugal to Set Mandatory Maximum Salt Levels in Bread. 2018. Available online: https://www.foodnavigator.com/Article/2018/07/23/Portugal-to-set-mandatory-maximum-salt-levels-in-bread# (accessed on 19 October 2018).
16. ICC. *Standard Methods of the International Association of Cereal Science and Technology*; The Association: Vienna, Austria, 2003.
17. AACC. *Approved methods of the American Association of Cereal Chemists*, 10th ed.; The Association: St. Paul, MN, USA, 2005.
18. Jafri, A.; El-Kardi, Y.; Derouiche, A. Sodium chloride composition of commercial white bread in Morocco. *East. Mediterr. Health J.* **2017**, *23*, 708–710. [CrossRef] [PubMed]
19. Al Jawaldeh, A.; Al-Khamaiseh, M. Assessment of salt concentration in bread commonly consumed in the Eastern Mediterranean region. *East. Mediterr. Health J.* **2018**, *24*, 18–24. [CrossRef] [PubMed]
20. Coyne, K.J.; Baldridge, A.S.; Huffman, M.D.; Jenner, K.; Xavier, D.; Dunford, E.K. Differences in the sodium content of bread products in the USA and UK: Implications for policy. *Public Health Nutr.* **2018**, *21*, 632–636. [CrossRef] [PubMed]
21. Pérez Farinós, N.; Santos nSanz, S.; Dal Re, M.-A.; Yusta Boyo, M.J.; Robledo, T.; Castrodeza, J.J.; Campos Amado, J.; Villar, C. Salt content in bread in Spain, 2014. *Nutr. Hosp.* **2018**, *35*, 650–654. [CrossRef] [PubMed]
22. Joossens, J.V.; Sasaki, S.; Kesteloot, H. Bread as a source of salt: an international comparison. *J. Am. Coll. Nutr.* **1994**, *13*, 179–183. [CrossRef] [PubMed]

18

Can *Zymomonas mobilis* Substitute *Saccharomyces cerevisiae* in Cereal Dough Leavening?

Alida Musatti, Chiara Mapelli, Manuela Rollini, Roberto Foschino and Claudia Picozzi *

Dipartimento di Scienze per gli Alimenti, la Nutrizione, l'Ambiente, Università degli Studi di Milano, 20133 Milan, Italy; alida.musatti@unimi.it (A.M.); chiara.mapelli1@unimi.it (C.M.); manuela.rollini@unimi.it (M.R.); roberto.foschino@unimi.it (R.F.)

* Correspondence: claudia.picozzi@unimi.it

Abstract: Baker's yeast intolerance is rising among Western populations, where *Saccharomyces cerevisiae* is spread in fermented food and food components. *Zymomonas mobilis* is a bacterium commonly used in tropical areas to produce alcoholic beverages, and it has only rarely been considered for dough leavening probably because it only ferments glucose, fructose and sucrose, which are scarcely present in flour. However, through alcoholic fermentation, similarly to *S. cerevisiae*, it provides an equimolar mixture of ethanol and CO_2 that can rise a dough. Here, we propose *Z. mobilis* as a new leavening agent, as an alternative to *S. cerevisiae*, overcoming its technological limit with different strategies: (1) adding glucose to the dough formulation; and (2) exploiting the maltose hydrolytic activity of *Lactobacillus sanfranciscensis* associated with *Z. mobilis*. CO_2 production, dough volume increase, pH value, microbial counts, sugars consumption and ethanol production were monitored. Results suggest that glucose addition to the dough lets *Z. mobilis* efficiently leaven a dough, while glucose released by *L. sanfranciscensis* is not so well fermented by *Z. mobilis*, probably due to the strong acidification. Nevertheless, the use of *Z. mobilis* as a leavening agent could contribute to increasing the variety of baked goods alternative to those leavened by *S. cerevisiae*.

Keywords: *Zymomonas mobilis*; *Lactobacillus sanfranciscensis*; sourdough; dough leavening; bakery products; *Saccharomyces cerevisiae*; anti-*S. cerevisiae* antibodies

---

1. Introduction

In the last decades, the research in human nutrition has aimed both at improving food safety and demonstrating new healthy properties of foods or ingredients. Particularly in the grain cereals area, great attention has been paid to the study of sourdough microbial ecology [1,2] and to the positive effects of lactic acid bacteria (LAB) and yeast fermentation on the technological characteristics of dough. Therefore, several contributions have led to the enhancement of baked products by using a sourdough technology, which also matches consumer's choices in terms of their preference towards the valorisation of traditional products that can be certified [3]. Organic acid production impacts on sourdough texture and product shelf-life, with acetic acid also displaying anti-ropiness and antifungal activities [4,5]. Acidification also helps to activate endogenous cereal proteases that release peptides and amino acids related to flavour formation [6]. The production of bacteriocins allows microorganisms to control the sourdough ecosystem [7], while the synthesis of homo-polysaccharides delays firmness and staling [6]. Sourdough fermentation can also have positive nutritional implications by biodegrading phytates, thus increasing mineral bioavailability, and by lowering the glycaemic response to the consumption of baked goods [6].

Nevertheless, adverse food reactions, such as baker's yeast intolerance, have recently been increasing among Western population [8]. Apart from in well-known alcoholic beverages, such as beer, wine and cider, and baked goods, *S. cerevisiae* is also used in savoury spreads, as a food supplement in 'multi-vitamin' preparations and 'probiotics' in animal feed [9], and even in vaccine production [10]. It is therefore clear that we are often exposed to yeast parietal components [11].

Several studies report that an adverse response to baker's yeast occurs in a proportion of patients with Inflammatory Bowel Disease (IBD). In particular, in patients with Crohn's disease (CD), *S. cerevisiae* is recognized as an antigen, and anti-*S. cerevisiae* antibodies (ASCAs), directed against the cell wall mannan (phosphopeptidomannan) of yeast, have been identified as an important serological marker of this pathogenesis. However, the determination of ASCAs is also reliable in other autoimmune disorders besides CD [12]. Environmental factors such as food antigens may play an important role in the pathogenesis of autoimmune disorders [10,13] and obesity [9]. Although there is scarce literature on allergy-hypersensitivity to yeasts, some clinical conditions might benefit from reduced exposure to these microorganisms [14].

Based on these considerations, the study of new microbial resources to be applied in leavened goods may be considered of actual relevance; in this context, the possibility of replacing *S. cerevisiae* is noteworthy. The use of *Zymonomas mobilis* as leavening agent can contribute to an increase in the variety of bakery products alternative to those leavened by yeast in order to meet the specific demands of consumers. *Z. mobilis* can therefore be an interesting candidate to create a new food area of yeast-free baked goods. This bacterium is commonly used in tropical areas as a fermenting agent of plant saps to obtain alcoholic beverages such as pulque [15]. *Z. mobilis* ferments only glucose, fructose and sucrose, and through alcoholic fermentation it provides an equimolar mixture of ethanol and CO_2 that can theoretically leaven a dough [16], just like *S. cerevisiae*. The narrow range of fermentable substrates is a technological limit of *Z. mobilis* vs *S. cerevisiae* that may be overcome by: (1) adding a fermentable sugar to the dough formulation; or (2) exploiting maltose hydrolytic activity of *Lactobacillus sanfranciscensis* associated with *Z. mobilis*. This unconventional association has been investigated as a model system (higher cell concentration and leavening temperature, shorter leavening time) in a previous paper [17]. The present research aims to compare *Z. mobilis* leavening performance when glucose is added to the dough both with its fermentative ability when *Z. mobilis* is in association with *L. sanfranciscensis* and in doughs formulated and processed similarly to a type I sourdough.

2. Materials and Methods

2.1. Microorganisms and Maintenance

Z. mobilis subs. *mobilis* type strain DSM 424 (DSMZ: Deutsche Sammlung von Mikroorganismen und Zellkulturen GmbH) and *L. sanfranciscensis* DSM 20663 were used in this study.

Z. mobilis was maintained in liquid DSM medium, while biomass production was carried out in liquid IC G20 medium (as previously reported) [16]. Both media contain bacto-peptone (Costantino SpA, Turin, Italy) 10 g/L and glucose (Sigma Aldrich, St. Louis, MO, USA) 20 g/L, while they differ for yeast extract (Costantino SpA) 10 g/L present in DSM medium and of casein enzymatic hydrolysate (Costantino SpA) 10 g/L in IC G20. For both media, the pH was set at 6.8, and sterilization occurred at 112 °C for 30 min.

L. sanfranciscensis was maintained and cultivated in MRSm medium as reported elsewhere [17]. Cultures were incubated at 30 °C in stationary conditions for 16–24 h. Stock cultures of both microorganisms were stored at −80 °C in the same media (DSM for *Z. mobilis* and MRSm for *L. sanfranciscensis*) added with 20% (*v*/*v*) glycerol (VWR International, Leuven, Belgium).

2.2. Biomass Production

Z. mobilis was cultured in 1 L flasks containing 600 mL of liquid IC G20 medium, inoculated with 5% (*v*/*v*) of a 9 h pre-culture grown in DSM medium. *L. sanfranciscensis* was grown in 1 L flasks containing 600 mL of MRSm medium, inoculated with 2% (*v*/*v*) of a 24 h pre-grown culture in the same medium. Cultures were incubated at 30 °C in stationary conditions for 16 h for *Z. mobilis* and 24 h for *L. sanfranciscensis*.

The determination of the cell biomass was performed by spectrophotometric measurement (OD 600 nm, 6705 UV-Vis Spectrophotometer, Jenway, UK). For each strain, at 16 h in the case of *Z. mobilis* and 24 h for *L. sanfranciscensis*, a calibration curve was built (OD 600 vs. CFU (colony-forming unit)/mL) to determine the proper culture volume to add in the dough preparation (cell concentration expressed as Log CFU/g dough).

2.3. Dough Production and Analytical Determinations

Doughs were prepared with 333 g of a commercial type 0 Manitoba wheat flour (Simec SpA, Santa Giusta, Oristano, Italy) and 167 mL of distilled water, with or without addition of 1 or 5% (*w*/*w* flour) glucose. *Z. mobilis* was added alone (7 Log CFU/g dough) or with *L. sanfranciscensis* (5 Log CFU/g dough) yielding to 100:1 ratio *Zymomonas*:*Lactobacillus* cells. Ingredients were mixed in a food mixer (CNUM5ST, Bosch, Stuttgart, Germany) at speed 1 for 6 min. The dough was divided into 3 sections, treated as follows and then incubated at 26 °C:

- 400 g, inserted into a 1 L graduate cylinder to evaluate the dough volume increase up to 24 h of leavening;
- 25 g, inserted into a double chamber flask connected with a graduate burette filled with acidified water, to evaluate the total amount of CO_2 produced during leavening [16];
- The remaining sample was left to leaven into a Becker; samples were taken at appropriate intervals to determine dough pH, microbial counts and to carry out HPLC (high performance liquid chromatography) analysis.

Each analysis was performed at 0, 8, 16 and 24 h of leavening time.

2.4. Evaluation of Dough Volume Increase and Total CO_2 Production

The increase in the dough volume (mL) was evaluated at appropriate time intervals through the record of the level reached by the dough inside the graduate cylinder. CO_2 production (mL) was monitored by measuring the level reached by the liquid present inside the burette connected to the double chamber flask.

2.5. Determination of the Microbial Populations in Doughs

Approximately 10 g of dough sample were decimally diluted in sterile peptone water (10 g/L Bacto-peptone (Costantino SpA), pH 6.8) and homogenized in a Stomacher 400 Circulator (Seward, Worthing, UK) for 5 min at 260 rpm. The appropriate dilutions were plated onto MRSm agar (MRSm broth added with agar 15 g/L) for the determination of *L. sanfranciscensis* population, as well as onto DSM agar (DSM broth added with agar 15 g/L) for *Z. mobilis*. Plates were incubated at 30 °C for 3 d in anaerobic conditions. Aerobic bacterial count (ABC) was determined by pour plating in Tryptic Soy Agar (TSA, Scharlab, Barcelona, Spain) after incubation at 30 °C for 48–72 h. The enumeration of yeasts and moulds were carried out in Yeast Glucose Chloramphenicol Agar (YGC-Scharlab, Barcelona, Spain) plates after incubating at 25 °C for 3–5 day.

2.6. HPLC Analyses and pH Monitoring

Maltose and glucose consumption, as well as ethanol production during leavening, were measured through an HPLC system (L 7000, Merck Hitachi, Tokyo, Japan) as reported by Musatti et al. [17]. Briefly, 4 mL of homogenized dough samples were centrifuged (Eppendorf 5804 (Hamburg, Germany), 10,600× *g*, 10 min) and supernatants were filtered (0.45 μm syringe filter, VWR International, Radnor, PA, USA) before HPLC analysis. Data refer to 1 g dough (mg/g dough).

Dough pH was monitored at different intervals on the integral undiluted dough sample (pH-meter Eutech Instruments pH 510, Toronto, ON, Canada).

2.7. *Statistical Analysis*

All samples were prepared and analysed at least in triplicate. The effect of two factors, such as % glucose addition or *L. sanfranciscensis* co-inoculation, on some fermentation parameters were investigated by ANOVA according to the general linear model. Results of microbiological counts were transformed in the respective decimal logarithms to match a normal distribution of values. Data were processed with Statgraphic R Plus 5.1 for Windows (StatPoint, Inc., Herndon, VA, USA). When the effect was significant ($p < 0.05$), differences between means were separated by LSD test of multiple comparisons.

3. Results and Discussion

3.1. *Trials with Glucose Addition into Dough*

Dough samples were prepared with or without glucose addition (1% and 5% *w/w*). When glucose was not added, *Z. mobilis* fermented only the glucose amount naturally present in the flour (around 2.01 $\pm$ 0.59 mg/g dough). However, even if there are some hydrolytic enzymatic activities in the dough due to the presence of endogenous amylases, the low glucose concentration does not allow adequate CO_2 production to obtain a suitable dough volume increase by *Zymomonas*, especially in the first times of incubation.

The need to add a fermentable carbon source to the flour, in order to obtain a leavening of the dough, had already been highlighted in a previous work [16]. Actually, the results confirmed that the addition of glucose increases the CO_2 production ($p = 0.001$), and that in the three tested conditions mean values became statistically different at 16 h leavening time ($p = 0.007$) (Figure 1). Similarly, the addition of glucose allowed the doubling of the dough volume within the considered incubation time. As expected, the highest CO_2 production is related to the highest dough volume increase; in particular, with 5% glucose, the mean value of dough volume reached more than 850 mL ($p = 0.019$) with respect to an average of 815 or 735 mL with 1% or without glucose addition, respectively. CO_2 production was also related to bacterial growth; when no glucose is added, *Z. mobilis* grew approximately 1.3 Log CFU/g in 24 h, and around 1.6–2 Log CFU/g in the presence of 1% and 5% glucose, respectively. The performances obtained in dough samples with the two glucose concentrations were not significantly different between them, but both were statistically different from those obtained without glucose ($p < 0.001$).

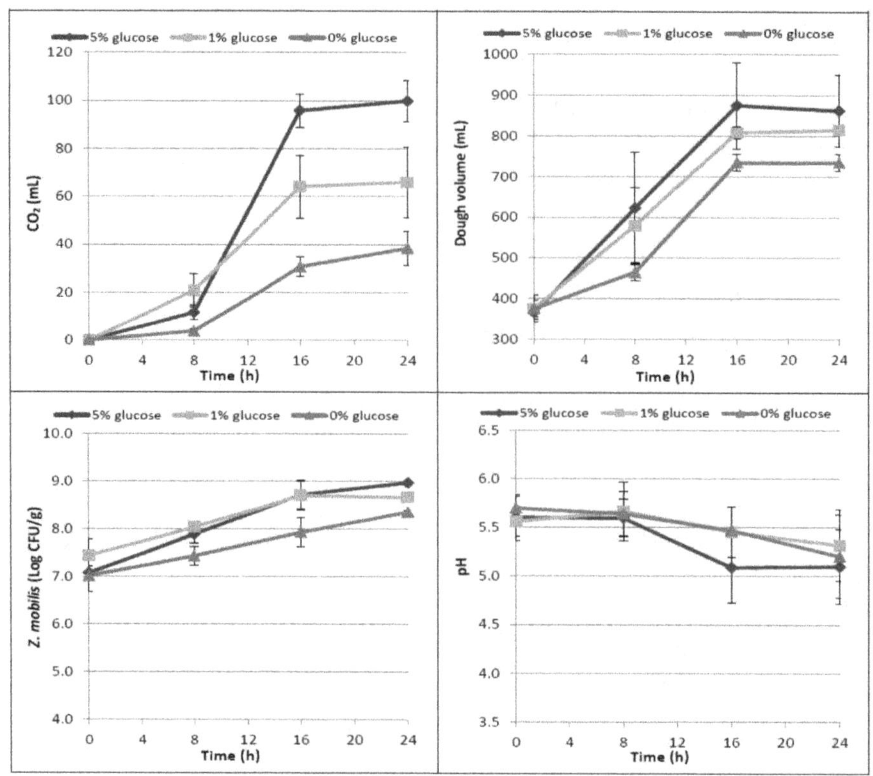

Figure 1. Time course of CO_2 production (mL), dough volume increase (mL), microbial growth of *Z. mobilis* (Log CFU/g) and dough pH in the three tested conditions (0%, 1%, 5% *w/w* glucose).

Results from HPLC analysis confirmed the increase of maltose during leavening time ($p < 0.001$) due to hydrolytic activity of the flour amylases and *Z. mobilis* inability to use this sugar (Table 1). At up to 8 h of incubation, the ethanol formation was not statistically different ($p = 0.414$), even if the three tested conditions had different levels of glucose. Then, glucose was mainly consumed between 8 and 16 h, producing CO_2 and ethanol in higher amounts in samples to which 5% glucose was added, as expected.

Table 1. Maltose, glucose and ethanol concentrations (expressed in terms of mg/g dough, mean and standard deviation (St. dev.)) present at 0, 8, 16 and 24 h in doughs leavened by *Z. mobilis* with 0%, 1%, 5% (*w/w*) of glucose added respect to the flour.

Glucose (% *w/w* flour)	Time (h)	Maltose (mg/g)		Glucose (mg/g)		Ethanol (mg/g)	
		Mean	St. dev.	Mean	St. dev.	Mean	St. dev.
0	0	10.50	0.96	1.96	0.06	0.00	0.00
	8	14.59	1.67	1.12	0.13	1.14	0.13
	16	17.71	3.16	0.23	0.33	2.79	0.49
	24	15.69	2.65	0.00	0.00	3.38	0.33
1	0	10.55	1.11	8.72	0.41	0.00	0.00
	8	15.48	5.22	3.42	0.62	1.84	0.41
	16	19.00	1.59	1.23	0.54	4.03	1.02
	24	21.43	4.49	0.92	0.44	3.96	0.77
5	0	8.33	0.95	35.72	2.95	0.00	0.00
	8	15.72	3.29	34.56	1.62	0.72	1.01
	16	18.57	2.84	2.66	1.48	9.73	0.13
	24	20.80	2.92	1.46	0.40	13.65	2.46

3.2. Bacterial Association *Z. mobilis-L. sanfranciscensis*

The association of *Zymomonas* with lactic acid bacteria has already been described in various food products, especially in some fermented drinks [18–21]. From this perspective, the possibility of obtaining a gradual glucose release in the dough exploiting the maltose hydrolytic activity of *Lactobacillus sanfranciscensis* was investigated [17].

When *L. sanfranciscensis* and *Z. mobilis* were inoculated together, the mean values of CO_2 production and dough volume increase did not significantly differ from those obtained with the use of *Z. mobilis* alone (Figure 2). Dealing with the single leavened samples, dough volumes at 16 and 24 h were found to be statistically different from those observed by using *L. sanfranciscensis* alone ($p = 0.023$ and 0.024, respectively). These results indicate that the contribution of the two microorganisms in association is not additive. Respect to the trials performed with glucose addition, in which the dough volumes nearly doubled in the first 8 h, the dough volume increased less than 20% in the case of the microbial association. As regards the trends of acidification and bacterial counts during the incubation time, the obtained data proved to be strongly affected by the presence of *L. sanfranciscensis*: the pH decreased to values of around 4 and the LAB growth (plus 4 Log CFU/g) was not influenced by the presence of *Zymomonas*. On the contrary, *Z. mobilis*, when grown in association with *L. sanfranciscensis*, statistically reduced ($p = 0.002$) its cell concentration from 16 h leavening onward. This behavior is probably due to the strong acidification of the medium produced by *L. sanfranciscensis*, able to affect both *Z. mobilis* vitality and fermentation ability.

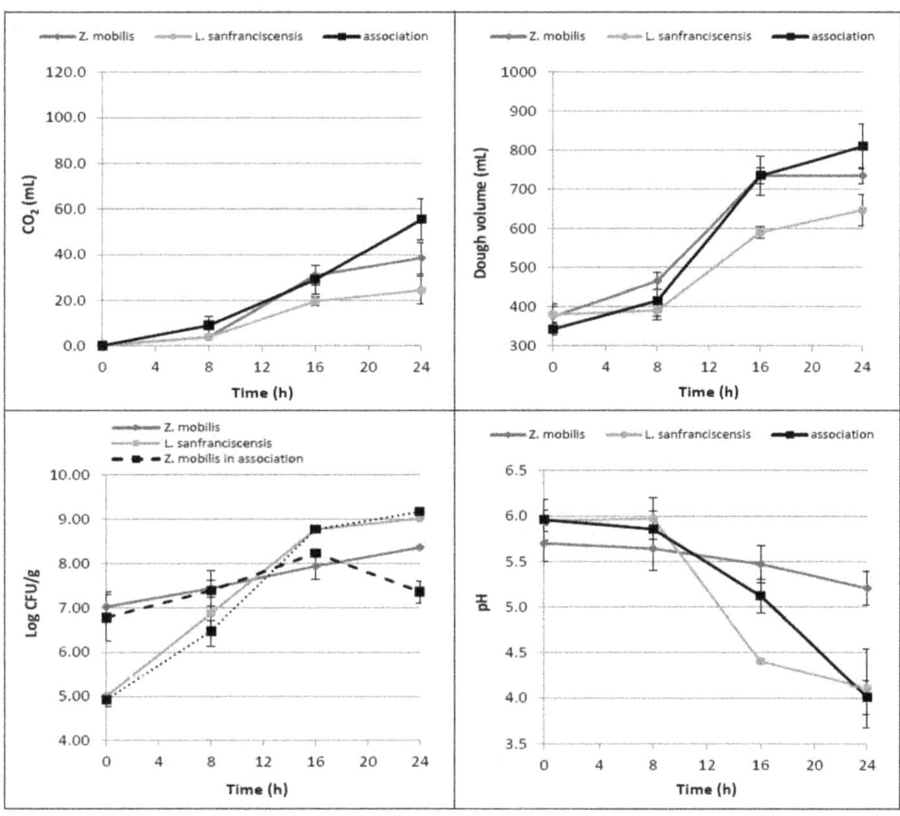

Figure 2. Time course of CO_2 production (mL), dough volume increase (mL), microbial growth (Log CFU/g) as well as dough pH, in doughs leavened by *Z. mobilis* and *L. sanfranciscensis* alone or by their association.

HPLC data confirmed that *L. sanfranciscensis* consumed maltose ($p = 0.012$) and released glucose ($p = 0.003$) in the dough [4], that it is not totally consumed by *Z. mobilis* (Table 2).

In summary, these results highlight that when inoculated alone, *Z. mobilis* is able to consume all the glucose present in a dough, while when coupled with *L. sanfranciscensis*, its fermentative performance decreases. Furthermore, the presence of *L. sanfranciscensis* did not lead to a significant ethanol yield increase, even if it can consume the available maltose in flour and release glucose.

Table 2. Maltose, glucose and ethanol concentrations (expressed in terms of mg/g dough, mean and standard deviation) present at 0, 8, 16 and 24 h in doughs leavened by *Z. mobilis*, *L. sanfranciscensis* and their association.

Microorganism	Time(h)	Maltose (mg/g)		Glucose (mg/g)		Ethanol (mg/g)	
		Mean	St. dev.	Mean	St. dev.	Mean	St. dev.
Lactobacillus sanfranciscensis (5 Log CFU/g)	0	11.33	1.46	2.08	1.01	0.00	0.00
	8	16.68	0.66	3.20	0.82	0.00	0.00
	16	9.43	0.60	4.01	0.28	0.00	0.00
	24	10.80	0.80	4.54	0.52	0.00	0.00
Zymomonas mobilis (7 Log CFU/g)	0	10.50	0.96	1.96	0.06	0.00	0.00
	8	14.59	1.67	1.12	0.13	1.14	0.13
	16	17.71	3.16	0.23	0.33	2.79	0.49
	24	15.69	2.65	0.00	0.00	3.38	0.33
L. sanfranciscensis coupled with *Z. mobilis* (5–7 Log CFU/g)	0	8.96	1.82	1.04	0.56	0.00	0.00
	8	14.21	2.70	0.92	0.31	0.75	0.28
	16	13.58	0.94	0.56	0.79	3.73	0.70
	24	12.33	2.76	0.82	0.35	4.91	1.23

4. Conclusions

The results obtained demonstrate that *Z. mobilis* is able to efficiently leaven a dough when glucose is present in the dough formulation. On the other hand, although the metabolic activities of LAB have positive effects on the structural and sensorial properties of the baked product [5,6], the traditional back-slopping sourdough technology [22] cannot be proposed due to the accelerated acidification of the dough impairing the growth of *Zymomonas*. In fact, preliminary trials have evidenced that, independently of the initial cell ratio between the two bacteria, *L. sanfranciscensis* always became the prevailing microbial population. This disproportion with *Z. mobilis* increased with refreshments, thus giving strongly acidified and poorly leavened doughs.

Future trials will be aimed at investigating microbial association with other LAB or the use of dough formulations naturally enriched of sugars fermentable by *Z. mobilis*. In this context, sucrose can also be considered an interesting alternative to glucose; nevertheless, the strain leavening performance with this carbon source has to be evaluated.

Acknowledgments: This work was founded by Bando Linea R&S per Aggregazioni, Regione Lombardia, Programma Operativo Regionale 2014–2020, Strategia "InnovaLombardia" (D.G.R. No. 2448/2014) Project number 145007.

Author Contributions: A.M. and C.P. conceived and designed the experiments; A.M. and C.M. performed the experiments; R.F. analysed the data; R.F. contributed reagents/materials/analysis tools; M.R. and C.P. wrote the paper.

References

1. Gobbetti, M. The sourdough microflora: Interactions of lactic acid bacteria and yeasts. *Food Sci. Technol.* **1998**, *9*, 267–274. [CrossRef]
2. De Vuyst, L.; Vrancken, G.; Ravyts, F.; Rimaux, T.; Weckx, S. Biodiversity, ecological determinants, and metabolic exploitation of sourdough microbiota. *Food Microbiol.* **2009**, *26*, 666–675. [CrossRef] [PubMed]

3. Picozzi, C.; D'Anchise, F.; Foschino, R. PCR detection of *Lactobacillus sanfranciscensis* in sourdough and Panettone baked product. *Eur. Food Res. Technol.* **2006**, *222*, 330–335. [CrossRef]
4. Gobbetti, M.; De Angelis, M.; Corsetti, A.; Di Cagno, R. Biochemistry and physiology of sourdough lactic acid bacteria. *Trends Food Sci. Technol.* **2005**, *16*, 57–69. [CrossRef]
5. Arendt, E.K.; Ryan, L.A.M.; Bello, F.D. Impact of sourdough on the texture of bread. *Food Microbiol.* **2007**, *24*, 165–174. [CrossRef] [PubMed]
6. Angioloni, A.; Romani, S.; Gaetano Pinnavaia, G.; Dalla Rosa, M. Characteristics of bread making doughs: Influence of sourdough fermentation on the fundamental rheological properties. *Eur. Food Res. Technol.* **2006**, *222*, 54–57. [CrossRef]
7. Messens, W.; De Vuyst, L. Inhibitory substances produced by Lactobacilli isolated from sourdoughs—A review. *Int. J. Food Microbiol.* **2002**, *72*, 31–43. [CrossRef]
8. Mansueto, P.; Montalto, G.; Pacor, M.L.; Esposito-Pellitteri, M.; Ditta, V.; Lo Bianco, C.; Leto-Barone, S.M.; Di Lorenzo, G. Food allergy in gastroenterologic diseases: Review of literature. *World J. Gastroenterol.* **2006**, *12*, 7744–7752. [CrossRef] [PubMed]
9. Salamati, S.; Martins, C.; Kulseng, B. Baker's yeast (*Saccharomyces cerevisiae*) antigen in obese and normal weight subjects. *Clin. Obes.* **2015**, *5*, 42–47. [CrossRef] [PubMed]
10. Rinaldi, M.; Perricone, R.; Blank, M.; Perricone, C.; Shoenfeld, Y. Anti-*Saccharomyces cerevisiae* autoantibodies in autoimmune diseases: From bread baking to autoimmunity. *Clin. Rev. Allergy Immunol.* **2013**, *45*, 152–161. [CrossRef] [PubMed]
11. Sicard, D.; Legras, J.-L. Bread, beer and wine: Yeast domestication in the *Saccharomyces sensu stricto* complex. *Comptes Rendus Biol.* **2011**, *334*, 229–236. [CrossRef] [PubMed]
12. Israeli, E.; Grotto, I.; Gilburd, B.; Balicer, R.D.; Goldin, E.; Wiik, A.; Shoenfeld, Y. Anti-*Saccharomyces cerevisiae* and antineutrophil cytoplasmic antibodies as predictors of inflammatory bowel disease. *Gut* **2005**, *54*, 1232–1236. [CrossRef] [PubMed]
13. Muratori, P.; Muratori, P.; Muratori, L.; Guidi, M.; Maccariello, S.; Pappas, G.; Ferrari, R.; Gionchetti, P.; Campieri, M.; Bianchi, F.B. Anti-Saccharomyces cerevisiae antibodies (ASCA) and autoimmune liver diseases. *Clin. Exp. Immunol.* **2003**, *132*, 473–476. [CrossRef] [PubMed]
14. Bansal, R.A.; Tadros, S.; Bansal, A.S. Beer, Cider, and Wine Allergy. *Case Rep. Immunol.* **2017**, *2017*, 7958924. [CrossRef] [PubMed]
15. Sahm, H.; Bringer-Meyer, S.; Sprenger, G.A. Proteobacteria: Alpha and Beta Subclasses. In *The Prokaryotes*, 3rd ed.; Dworkin, M., Falkow, S., Rosenberg, E., Schleifer, K.-H., Stackebrandt, E., Eds.; Springer: Berlin, Germany, 2006; Volume 5, ISBN 978-0-387-25476-0.
16. Musatti, A.; Rollini, M.; Sambusiti, C.; Manzoni, M. *Zymomonas mobilis*: Biomass production and use as a dough leavening agent. *Ann. Microbiol.* **2015**, *65*, 1583–1589. [CrossRef]
17. Musatti, A.; Mapelli, C.; Foschino, R.; Picozzi, C.; Rollini, M. Unconventional bacterial association for dough leavening. *Int. J. Food Microbiol.* **2016**, *237*, 28–34. [CrossRef] [PubMed]
18. Alcántara-Hernández, R.J.; Rodríguez-Álvarez, J.A.; Valenzuela-Encinas, C.; Gutiérrez-Miceli, F.A.; Castañón-González, H.; Marsch, R.; Ayora-Talavera, T.; Dendooven, L. The bacterial community in "taberna" a traditional beverage of Southern Mexico. *Lett. Appl. Microbiol.* **2010**, *51*, 558–563. [CrossRef] [PubMed]
19. Escalante, A.; Giles-Gómez, M.; Hernández, G.; Córdova-Aguilar, M.S.; López-Munguía, A.; Gosset, G.; Bolívar, F. Analysis of bacterial community during the fermentation of pulque, a traditional Mexican alcoholic beverage, using a polyphasic approach. *Int. J. Food Microbiol.* **2008**, *124*, 126–134. [CrossRef] [PubMed]
20. Nwachukwu, I.N.; Ibekwe, V.I.; Anyanwu, B.N. Investigation of some physicochemical and microbial succession parameters of palm wine. *J. Food Technol.* **2006**, *4*, 308–312.
21. Valadez-Blanco, R.; Bravo-Villa, G.; Santos-Sánchez, N.F.; Velasco-Almendarez, S.I.; Montville, T.J. The Artisanal Production of Pulque, a Traditional Beverage of the Mexican Highlands. *Probiotics Antimicrob. Proteins* **2012**, *4*, 140–144. [CrossRef] [PubMed]
22. Vogelmann, S.A.; Hertel, C. Impact of ecological factors on the stability of microbial associations in sourdough fermentation. *Food Microbiol.* **2011**, *28*, 583–589. [CrossRef] [PubMed]

Permissions

All chapters in this book were first published in MDPI; hereby published with permission under the Creative Commons Attribution License or equivalent. Every chapter published in this book has been scrutinized by our experts. Their significance has been extensively debated. The topics covered herein carry significant findings which will fuel the growth of the discipline. They may even be implemented as practical applications or may be referred to as a beginning point for another development.

The contributors of this book come from diverse backgrounds, making this book a truly international effort. This book will bring forth new frontiers with its revolutionizing research information and detailed analysis of the nascent developments around the world.

We would like to thank all the contributing authors for lending their expertise to make the book truly unique. They have played a crucial role in the development of this book. Without their invaluable contributions this book wouldn't have been possible. They have made vital efforts to compile up to date information on the varied aspects of this subject to make this book a valuable addition to the collection of many professionals and students.

This book was conceptualized with the vision of imparting up-to-date information and advanced data in this field. To ensure the same, a matchless editorial board was set up. Every individual on the board went through rigorous rounds of assessment to prove their worth. After which they invested a large part of their time researching and compiling the most relevant data for our readers.

The editorial board has been involved in producing this book since its inception. They have spent rigorous hours researching and exploring the diverse topics which have resulted in the successful publishing of this book. They have passed on their knowledge of decades through this book. To expedite this challenging task, the publisher supported the team at every step. A small team of assistant editors was also appointed to further simplify the editing procedure and attain best results for the readers.

Apart from the editorial board, the designing team has also invested a significant amount of their time in understanding the subject and creating the most relevant covers. They scrutinized every image to scout for the most suitable representation of the subject and create an appropriate cover for the book.

The publishing team has been an ardent support to the editorial, designing and production team. Their endless efforts to recruit the best for this project, has resulted in the accomplishment of this book. They are a veteran in the field of academics and their pool of knowledge is as vast as their experience in printing. Their expertise and guidance has proved useful at every step. Their uncompromising quality standards have made this book an exceptional effort. Their encouragement from time to time has been an inspiration for everyone.

The publisher and the editorial board hope that this book will prove to be a valuable piece of knowledge for researchers, students, practitioners and scholars across the globe.

List of Contributors

Przemysław Łukasz Kowalczewski
Institute of Food Technology of Plant Origin, Poznań University of Life Sciences, 60-624 Poznań, Poland

Katarzyna Walkowiak, Łukasz Masewic and Hanna Maria Baranowska
Department of Physics and Biophysics, Poznań University of Life Sciences, 60-637 Poznań, Poland

Olga Bartczak
Students' Scientific Club of Food Technologists, Poznań University of Life Sciences, 60-624 Poznań, Poland

Jacek Lewandowicz
Chair of Production Engineering and Logistics, Poznań University of Technology, 60-965 Poznań, Poland

Piotr Kubiak
Department of Biotechnology and Food Microbiology, Poznań University of Life Sciences, 60-627 Poznań, Poland

Loreto Alonso-Miravalles and James A. O'Mahony
School of Food and Nutritional Sciences, University College Cork, Cork T12 Y337, Ireland

Jingrong Gao
School of Food Science and Engineering, South China University of Technology, Guangzhou 510640, China
Department of Wine, Food and Molecular Biosciences, Lincoln University, Christchurch 7647, New Zealand
Riddet Research Institute, Palmerston North 4442, New Zealand

Xinbo Guo and Xin-An Zeng
School of Food Science and Engineering, South China University of Technology, Guangzhou 510640, China
Overseas Expertise Introduction Center for Discipline Innovation of Food Nutrition and Human Health (111 Center), Guangzhou 510640, China

Margaret A. Brennan
Department of Wine, Food and Molecular Biosciences, Lincoln University, Christchurch 7647, New Zealand
Riddet Research Institute, Palmerston North 4442, New Zealand

Susan L. Mason
Department of Wine, Food and Molecular Biosciences, Lincoln University, Christchurch 7647, New Zealand

Charles S. Brennan
School of Food Science and Engineering, South China University of Technology, Guangzhou 510640, China
Department of Wine, Food and Molecular Biosciences, Lincoln University, Christchurch 7647, New Zealand
Riddet Research Institute, Palmerston North 4442, New Zealand
Overseas Expertise Introduction Center for Discipline Innovation of Food Nutrition and Human Health (111 Center), Guangzhou 510640, China

A. K. M. Mofasser Hossain and Charles S. Brennan
Centre for Food Research and Innovation, Department of Wine, Food and Molecular Biosciences, Lincoln University, Lincoln 7647, New Zealand
Riddet Institute, Palmerston North 4442, New Zealand

Margaret A. Brennan and Susan L. Mason
Centre for Food Research and Innovation, Department of Wine, Food and Molecular Biosciences, Lincoln University, Lincoln 7647, New Zealand

Xinbo Guo
School of Food Science and Engineering, South China University of Technology, Guangzhou 510640, China

Xin An Zeng
School of Food Science and Engineering, South China University of Technology, Guangzhou 510640, China

Valentina Narducci, Enrico Finotti, Vincenzo Galli and Marina Carcea
Research Centre for Food and Nutrition, Council for Agricultural Research and Economics (CREA), Via Ardeatina 546, 00178 Rome, Italy

Maryke Labuschagne, Angeline van Biljon and Nomcebo Mkhatywa
Department of Plant Sciences, University of the Free State, Bloemfontein 9300, South Africa

Eva Johansson
Department of Plant Breeding, The Swedish University of Agricultural Sciences, SE-230 53 Alnarp, Sweden

Barend Wentzel
Small Grains Institute, Bethlehem 9700, South Africa

Idoia Larretxi , Itziar Txurruka, Virginia Navarro, Arrate Lasa, Edurne Simón and Jonatan Miranda
Gluten Analysis Laboratory of the University of the Basque Country, Department of Nutrition and Food Science, University of the Basque Country, UPV/EHU, 01006 Vitoria, Spain
GLUTEN3S research group, Department of Nutrition and Food Science, University of the Basque Country, UPV/EHU, 01006 Vitoria, Spain

María Ángeles Bustamante and María del Pilar Fernández-Gil
Gluten Analysis Laboratory of the University of the Basque Country, Department of Nutrition and Food Science, University of the Basque Country, UPV/EHU, 01006 Vitoria, Spain

Marcus Schmidt and Emanuele Zannini
School of Food and Nutritional Sciences, University College Cork, Western Road, T12 Y337 Cork, Ireland

Elke K. Arendt
School of Food and Nutritional Sciences, University College Cork, Western Road, T12 Y337 Cork, Ireland
Alimentary Pharmabotic Centre Microbiome Institute, University College Cork, T12 Y337 Cork, Ireland

Kathryn Colla, Andrew Costanzo and Shirani Gamlath
Centre for Advanced Sensory Sciences, School of Exercise and Nutrition Sciences, Deakin University, 1 Gheringhap Street, Geelong 3220, Australia

Shirin Pourafshar and Padmanaban G. Krishnan
Dairy and Food Science Department, South Dakota State University, Brookings, SD 57007, USA

Kurt A. Rosentrater
Department of Agriculture and Biosystems Engineering, Iowa State University, Ames, IA 50011, USA
Department of Food Science and Human Nutrition, Iowa State University, Ames, IA 50011, USA

Serena Niro, Annacristina D'Agostino, Alessandra Fratianni and Gianfranco Panfili
Dipartimento di Agricoltura, Ambiente e Alimenti, Università degli Studi del Molise, Via De Sanctis, 86100 Campobasso, Italy

Luciano Cinquanta
Dipartimento Scienze Agrarie, Alimentari e Forestali, Università di Palermo, Viale delle Scienze 4, 90128 Palermo, Italy

Markus C. E. Belz, Claudia Axel, Jonathan, Emanuele Zannini and Elke K. Arendt
School of Food and Nutritional Sciences, University College Cork, National University of Ireland, College Road, T12 Y337 Cork, Ireland

Jonathan Beauchamp and Michael Czerny
Department of Sensory Analytics, Fraunhofer Institute for Process Engineering and Packaging IVV, 85354 Freising, Germany

Marina Carcea, Valeria Turfani, Valentina Narducci, Alessandra Durazzo, Alberto Finamore, Marianna Roselli and Rita Rami
Research Centre for Food and Nutrition, Council for Agricultural Research and Economics (CREA), via Ardeatina 546, 00178 Roma, Italy

Jussi Loponen
Fazer Group, 01230 Vantaa, Finland

Michael G. Gänzle
Department of Agricultural, Food and Nutritional Science, University of Alberta, Edmonton, AB T6G 2P5, Canada

Felicity Curtain
Grains & Legumes Nutrition Council, Mount Street, North Sydney 2060, Australia

Sara Grafenauer
Grains & Legumes Nutrition Council, Mount Street, North Sydney 2060, Australia
School of Medicine, University of Wollongong, Northfields Avenue, Wollongong 2522, Australia

Elena Mellado-Ortega and Dámaso Hornero-Méndez
Chemistry and Biochemistry of Pigments Group, Food Phytochemistry Department, Instituto de la Grasa (CSIC), Campus Universidad Pablo de Olavide, Ctra. de Utrera km. 1, 41013 Seville, Spain

Marina Carcea, Valentina Narducci, Valeria Turfani and Altero Aguzzi
Research Centre for Food and Nutrition, Council for Agricultural Research and Economics (CREA-AN), Via Ardeatina 546, 00178 Roma, Italy

Alida Musatti, Chiara Mapelli, Manuela Rollini, Roberto Foschino and Claudia Picozzi
Dipartimento di Scienze per gli Alimenti, la Nutrizione, l'Ambiente, Università degli Studi di Milano, 20133 Milan, Italy

Index

Printed in the USA
CPSIA information can be obtained
at www.ICGtesting.com
JSHW051405091023
49903JS00006B/291